the momentum of folly

———

robert p johnson

Copyright © 2011 Robert P Johnson
All rights reserved.

ISBN: 0615480438
ISBN-13: 9780615480435
Library of Congress Control Number: 2011941429
Just Two, Santa Barbara, CA

Dedication

This book is dedicated to the hope that the dire consequences of our rampant population growth becomes universally acknowledged regardless of religion, nationality, or ethnicity, so our numbers can be voluntarily tapered-back to a sustainable level before we thoroughly trash this beautiful planet upon which we had the good fortune to be born.

✽ ✽ ✽

"Just two kids, just two billion; we can live with that."

```
   0    ---   170 million
 1805   --    one billion
 1928   --    two billion
 1961   --    three billion
 1974   --    four billion
 1987   --    five billion
```
1999 -- six billion
2011 -- seven billion

Teller Mission, Alaska. February 2010.

Above... the Aurora Borealis shifts and dances in the otherwise pitch-black sky of the eighty-eight day long night. To the naïve it's a beautiful display of color and wonder, perhaps even a nod to the *Miracle*. But for those few who know better, it's merely the violent blasts of solar radiation the atmosphere barely manages to stave off; that radiation being just one of the many corrosive forces trying to crush this anomaly called "life" from Earth once and for all and return the universe to its pulse-less normalcy, and time is on their side.

Below... amidst the blowing ice and snow a team of five labors under portable construction lights, their identities concealed beneath thickly insulated biohazard suits, their generators adding to the natural din of the howling elements.

They are excavating. One cuts at the permafrost with a hissing steam hose, slowly changing what was frozen solid to a boggy muck. Another chips down through a century's depth of ice with a pneumatic jackhammer, while another, awkwardly wrestling a snow blower, tries to clear away the progress. When particularly stubborn spots are encountered, dynamite is slid into holes drilled into the ice, fuses are lit with flares, and warnings – at times in French, at times in Japanese or Spanish or English – are shouted: *"Stand clear!" "Fire in the hole!" "Hit the deck!"* And then comes the muffled explosion – *Fffmmmpht!* – to be followed by more tedious snow blowing, jack hammering and steam cutting.

The work site is about the dimensions of a large school bus carved out of the Arctic ice. At either end of the rectangular pit two whalebone crucifixes stand tall and defiant against the wind. Upon closer inspection, a few Eskimo necklaces and festoons still cling tenuously from one of the crucifix's crossbars, though the lion's share of such adornments has been ripped away by the howling winds of winters past.

Just outside the excavation site a wooden headstone sticks up at a slant through the snow. Credit efficiency in the face of what must have been a frantic

the momentum of folly

evacuation, for the single headstone is inscribed with seventy-two names beneath the vague date of "November 1918."

The guy working the jackhammer is in over his head by now and still digging. He pauses, then, laying the jackhammer aside, bends over to the spot where his blade had just been chipping. With a gloved hand he brushes aside the loose ice chips, slowly at first, then with ever increasing anxiousness. Spotting something, he shouts out to his confederates – in English with a Japanese accent – and excitedly enough to be heard over the wind, "Over here! Over here, I found one!"

As the other workers toss down their tools and rush towards the discovery, the jackhammer guy keeps brushing aside the ice chips until the frozen face of a young Eskimo girl can be made out, her features preserved under another few centimeters of ice, her body still wearing the light fuchsia dress in which she was buried. And submerged beneath her, as deeply as the construction light can penetrate into the otherwise dark ice, the clothing and hair and discolored skin of more bodies can be detected – many more.

One of the whalebone crucifixes creaks in the shifting wind. There, on a crossbar, one last feather clings to a tattered necklace being whipped about by each new gust. And it perseveres for another few seconds or so, until it too is ripped away by the wind.

Tijuana, Mexico. Late Spring 2010.

A lean mosquito patiently descends, following a wafting trail of carbon dioxide down towards its prey, its trademark pesky buzzing augmented by the faint strains of Mariachi music — guitars, bass, muted trumpets, and chirping accordion — seeping through some cheap walls from some cheaper radio, and the very distant laughter and shouts and mirthful screams of children at play. But the mosquito dutifully ignores all those human-made distractions, focusing instead on the task at hand as she follows her nose and 165 million years of evolutionary refinement down to a bare patch of white skin.

Scarcely believing her luck, the parasite balances on the front four of its six legs and lowers its proboscis towards a skin pore. After injecting a mild analgesic, she begins tanking up with the supplemental blood protein she'll need to develop her eggs in the coming days. As her abdomen begins to swell translucent red, a pair of human voices — a male's from nearby, and a female's from some adjoining room — rekindle a conversation.

The male: "... E coli, herpes, influenza...."

The female: "It's all fine by me."

"But it's Level Two."

"So?"

"So, it's not something to *aspire* to; it's something you *settle* for."

"Oh, please..."

Tanked up, the mosquito retracts her proboscis, cleans it off a bit with her front legs, then, with a relatively Herculean effort, takes to wing.

Watching all this with scientific detachment is Dr. Carl Sims. He lightly scratches the spot on his stomach from where the mosquito fed but otherwise seems unaffected by it all. He lays atop a no-frills bed in his boxer shorts, propped up so he can read one of the many infectious disease journals scattered beside him. Though accurate, the "doctor" title doesn't seem to fit him. For being twenty-seven he seems not only too young for such a serious profession, but also too "jockey" – his tanned, taut build seeming to be more testimony to countless hours of pick-up basketball and ultimate Frisbee than to the requisite study time demanded by a medical career, but accurate it is.

"So, what if they don't offer you the promotion?" the female's voice calls out from the adjoining room.

"Why wouldn't they?" asks Carl, revealing a confidence that doesn't allow much room for self-doubt.

That female voice, as it turns out, belongs to Angela Varella, twenty-eight and change. She stands in front of a mirror in her bra and panties as she applies a generous coat of red lipstick to what Nature had already made pretty close to perfect.

"Oh, I don't know: maybe because every other virologist at the CDC has more seniority than you," she replies, with wry sarcasm.

"Oh, that."

"Don't see why anyone would *aspire* to do Level Four research in the first place."

Carl hops off the bed and crosses the budget hotel room, sauntering past scores of stacked boxes labeled "Influenza Vaccine" and "Sterile Injectors" and "Trivalent A/Brisbane/59/2007(H1N1)-like virus, A/Brisbane/10/2007 (H3N2)-like virus, B/Brisbane/60/2008-like antigens" as he heads towards the open bathroom door. It's the very end of the flu season for the Northern Hemisphere – indeed, under normal circumstances vaccination campaigns would have ended well before now – but the sundry health agencies don't want to take any chances with that pesky H1N1 mutating and coming back. So, here they are.

"C'mon, it's the big leagues, baby. Every virologist yearns to do BSL-4. It's sexy."

Leaning in towards the mirror with her eyeliner brush, Angela demonstrates her knack for scoffing sans even the slightest inflection. "Hanging out in stuffy labs all day with a bunch of nerds in biosafety suits, watching monkeys die of machupo, ebola, anthrax; call me old-fashioned, but that ain't my idea of sexy."

Carl snuggles up from behind, wrapping his arms around her. "No? Then what is?"

"The first job my headhunter finds me doing lowly Biosafety Level Two influenza research at some big-ass, publicly-traded pharmaceutical company, that's what."

And now Carl demonstrates his knack for wrapping a single word with disapproval. "Money."

"Mama didn't raise no fool."

In the mirror, Carl watches as Angela now applies an extra long streak of eyebrow pencil, as she adds rhetorically, "Muy Latina, si?"

"Si, muy Latina."

The sounds of the children playing outside wend their way through the closed bathroom windows. Carl pushes the curtains aside and opens the windows. After his eyes adjust to the harsh glare of sunlight he gazes out across the seemingly endless scar of ramshackle houses, slapped together from scrap plywood, cardboard and tin. Not far from their hotel window, children – dressed in rags, if that – splash in a stream that doubles as an open sewer and public dump. In the muddy center of the arroyo, one child, bereft of legs, sits splashing in a discarded truck tire.

"Good morning, Tijuana," Carl mutters wistfully.

"Close it."

Heeding Angela's request, Carl pulls the windows closed.

La Clinica de los Niños has a concrete floor, cinder block walls, and a corrugated metal roof, making it the veritable Palace of Versailles in comparison to the neighborhood's surrounding architecture. Except for the church, of course. Outside the clinic a queue of more than a hundred Mexicans – greater Tijuana's poorest of the poor – stretches well out into the street. Their anxiety—especially the children's, especially the closer they creep towards the clinic's front double-doors – is not only palpable but understandable considering only about six percent of them have ever received a vaccination before.

Inside the clinic the queue splits into two lines, cleaved by a local nurse at a reception table who takes down the patients' names. And further in still, two more nurses prepare the recipients' left shoulders by rolling up their sleeves and cleaning the skin with an alcohol wipe, and assuaging any concerns with a smile and quiet words of assurance.

the momentum of folly

Seemingly incongruous to this orderly setting, Carl's voice booms loudly, filling the room with a language comprehended only by Angela and maybe a couple of the nurses.

"431 BC. Athens, Greece. Forty-five percent mortality rate. Pathogen unknown though recent evidence suggests ebola...."

Angela gives a shot to a young girl, smiles reassuringly, and then hands her a lemon lollipop as reward.

Carl, behaving more like an assembly line robot than a caring health official, doesn't even interrupt his monologue as he gives a boy a shot, disposes of the needle, and unwraps another. The boy, uncertain of the protocol, takes a green lollipop from the open box and, since Carl seems wholly disinterested, snatches a handful more.

"590 AD. Yesinia pestis; Justinian's Plague, returning in 1348 as The Black Death or Bubonic Plague with a thirty percent mortality rate that killed nearly a third of Europe, or an estimated 100 million in a time when there were only 450 million on the planet."

The man to whom Angela is giving a shot, nods towards Carl as he asks her with concern, "El medico; poco loco?"

Angela laughs, adding facetiously, "Si, verdad. Verdad!"

Carl unwraps another needle, inoculates another patient, as he continues with his recounting of the known great plagues of human history. "1818 through 1832. Vibrio cholerae – cholera. Sixty percent mortality from Calcutta to Moscow to London."

Angela smiles and shakes her head again, hands out another lollipop, tosses out the spent injector, begins unwrapping yet another, then takes a deep breath and sighs before mustering another disingenuously reassuring smile. And it probably doesn't help to know her efforts here are but a frail finger in a hopelessly crumbling dike, what with antibiotic-resistant pneumonia, tuberculosis, staph, AIDS, et al, so on the rise. And it certainly doesn't help that she knows also that the efforts of this tiny clinic and the hundreds of thousands of clinics just like it, trying to dig feeble trenches of resistance the world 'round, are ultimately futile owing to the double-whammy-esque trends of waxing global malnutrition and waning funding; those trends combining to overwhelm the only recently-organized infrastructure of national and international health organizations and turn it towards the incipient state of collapse it is in today. Verily, the dashed hopes of all those like Angela who had dreamed of a new, healthy era for humanity can be epitomized by that endless trickle of frail adults and doe-eyed children stretching beyond *La Clinica's* double doors, their ranks being added to faster than she and others like her can vaccinate them. Where does that queue end? Does it end? – that incessant trickle, cum stream, cum river, cum flood of humanity, ever-shuffling, ever-leaning, ever-pushing forth. *The momentum of folly*; that's the term she had heard Carl use, quoting his deceased father's attempt to describe humanity's blind march towards self-destruction. *The momentum of folly*. Surely someday this human trickle will gasp its last, whether by its own doing or Nature's, but when?

A slight disturbance at the registration table lifts Angela's attention. There the local Priest and a handful of his flock of rural parishioners have cut in line and are pushing through the doorway. These happen to be Catholics, one of the more than 1,500 religions dreamed up in the 170 thousand years since modern humans first looked up from the earth to the sky, but it could as well be any persuasion. The Priest, as demarked by his black tunic and white collar, seems particularly edgy, clearly the rabble-rouser of the bunch. He's now in the face of the registration nurse, and raising his voice in an obvious attempt to infect the others with his outrage.

The two other nurses look to Angela for guidance. After some hesitation she nods for them to help the registration nurse in calming the Priest and his mob as she finishes up with her current patient.

Carl, his vaccination station positioned so that he doesn't quite face the doors, prattles on, oblivious to the brewing consternation.

"1918. The Spanish Flu, though not really from Spain at all. This strain of influenza – this one right here –" Carl says, referring to the injector he holds above him – "H1N1; this little virus killed more people in a shorter time frame than any other disease ever; as many as 100 million in that single year, or more than World Wars One and Two, Korea, Vietnam and Iraq combined. As you may know, it then vanished without a trace with its last gasping victim; lying dormant for the next 91 years before reincarnating just last spring as a mere shadow of its former self known to all as The Swine Flu."

But as the Priest's shout's become louder – and the heads of those in the queues now pull towards him with the same conflicted look, of being torn between two authority figures — now even Carl interrupts his monologue to turn to see what the hell is going on.

The Priest locks eyes with Carl and shouts angrily at him in Spanish, "We know what you are doing. We are not as stupid as you think!"

Not understanding the Priest, Carl turns towards Angela for the translation, "What's his problem?"

But Angela can only shake her head, herself puzzled and worried.

The Priest yanks an injector out of one of the nurse's hands and begins shaking it angrily as he moves to the center of the room — center stage — shouting in Spanish to all those waiting to be vaccinated, "They don't want us having children. They don't want any more brown people invading their country!"

"Oh, God," Angela gasps quietly.

"What is it?" Carl asks.

"He thinks we're trying to sterilize them."

"No way," Carl scoffs.

But Angela nods back, "Way."

"Fucking moron. Can't you explain to him what we're doing?"

Angela shrugs, "I don't know; there's kind of a long history to Latino distrust of Gringo generosity. And this sterilization thing goes way back, kind of like the urban myth of harvesting for organs. Gotta admit, altruism kind of flies in the face of human nature."

The Priest is ranting now like a televangelist, "You see, they don't mind us cleaning their toilets, they just don't want us taking back the land that was once ours!" — many of his audience are now nodding in agreement.

"Shit!" Carl mutters, shaking his head in disbelief. "You've gotta fix this before he fucks it all up!" he tells Angela.

Angela glances at Carl, then back to the Priest. After a strategizing beat, she crosses towards the Priest, summoning up her most reassuring countenance as she tries to explain the reality of the situation to him.

"Padre, por favor. Esta vacuna por la influenza solamente."

But her efforts only cause the Priest to doubt her the more. He shakes his head, staring daggers at her as he explains the situation as he sees it in Spanish to his people: "Brothers and sisters, what she says is a lie. This is not true. She is lying to you. Look…" The Priest lifts one of the unopened boxes of injectors to one shoulder, rotating as he points to the words *Sterile Injectors* printed on the label to his audience of frightened Mexicans. "See? – *sterilization!* Do you know what *sterilization* means? Yes, all of you? Good, then you know it is not God's word. And that which is not God's word is el Diablo's!" And with that the Priest throws the box to the floor with disdain. "Come, my people, let us leave this place of sin."

With that many of the Mexicans begin to heed the Priest's edict by falling out of line and moving sheepishly towards the exit.

"Idiots," Carl mutters.

In an attempt to quell the exodus Angela calls out in Spanish to the people heading for the doors, "People, please. You will get sick. It is not true what the Priest says. He does not understand!"

Fuming, the Priest gets right into Angela's face, shouting, "Not true, you say?" The Priest then grabs an injector off the table and dares Angela to vaccinate herself with it. "Then let's see you do it. *Sterilize* yourself. It's a good thing, right? Then go on, you do it!"

With that the Priest slaps the injector into Angela's open palm then wraps her fingers around it. Already trembling, Angela holds the injector, clearly hesitant to vaccinate herself.

Carl is perplexed by the standoff. "What's he want?"

"He wants me to immunize myself."

"So do it!"

Angel shakes her head; dreading what she'll probably have to admit to him, already fighting back tears.

"Stick yourself! What's the problem?" he presses.

Despite her reluctance, Angela caves, "I'm pregnant."

Carl stares at her, as shocked by the news as he is confused. "Why didn't you tell me?"

But rather than answering him – verbally, at least – Angela merely turns her wet eyes towards him, and stares with a steely resolve he had never before witnessed. And clearly Carl is shaken by it.

Meanwhile, the Priest has taken hold of a fistful of injectors from an opened box and, holding them up as prop for his ad hoc sermon, he begins to extemporize to his cowering flock.

"It is written: idle hands are the Devil's tools!"

the momentum of folly

After allowing the saying to sink in, the Priest lets the needles fall from his hands then begins crushing them on the floor with his shoes.

"Hey! What the hell are you doing?" Carl shouts, angrily but ineffectually. Ignoring Carl, the Priest then dramatically hoists the entire opened box high above his head asking rhetorically to all, "And what did our Jesus do when he confronted the moneychangers in the Lord's temple?"

Sensing that things are spiraling out of control, Carl mutters, "Fuck this," and begins towards the Priest with destructive intent.

"Carl, don't!" Angela pleads.

But Carl isn't about to listen. Instead he ramps up his gait to a determined charge, fully committing himself to a head-on tackle of the Priest until a trio of townsfolk leap into his path to prevent him, the collision bringing all four to the floor in an entangled heap.

"Fucking morons, let me go!" Carl shouts at them, struggling to extricate himself. But the trio maintains their hold on the kicking and squirming Carl, allowing the Priest to hurl the box against a wall, and thereby initiate the destructive chaos to follow.

Across the room a table crashes, purposely tipped by one of the Priest's followers, opened boxes of vaccine spilling their contents across the floor. And off in an opposite corner a tower of boxes, stacked to the ceiling, is pushed over by an elderly female on a newly inspired holy mission, while some kids make off with the boxes of candy.

Carl shakes free of his restrainers, picks up a pair of injectors and quickly unwraps them, shouting out to a group of a dozen or so he has cornered in one side of the room, "What is it you want? You want proof?" Exhibiting a bit of theatre himself, Carl injects himself in both shoulders simultaneously. "There. Did that do it for you?"

Just getting warmed up, he rips open another pair of injectors and, turning towards another huddled mass of rapt if unwilling audience members, he shouts angrily, "And how about you people over here; need proof that evil man from *el Norte* isn't trying to sterilize you?" then shoots himself up in both forearms. "There. Convinced?"

Through his extreme antics Carl manages to snag enough of the room's attention to effectively diffuse the destructive uprising and perhaps even convince a slight majority of the Mexicans he means them no harm. But still he's not finished. Grabbing another pair of injectors and ripping them open, he turns now towards the Priest. "How 'bout you, Padre? Looks like you still need more proof. *Verdad?*" Carl holds the needles in his teeth as he undoes his belt and pulls down his pants. "Well, here it is..." And with this, Carl turns his bared ass towards the Priest and injects himself in both buttocks. "There you go, Padre. Satisfied? Happy now? Hey, that kind of smarted; would you mind kissing it for me? Kiss my ass, pretty please?"

Seething at Carl's taunting, the Priest turns to leave, shouting out to his reeling flock as he does, "You do not need this. God heals all. Let *His* grace be your only medicine!"

The Priest then crushes a last small pile of injectors with an angry stomp as he exits, his same small entourage, and maybe a few new enlistees in tow.

Two of the Red Cross nurses begin to right the tipped table and restack the undamaged boxes, as the other nurse politely herds the patients back into their original queues.

Getting back to business, Carl turns towards Angela.

But Angela only returns his stare, saying nothing.

Centers for Disease Control. Atlanta, Georgia

―――

A cake — one whose shape can only be described as *blobular* — is being pushed down a corridor on a squeaky-wheeled gurney, candles ablaze. Angela is the engine behind this effort, in both the figurative and literal sense. Accompanying her is a rag-tag team of research scientists, laboratory technicians, and CDC staffers; basically anyone tugged from their offices by the passing cake's gravitational pull and its promise of a snack and some welcomed yucks. Any excuse to get them through those late-afternoon doldrums.

And there's some "brass" sprinkled in the pack as well; evidence, to some degree, of the modest importance of the event. One such notable is the Facility Manager for the National Center of Preparedness, Detection, and Control of Infectious Diseases *(aka* the NCPDCID) Ross Corman, whose egoless joviality makes him the ideal nexus between the Shipping and Receiving grunts, lab techs, and cranky scientists alike. Fortunately or not, Ross is a hands-on kind of manager who tries his best to give everything on his "To Do" list top priority, be it a ventilation pump in urgent need of replacement in the P-4 lab's Marburg-infected primate cages or the basketball hoop out back in the loading dock in need of a proper net. In either scenario Ross is on it 24/7 either unseen and overhead somewhere, sweating in his biosafety suit, dragging a toolbox through the air ducts, or up there on the step ladder, cutting down the frayed old net and replacing it with a shiny new one. He is, indeed, the veritable nerd who has no life of his own and, ergo, the perfect CDC employee.

Also to be found in the party entourage is Hans "Hank" Bruckner — the former head of the Division of Emerging Infections and Surveillance Services (DEISS) whose job was renamed and reconfigured to appease the new paradigm of fear that swept into so many government agencies in the wake of 9/11. He now officially heads up the CDC's Division of Bioterrorism Preparedness and

the momentum of folly

Response (DBPR), though the only thing that has really changed is the placard on his office door. "Bioterrorism? – gimme a fuckin' break!" were rumored to be Hank's spiteful words straight to the faces of the Directors of both the CDC and Department of Homeland Security upon receiving the "promotion." And though such an indignant reaction might be cause for dismissal for most anyone else, Hank's compulsive tenacity coupled with his twenty-five years of experience made him just too valuable not to have around. So the directors sucked-up Hank's indignation, got him a new chair and placard for his desk and held on to him; knowing full well that in a system that too-often can get mired in protocol, and with nasty pathogens being what they are, it's vital to have someone who knows the tedious but time-proven procedures by rote, someone who knows how to grease the wheels and cut through the bureaucratic crap, someone who plain and simply can get things done. And that's Hank.

And, up there near the very top of the CDC's befuddling food chain – which falls under the jurisdiction of the Federal government's Department of Heath and Human Services, and includes a Hydra-esque snarl of six main "Coordinating Centers" consisting of: the Coordinating Center for Environmental Health and Injury Prevention (CCEHIP), the Coordinating Center for Health Information and Service, the Coordinating Center for Health Promotion (CCHP), Coordinating Center for Global Health (CCGH), the Coordinating Center for Terrorism Preparedness and Emergency Response (CCTPER), and the one responsible for this particular group of buildings, the Coordinating Center for Infectious Diseases (CCID) – is Dr. Bronwyn Galloway, head of one of the four subdivisions of the CCID, the National Center for Immunization and Respiratory Diseases (NCIRD). Despite the plethora of departments and centers and divisions of the CDC, whenever the subject of its future is pondered, Dr. Galloway's name is often mentioned as heir apparent for the Director position. This is part of the current trend of actually placing *competent* persons at the helm of the sundry Federal agencies, which is in response to the trend of corruption, nepotism and incompetence of the previous decade's appointees, as revealed by the debacles and failures of FEMA, the USFS, EPA, and CIA, to name a few. But the fact of the matter is it will never happen: Dr. Galloway will never be appointed Director of the CDC because she is simply too good at what she does, and what she does best is managing emerging infectious diseases. So here at the NCIRD is probably where she'll stay for the remainder of her working years, with only the remote possibility of being bumped-up an echelon to Director of the CCID, even though, as she has confided with friends, such a promotion might supersede both her expertise and interest.

Bronwyn checks her watch then calls from the back of the pack up to Angela, "I've got a Senate to try to squeeze funding out of; you sure he's even here, Angela?"

"Yep, just spoke with his lab partner," Angela assures her.

"So, why don't I ever get a birthday cake?" Ross asks, mostly in jest.

"It's not a birthday cake, Ross," replies Angela.

"Sure looks like a birthday cake."

"It's a going-away cake," chimes in Hank.

"Ah. Is there a difference?"

"Birthday cakes say, Happy Birthday on them."

"No shit?"

"No shit."

"So, where's he going away to, Angela?"

Ross's question is met with a hesitant pause. Eyes dart. The gurney's wheels squeak onward. This will be Bronwyn's call: "China."

"China? Influenza reconnaissance? " Hank asks, his surprise obvious.

"Yep."

"Does he know?"

More silence. More darting eyes. Eventually Angela, with an ever so slight smirk, shakes her head.

"Hah! Cool!' Ross remarks facetiously, clapping his hands and laughing. "Not that I'd ever want you guys to do that to me."

"So, when's he suppose to leave?" Hank asks, thinking more about the available lab space he'll have to fill.

"Tomorrow," Bronwyn replies.

"*Tomorrow!* And he doesn't even know?" Ross laughs. "He'll shit! What do you think, Hank?"

Hank shakes his head. "Oh, he'll shit alright."

"Hah, Guangdong Province: he won't be happy."

"Why won't he be happy?" Bronwyn asks.

"He just got back from your dispatching him to Tijuana; from one smelly armpit right into the other. Trust me: he won't."

"Guangdong and Tijuana aren't so bad," Bronwyn argues.

"What're ya talking about? They're the armpits of the world!"

"*Phffft*, what's that make Calcutta, San Paulo, Lagos, Islamabad, Jakarta, et cetera."

"Armpits as well. Like the Goddess Shiva, the Earth has many armpits," Ross sums it up.

"*Sssh!*" Angela hisses, trying to quiet them all as she pushes the cake around a corner and onward down a corridor of laboratories.

In one such lab not so very far away, Carl is bent over a sink, throwing up. Closer inspection would also show him to be sweating profusely, with skin color somewhere between pale and green.

Across a lab counter a comfortable distance away, Carl's labmate and housemate Stuart Chew chuckles heartlessly as he balances on the rear wheels of his wheelchair.

"You deserve it, ya know," Stuart is saying, "Dead virus or not, you can always count on an immune reaction, fool. Wanna know the trippy part?" Stuart spins about 360° in his wheelchair, glancing at Carl dry hurling again into their lab sink. "Sure you do: the trippy part is, most all those symptoms – the aches and pains, the inflammation, the pounding headache, the diarrhea, the fever – that ain't the virus; that's just your immune system dumping all the toxic wastes in its arsenal *at* the virus. Dig it; if not for your immune response you might not even know you had the flu. The inflammation? – that's just your white blood cells releasing cytokines, which are the same proteins responsible for your fever, all because they happen to bind with receptors in your hypothalamus which regulates your body temperature, hence the sweaty delirium. As for those influenza-intrinsic aches and pains in your joints and bones; that's the GM CSF factor at work; other cytokines stimulating production of yet more white cells – macrophages and granulocytes in particular – deep down in the marrow of your bones. In fact, only a handful of your white cell types and interferon and some really, really nastily toxic stuff called TNF actually attack the virus itself. But most of the time the agony associated with influenza is just your body's overly zealous response to the virus. Factoid: a sizeable percentage of the flu deaths each year are caused, not by the flu per se, but by the immune system's *friendly fire*, if you will. That's why often, unlike other pathogens which predictably cull the young or the old and infirmed, particularly lethal strains of flu will strike the twenty to forty-year-old range hardest because they're the part of the Bell Curve with the healthiest immune systems." Stuart spins again on the rear wheels of his wheelchair, blurting out sarcastically to Carl, "Hey, that's you! Ironic, eh?"

Carl dry heaves into the sink again, wipes his mouth with the tail of his otherwise white lab smock, then musters the strength to utter, "Stu, please shut the fuck up."

Tight friends since their first day of Chem 1A at the University of California, Santa Barbara, Stuart and Carl have roomed together, with the exception of only a few transitory months here and there, for the past decade. Stuart, as his surname *Chew* implies, is of Asian descent, though any affinity for his Orient homeland is hopelessly buried beneath too many generations of American births for him to know anything about those roots. About all he knows is that some distant great-great-grandfather came to the States as a slave. Working shoulder to shoulder with teams of his countrymen, that forefather chipped and drilled and dynamited a winding path through the high Sierra Nevada granite for the Transcontinental Railroad, with only opium pipes and spectacular scenery and trout fishing in crystalline rivers to help them forget about their homeland. And when the railroad was completed, and with it his release from servitude, that great-great-grandfather and some of his buddies jumped into the Gold Rush, doing just well enough to call over a mail-order bride from China whom he had never met and impregnate her on their perfunctory wedding night. Over the next few months they lived in a placer mining camp on the southern bank of the American River, the mail-order bride and others like her doing the fishing and cooking and child-rearing as their men sluiced the sandbars for the "yellow metal that makes the white man crazy." And on one such day – a particularly warm one, in late April 1851 – the mild heat wave had caused the heavy winter's snow pact to begin melting rapidly and the river to swell to several thousand cubic feet per second through narrow Humbug Canyon. And as bad luck would have it, the high water brought a trio of Maidu Indian braves downstream in order to use a "Dutchman" cable cart strung across the river by a company of White miners. What happened next is only known because it happened to be witnessed and recorded in the journal of a barely-literate White miner working just across the river on its north bank. To wit: the trio of braves happened upon Stuart's great-great-grandfather and a co-worker as they squatted on a rock ledge above the raging river, panning down the various metals they had caught in their sluice box so far that morning. And according to that White miner, squinting, as he probably was into the morning sun from across the river, he sensed a bit of tension as the three braves stepped up to the two nervous Asians. And though the White miner remarked how similar the five looked, what with their narrow eyes and jet black hair, apparently the Indians thought otherwise; so much so in fact that they weren't quite convinced the "Chinamen" were even human. Thus, as some sort of sink-or-swim test, one of the braves pushed Stuart's great-great-grandfather off the ledge and into the rapids; a random act in a clash of cultures that resulted in the great-great-grandfather's never being seen again. Stuart's great-great-grandmother, watching this from the camp some fifty meters above, screamed and sobbed for the man she had "known" but once. Be that as it may, the seed was planted, and thus Stuart's great-grandmother was begat, and thus Stuart's lineage was tenuously connected so that he would be here today, doing a wheelie in his chair, a wispy-bearded, pony-tailed research epidemiologist with the CDC.

Carl wretches again, but it's all dry heaves at this point due to the fact that he's been at it for some hours now.

"Just desserts, bro. You fucked up. Just desserts."

Carl splashes water on his face, rinses out his mouth then the sink, combs his longish hair back with wet fingers, then slings his laptop case over a shoulder announcing, "I'm outta here."

"Well, pack the bong, I'll be home soon."

Carl is just pulling open the door when it happens; into the lab rolls the gurney featuring the blobular-shaped, going-away cake with candles, and even a few sparklers ablaze, Angela still at the helm with her entourage of CDC geeks all shouting in not quite unison, "Surprise!"

Carl holds the door open for them and steps back, assuming the cake must be for Stuart. "Did I forget your birthday?"

In on the surprise, Stuart grins, "This ain't about me."

"Is it *my* birthday?" Carl asks, proving he's not so good when it comes to such things.

"Your birthday is in February, dorko. This is June," Angela replies, almost embarrassed for him.

If not a birthday cake, then what can it be? Carl ponders. Thoroughly perplexed he looks up at Angela – beaming, hands covering her mouth to keep from laughing. *So, might this be some sort of female celebration for their so-very-inconvenient pregnancy? Not likely, not with Angela anyway. Another expecting mother might publicly celebrate such a thing, but not her!* – Carl ponders, all in about two milliseconds' time. *Then what can this be about?*

"My promotion?" he guesses timidly.

Angela shrugs, toying with him. She turns to Bronwyn, "Promotion?"

Bronwyn toggles her head from side to side musing it over, "Sort of. Maybe. Still G-8, so no pay raise, if that's any help."

This only adds to Carl's befuddlement.

Stuart points at the sparkling blob with a pair of emphatic index fingers. "The cake, you moron. The cake!"

"What, this is a *clue*?" Carl asks incredulously.

"Maybe not to the layperson out there on the street, but to you it should be," Ross hints, adding for his cohorts, "Let's hope so anyway."

Carl turns back to the cake, now perusing it much more closely. He checks the frosting, but there's nothing legible written there, just a seemingly random artwork of colors and odd appendages and – "Ah, I get it; this messed-up design is intentional!"

"Of course it's intentional," Angela avers.

"Sorry, I figured you just must've dropped it on the way in."

"Hey!" scolds Angela, feigning hurt feelings.

"Yeah, show a little gratitude, smartass. This cake took us several taxpayer-sponsored minutes to decorate just right." Hank quips wryly.

"Several minutes with blunt instruments," Ross adds.

"And even blunter brains!"

"With Angela riding our collective ass the whole time: *No, that's not the right color, this goes here, blah-blah-blah!*"

"Okay, I get it," Carl laughs, finally coming to some sort of understanding. "So, we're talkin' some sort of pathogen here. Well, it's cute. Good work. Let's eat it."

"Whoa, whoa – there's a lot more to it than just some pathogen!" Angela says.

"Yeah, put some effort into it, dumbshit," Stuart chides.

"Smartass, dumbshit; with friends like you guys, who needs critical parents?" Carl quips, focusing his scrutiny back to the cake. "Okay, okay, now I'm getting it. It's a pathogen but not bacterial, judging by the stringy looks of it. Viral? It's a virus?"

"He's brilliant. See? – I told you he was brilliant!" Ross quips to Angela, her eyes rolling.

"Sure, but what *kind* of virus?" presses Stuart.

"There's more? Geez, I thought you guys had jobs."

"They *used* to," Bronwyn can't resist.

As the others react to Bronwyn's subtle jab – *Oooh! Ouch! Ah, Homeland Security is better funded anyway...* – Carl leans over the cake more closely, pulling out details he hadn't noticed before. "Wow, you guys really put both your brain synapses into this. This is cool!" Carl is getting excited, in that way only an obsessed virologist can get excited. "Okay, this red crap here is RNA, right?"

"Yep," Stuart confirms, "But it's not crap, it's actually this stuff called *frosting*. Am I right, Angela? – frosting right, not crap?"

"That's right, Stuart," Angela answers just as sarcastically, suppressing her exasperation.

"What? It's not real crap? Then why'd you have me scrape out the monkey cages?" Ross quips.

"Now that's disgusting," Hank tells him.

"And, ergo, funny."

Bronwyn shakes her head, prodding them along, "Did I mention I have the *U.S. Senate* to prepare for?"

Ignoring them, Carl narrows his study of the cake further. "Six, seven, eight strands of RNA; clearly an orthomyxovirus; rules out Ebola."

Ross turns a glance to Bronwyn, a subtle raised brow confirming what they both are thinking – *He's good.*

"Looks like it could be airborne?" Carl suggests, taking a bit of an intuitive leap.

"Da, Kimosabe, airborne," Stuart confirms.

"Coronavirus?"

Both Carl and Ross react immediately to Carl's bad guess; Ross with a fair mimicking of a game show buzzer's *"Eeeent!"* and Stuart burying his face in his hands while feigning shame, "I'm so embarrassed! Who knew my roommate was from Dumbfuckistan?"

"Alright, alright; the coconut shavings threw me, thought it was sheathing."

"Nope, merely coconut," Angela clarifies.

Carl rubs his chin, thinking even harder, mentally scanning the thousands of viruses he's perused under electronic microscopes for a match. "Measles? Mumps? RSV?"

"He's getting warmer," Hank encourages.

"He is?" quips Ross.

"Well, by virtue of the process of elimination."

"Ah, yes; the scientific method."

"He better be getting warmer, the candles are melting," Stuart moans.

"*MacArthur Park is melting in the dark, all the sweet cream icing flowing down....*" Ross has broken into song, showing he's the kind of guy whom will exit onto any segue, no matter how frail.

"CDC: the musical," Hanks comments. "You'll laugh, you'll cry, you'll doze off for a bit, then you'll cry some more…"

"*And I don't think that I can take it, 'cause it took so long to bake it, and I'll never have that recipe again, oh, no!...*"

Carl leans away from the cake with a big grin.

"C'mon, Carl, put some effort into it," Angela urges.

"No need to, I know what it is."

"Yeah, right."

"I do."

"You're just not going to say, right?"

"What's the point?" Carl teases, "I mean, you know what it is, I know what it is, so, why waste the time when we could be eating it?"

"Now *that* was an extraordinarily lame attempt to cover the fact you don't know what type of virus it is," Ross challenges.

"I'm assuming that, as a betting man, you're willing to put money where your mouth is."

Ross nods, "Damn tootin'. Ten bucks, baby."

"How 'bout double or nothing what you owe me from basketball?"

"Normally I try not to mix sports betting with science betting, but I'm willing to make an exception. Forty bucks it is."

the momentum of folly

Ross and Carl shake on it. Then Carl stoically answers, "Influenza."

"Yes!" Angela shouts, causing Ross to immediately recoil in the anguish of a lost bet.

Angela then turns to Stuart, "Stuart Chew, please tell our contestant what he has won."

With that, Stuart musters his best game show host M.C. impersonation, "Color coordinated Samsonite luggage, a handsome blue windbreaker with CDC printed in tasteful yet bold yellow lettering across the back to keep you from getting shot by one of the other fifty-four Federal Agencies licensed to carry firearms, *and* – but wait, that's not all – round-trip airfare for one to Guangdong Province, China! Please give it up for Dr. Sims!"

As the others applaud and prepare to divvy up the cake, the reason for this celebration suddenly hits Carl.

"Wait a minute – *Guangdong?*" Carl turns towards Bronwyn. "You're sending me on flu re-con?"

Bronwyn smiles. "Yep, Dr. Jenna Williams specifically requested you."

Carl goes silent, already smoldering.

"Uh-oh, I sense a modicum of disappointment," Ross mutters, aside to Angela.

"You know the only reason I joined the CDC was to work P-4. I told you that at my interview!" Carl says.

Bronwyn nods, "And I also know you've barely been here two years, giving you plenty of time to move up."

"Sure, that's always the carrot. But the fact is you get typecast in whatever virus you start in here. A few months of flu vaccinations and I'm already trapped in the influenza closet."

"But you've been bumped up to recognizance, dude; hell, that's about as exciting as CDC work gets!" Stuart retorts, trying to assuage Carl's rage.

"It's still only P-2," Carl explains, still eye-locked with Bronwyn, "I'll have to quit, ya know."

Losing her patience, Bronwyn levels a glower at Carl, "Considering I just received an official complaint from the Mexican embassy stating you told a priest to kiss your... *rear end*, I'm alright with your quitting." And with that, Bronwyn turns away, leaving an angry vacuum as she pushes through the lab door and exits.

Carl swallows hard, sensing he may have overreacted.

And Angela's analysis doesn't help, "You dumbfuck! You go apologize to her before she reaches her office, and *beg* her for your job back!"

From somewhere just behind Carl and Angela's all-so-serious discussion about careers and life and pecking-orders, Stuart incongruously shouts out as he cuts into the cake: "People, let us party!"

With the exceptions of a few kitchen fires, Health Department lockdowns, and police crime scene closures for drunken stabbings and whatnot, The Juke Joint has been open for business every day since Robert Johnson and Son House first played there back in the late 1920's, the success of its longevity owed to its unwillingness – more out of laziness rather than stubbornness – to mutate with each new fad. It was never a speakeasy. It was never a den. It was never a shindig. It was never a disco. It was never an overpriced and exclusive salon featuring oxygen tanks and green tea elixirs. It was just a juke joint down by the tracks that never found the time to give itself a proper name. People just called it the Juke Joint and that was good enough. And for nearly a century now it's served up just two things: its signature supper special – barbeque ribs or chicken, baked beans, cole slaw, and corn bread – and straight-up, unpretentious music, which most commonly meant Blues.

And tonight is no exception, with some tip-jar band of fifty-somethin's playing a faithful cover of an obscure Leonard Cohen song peppered with all the requisite heartbreak and poetic musings and driving beat necessary to have most everyone out of their chairs and dancing. In a room not much bigger than a prison handball court, the band, crammed in a corner, can scarcely be seen beyond the bouncing, spinning heads of the sixty or more CDC geeks that have dragged themselves from their microscopes and computer screens in order to send Carl off to the Asian hinterlands in a manner befitting and enjoyable for all. It's loud. There's no shortage of alcohol. And there's nearly as many dance styles being resurrected as there are dancers, including, of course, the few-too-many-tequila-shots guy attempting the Worm down there on the floor, mopping up the spilled beer with his flannel shirt and jeans. He'll regret it in the morning when he's trying to isolate methicillin resistant staph aureus bacterium from tens of thousands of blood samples. But for now, for this fractional slice of eternity, he's doing the coolest thing imaginable: what woman in her

the momentum of folly

right mind could resist this courtship presentation? Well, fortunately for him, there aren't too many women in their right minds here tonight, leading them to momentarily think his efforts are funny or cool enough that they might consider letting him father their child, or at least perform the act. *How?* — you ask incredulously. Suffice it to say, trying to understand the 2.3 million years-old socio-biological dynamics of it all can make one's head spin every bit as much as the margaritas flowing here tonight, or the foreboding if inscrutable lyrics reverberating throughout the room as bellowed by that old, gray-pated beatnik somewhere up in the corner:

>*Your servant here, he has been told*
>*To say it clear, to say it cold:*
>>*It's over, it ain't goin' any further.*
>*And now the wheels of Heaven stop*
>>*You feel the Devil's riding crop*
>*Get ready for the future,*
>>*It is murder...."*

Carl is in the middle of the moshpit, still upright for the time being, "dancing" whenever some drunker guy throws a body slam at him, teetering whenever someone shoves another going-away beer in his hand and toasts him. Pale and sweating, Carl takes the drink and the *good luck* slap on the back with ne'r an acknowledgement and angrily guzzles it down, not even bothering to wipe the froth from his face as he joins in with the girl back-up singers and the other drunks for the refrain:

>*When they said:*
>*Repent! Repent! Repent!*
>>*I wondered what they meant.*
>*When they said:*
>>*Repent! Repent! Repent!*
>*I wondered what they meant....*

1414 Peach Lane, Atlanta, Georgia

The bungalow Carl and Stuart call *Mi Casa* is in one of Atlanta's post-WWII housing tracks; *bungalow* being a realtor euphemism for too small for anyone other than a couple of guys with some serious student loan debt. *Crack house* might be a more accurate description but even that might be gilding the lily a bit. The one remarkable feature — well, aside from the years-old and year-'round Christmas and Halloween and Fourth of July decorations — is the old and warped piece of OSB plywood tossed over the three steps rising from the walkway onto the porch. That's Stuart's no-frills wheelchair ramp. Carl threw it together just to help facilitate their move-in almost three years ago now, but, remarkably, it's held up, so there's really no need to mess with it. Clearly these occupants operate under the *If it ain't broke, don't fix it* philosophy.

Inside, within the bungalow's proportionately tiny living room, the distinctive gurglings of a bong can be heard. Smoke tumbles languidly within the bong's cylindrical, translucent purple plastic chamber for a few peaceful seconds until being violently sucked out via inhalation. Stuart is the cause of this: he holds the hit in his lungs for a few burning seconds, releasing in measured syllables as he calls out across the room, continuing a discussion of the sudden twist put in Carl's career path just this afternoon:

"Dr. Jenna Williams, former Dean of Epidemiology, U.C. Berkeley, former head of influenza research for the World Health Organization, not to mention *Nobel Laureate*: dude, I don't get it; you should be, like, stoked!"

Across the room Carl stuffs clothes into a backpack. He still looks sick though it's difficult to say if his clammy pallor and perspiration is still in reaction to his self-inflicted vaccine overdose or merely to last night's going-away binge. Carl considers packing a jacket for a moment, then tosses it back in the closet, as Stuart adds:

"And she's foxy too; kind of like Miss Black America's better-looking sister, and in a lab coat no less!"

the momentum of folly

"Is that supposed to entice me?"

Stuart repacks the bong then wheels it over to where Carl is packing. "Shit, yeah; I'd follow that ass through the Valley of the Shadow of Death, and with a smile on my face! *Oooh* – tight khaki jungle shorts! Can't you see it? – she's just up ahead, all taut and sweaty, hacking away the vines with a machete – and you're following a few steps behind…" Stuart pants like a dog. "But, you know, to each his own, dude."

Stuart offers the bong to Carl.

Carl shakes his head.

"Chicken."

Caving to the formidable pressure heaped upon him by his peer, Carl grabs hold of the bong. Stuart lights it. And Carl takes a hit.

"So, I take it you've never met her."

Carl shakes his head as he holds in the burning smoke, "Supposed to on the plane."

Carl tosses his airplane tickets onto Stuart's lap. Stuart pulls the tickets from their envelope and peruses them, his eyes popping when he notices that they are First Class.

"First Class? Dude!"

"Yeah. Go figure, huh."

"What is that; some WHO perk?"

Carl shrugs as he exhales, "Dunno."

"Shit, the cheap-ass CDC doesn't fly anyone First Class, not even Bronwyn. It's probably a mistake."

"Well, you know what they say: Don't horse gift a look in the mouth."

"Dude, I, like, learn so much from you," Stuart wryly quips, just before lighting his next bong hit. He sucks it in, then, "Ooh, and warm chocolate chip cookies!"

"Yeah, well, that's why I agreed to go," Carl quips back as he stuffs his CDC windbreaker into a side pouch then zips his pack.

Stuart releases the cloud of smoke, then, "So, need a lift to the airport?"

"Naw, Angela's coming by. Says she's got a *surprise* for me."

"Thought she already gave you that, *a-hem*, surprise."

Carl pauses to look Stuart in the eye, "That goes nowhere, alright? Promise?"

"For sure; cross my, you know, whatever."

"After all, she wasn't even going to tell *me*."

Stuart summons up a Jamaican accent, "No worries, mon. Me lips are like supper-glued."

Carl drags his backpack across the living room, out the open front door, and sets it out on the porch. Stuart spins his wheelchair about, following Carl like a radar dish, then posing the burning question:

"So, if you don't mind my asking, what're you guys gonna do; you know, *para el niño?*"

Shamed, Carl ponders the dilemma for a bit then admits, "I don't know."

Angela walks behind a blindfolded Carl, guiding him, a hand on either shoulder, down the flimsy wheelchair ramp and off the bungalow's front porch.

"Is the blindfold really necessary? I mean, I could just simply keep my eyes closed," he suggests, as she reties the spaghetti sauce-stained dishtowel serving as the blindfold for the third time.

"Nope. I don't trust you," Angela explains.

"But if it's *my* surprise—"

She leads him out the broken front gate and onto the sidewalk, "Turning right."

"... shouldn't it, like, be up to me to spoil or not?"

"What is it with you anyway? Every present has to be secretly opened. If you even suspect someone might be throwing you a surprise party, you have to interrogate all your friends into divulging the plot. I bet yours was one of those families that tell one another what to buy them for Christmas. What's up with that?"

"Maybe I don't like surprises."

"Maybe you don't like not being in control."

"Hah! Maybe you should try asking some objective passersby – someone watching *me* obsequiously allowing *you* to lead me blindly through a bad neighborhood – which one of us they think has the control issues here!"

"Appearances can be deceiving."

"Yeah, well, they can also be revealing."

"Well, maybe, just maybe this time it's *my* surprise and not yours. Did you ever think of that?" she asks, with some edge in her voice by now as she guides him past the driveway where Stuart's hippy-painted VW van is parked. "Probably not, is my guess."

"Alright, alright. I'm sorry."

Angela sighs, as she brings Carl to a stop and adds, now joylessly, "You may now remove your blindfold."

And Carl does but, after a bit of looking about, sees nothing that fits the definition of surprise; not even the brand, spanking-new Lincoln Navigator SUV parked at the curb directly in front of him. It's not that he doesn't see it of course; it's just that it doesn't register, it being so far out of the realm of possibilities.

"So, where's the surprise?"

Angela alludes with a beaming nod to the shiny Navigator.

"That gas-hog there?" Carl asks disdainfully.

"Yes, that gas-hog," Angela replies, trying to keep a smile on her face.

"Well, what about it? Who's the dickhead who owns it?"

Angela's pent-up ire immediately takes to wing. "Fuck you! Fuck you *and* go to Hell! I'm so fucking tired of this shit!"

"What shit?"

"Your sanctimonious, groveling, environmentalist, disapproval shit!"

"What are you saying?" Then it occurs to Carl, "Ohmygod, this is *your* car?" he says almost laughing with incredulity.

"Fuck you!"

"What was wrong with your Geo? It was a little old but –"

Angela is screaming now, "Fuck that. I'm the only kid in my family ever to finish college, and it nearly bankrupted my parents. And do you know what? They cried when they saw this car. Yeah; they were that proud of me, they *cried*!"

"Yeah, but you know better, Angela."

Angela shakes her head, hurt and livid, "Naw, naw, don't try laying that guilt trip crap on me. I'm not like you, I've lived hand-to-mouth long enough and I don't like it!"

Carl considers the rage in Angela's glower. He's seen it before, too many times in the mere year and some they've been together. That glower, bearing down on him like a locomotive. Realizing there's no stopping it – or maybe momentarily lacking the energy to try – Carl decides, prudently, to step off the tracks. It's not like he's consciously trying to change the subject; he's merely switching it over on to a sidetrack for the time being. Leaning towards the manufacturer's sticker still adhered to a back window; he decides not to broach the 15-mpg highway estimate issue, or the $56, 965 MSR, or the beverage cup warmers – "standard." Instead he asks the obvious question:

"So, looks as if your headhunter found you that big-assed, publicly-traded pharmaceutical company you so longed for. Which d'ya go with?"

"Aegis."

Carl keeps what he's thinking to himself; about Aegis being the least ethical of a morally bankrupt industry. Why, weren't they one of the companies leading the charge in the Medicare Prescription Drug Bill debacle; bilking US taxpayers for more than $18 billion in nonnegotiable drug costs? He's sure they were, but that's just their business side; every pharmaceutical has that evil alter ego. But for Carl, his big complaint has more to do with their antiviral research; their unique style wrapped up for the stockholders in their specious mission statement ripped off from the Boy Scouts – *Be prepared.* Those fuckers. But again, prudently, Carl keeps these thoughts to himself.

"I know what you're thinking, Carl, but it's not like that. The CEO is actually a really good guy."

"You've already met the CEO?" Carl asks, already suspicious. "What am I saying'? – of course you have. Bet that was one *stimulating* interview. Yeah, like to see the YouTube of that!"

Hurt more than angered, Angela doesn't even dignify the accusation with a reply.

Carl decides to lighten the topic some. "Sorry, I – So, what department, division, cellblock, whatever, will you be working in: vaccines?"

Angela shakes her head. "Antivirals."

"Antivirals? – they obviously don't know you're pregnant."

Again, Angela says nothing.

Carl nods. "Don't suppose they have lab here in Atlanta?"

Angela doesn't bother shaking her head this time. "L.A."

If Carl didn't sense it before he does now; that sinking feeling of being dumped. No matter how bad the relationship, nor whether the dumper or the dumpee, it hurts.

"I see. Well, nice while it lasted, eh? Kinda like *In one year and out the other*," he adds, spitefully.

"You'll be gone a few weeks; should give us time to think things over."

"Oh, I don't know; sounds like you already did our *thinking* for us."

Angela stares at him for a beat, not so much angry as just plain spent. "So, how do you want to hear it; all at once? 'Cause I was thinking the more time-released, *Honey-I-had-a-miscarriage-Level-Two/Level-Five-Los-Angeles/Atlanta-You-know-maybe-we're-just-geographically-undesirable-at-this-point-in-our-lives-anyway* approach would be easier on you. But, hey, your choice."

And, then again, that glare.

Shiny-new or not, the Navigator is mired in the same James Wendell George Parkway southbound, late-morning, stop-and-go traffic as everyone else. Some of it, like Angela and Carl, is airport-bound traffic. Some of it is homebound night-shifters. Others, the trucks mostly, are out-of-town bound freight. But all of it is ostensibly due simply to the fluid dynamics of an overburdened, half-century old infrastructure designed for a populace less than half its current size. Businesses have tried to stagger their workdays, which worked for a while, but now the congestion is like this almost around the clock. And Atlanta isn't alone: in most every city, nationwide, worldwide, this is the case. Overcrowding. Under-funding. Stress. Didn't use to be like this.

"Take the 85," Carl says, pointing to the off-ramp they are just about to creep past. But Angela, whether intentionally ignoring him or simply too busy with her ear-mounted cell phone conversation, drives past the exit and its promise of lighter traffic. Exasperated, Carl leans back against the headrest, groaning as Angela prattles on into her phone.

"... Predominantly PB1 and PB2 genes... in H9N2... Well, H5N2, H9N2 and H6N1 are the other avian viruses known to encode internal proteins.... Canine kidney cells...."

Carl opens his beaten but trusty field laptop computer and boots it up. Still sweating, still hung over, still waging that immuno battle against the dead vaccine on the cellular level, he rolls down his passenger window in the hopes of catching some puffs of breeze. And now that the Navigator is moving again, just such a breeze comes through; not a cool breeze by any measure, but due to the principle that evaporation causes cooling, it suffices, softly dabbing, as it were, the tiny beads of perspiration from his forehead. Carl closes his eyes, enjoying the brief respite from the ongoing swelter, the breeze being the first bit of relief he's felt in days. But, oblivious of all this, Angela touches the button on her master control console and rolls Carl's window back up, eliciting another frustrated groan out of him.

He switches on the air conditioning.

She switches it off.

He turns on the radio.

She turns it off, continuing into her phone: "... We're currently doing trials with a neuraminidase inhibitor.... No, intranasal at ten milligrams...."

Exasperated, Carl slips on a pair of headphones and goes online. Clicking on the National Public Radio website, he catches the end of a live interview with internationally acclaimed biologist, Dr. Henri LaFond.

"... as events unfold even more quickly than biologists had feared. Dr. LaFond, so what are we witnessing here?" the NPR Reporter is asking.

"This is a spotted tree frog – *Litoria castanea* – believed to be the very last of his species."

"*Very last* in the wild, I assume; meaning there are still some tucked away in zoos and whatnot, right?"

"I wish that were the case."

"You're telling us if – *when* this frog dies this species is extinct?" the reporter asks with concern.

"As much as it troubles me to say it, yes, we believe that to be the case. Some twenty years ago we witnessed the extinction of the Golden Toad here also on Monte Verde. Back then we were skeptical. *Surely there must be others of its species somewhere. Could this really be it?* Turns out it was."

His interest piqued, Carl clicks on for the live video feed for the story. Within a few seconds his computer screen shows the grainy image of the frog being discussed, the caption *Live from Costa Rica* printed in a lower corner. The frog looks distressed, barely alive, though its immediate environs appear lush and sustaining. From time to time, the latex-gloved hand of Dr. Henri LaFond appears on the screen, carefully touching the amphibian as he explains his theory regarding the frog's demise in his thick Parisian accent.

"As recently as twenty-four hours ago there were still six frogs alive in this stream, five of which died by morning, each with the same symptoms; lethargy, taut-dry skin, dehydration."

The web cam slowly zooms in on the frog until only its head fills the screen.

the momentum of folly

"Help us understand: if dehydration is the problem here, why doesn't it simply hop back into the water? – assuming it had the energy to do so," asks the NPR Reporter.

"Simply put: it would drown, since frogs breathe through their sensitive skin. For whatever reasons, this species has been unable to process oxygen as it normally should. Essentially, it cannot breathe effectively. Unfortunately this phenomenon isn't unique to this guy here; we're already seeing rapid die-offs in almost half of the six thousand plus species worldwide. And many of us believe this is just the beginning of the end."

"So, we're talking about the likelihood of all frogs becoming extinct."

"That's right."

"Any idea how soon?"

"No. No one knows; the world is still a big place. But I'd be surprised if it doesn't happen in our lifetimes. In fact, I'd be very surprised."

"So, what has brought about this rapid decline?"

"Theories abound; from increased ultraviolet light penetration due to erosion of the ozone layer, to some as yet undetected viral infection, to toxic chemicals – fertilizers, herbicides, insecticides, dioxins – gradually working their way up the frogs' food chain. But certainly habitat loss is a big factor, as is chytrid."

"Chytrid; what's that?"

"A type of fungus pretty much ubiquitous and flourishing these days of global warming. Once chytrid hits an area – say, Costa Rica – most of the species therein – and we have some forty species here – will go extinct within six months."

"So, is the fungus the reason for this frog's demise?"

"His siblings all tested negative for it, so we don't know what exactly is causing it. All we can state unequivocally is that it *is* happening."

Feeling an anxious knot in his stomach, Carl pulls his eyes from the computer screen. He glances at his hand – shaking. He averts his attention out to the snarled rivers of traffic; heading off in all directions, pumping tons of emissions into the already stifling, oxygen-starved atmosphere. *What is this feeling; this deep sense of malaise, this profound hopelessness?* he is asking himself, though not with words as Dr. LaFond's voice pulls his attention back to the computer screen.

"Here in Costa Rica the impact of global warming is causing more dry days and warmer nights. This benefits some species over others. Toucans like it, Resplendent Quetzals don't. Though the two live in precisely the same niche, they eat different things, thus only one will survive the coming decade. That's the other side of the climate change *coin*, if you will – starvation."

"So, unlike the fate facing the Quetzal, this frog's demise wasn't brought on by a competition for food; rather, it is literally suffocating, right?"

"Yes. It might as well be in a plastic bag," Dr. LaFond explains.

"How does this bode for amphibians in general?"

"Not well. Turtles are certainly on the decline. I doubt if they'll see out this century as well. Then again, most every species – except humans and crows and cockroaches and such – seem to be on the decline: currently we're losing on the average of one species of plant or animal every twenty minutes, or some 27,000 each year."

"So, is this frog here the proverbial canary in the coal mine?"

"Generally speaking, scientists are too specialized in their fields of study to be able to make such a grand unifying hypothesis. That said, if this frog *isn't* your proverbial canary, it is certainly cause for grave concern."

The camera is now pulled into an extreme close up of the frog, its otherwise vibrant coloration fading before Carl's eyes. After one last feeble gasp of air, it becomes perfectly still. Its still-shiny eyes taking on that lifeless stare into the unknown.

Over this image the reporter whispers, reverently, fearfully, "Is that it?"

Dr. LaFond takes a breath, hesitant, wishing he didn't really know the answer to the question. But he does: "It seems so."

Carl closes his computer. He swallows at the lump in his throat, then turns his squinting eyes towards the smoggy glare outside.

It's raining, pouring out of the sky in buckets and onto the busiest airport in the United States – Hartsfield-Jackson International. It's still only June yet, another week of this will break the record for annual precipitation. None dare call it monsoon. And to think it was just last year that Georgia suffered its worst drought ever. Abnormal weather, it seems, has become the norm.

the momentum of folly

Just above a sign demarcating the area for "Departures" there's an obscenely large flat-screen television, mounted on the exterior concrete wall of the airport terminal. And every fifty meters or so there's another one of these; blurting out in perfect synchronicity their oh-so-important messages to the masses — wall art for the new "connected" era. And like all the other flat-screen televisions, this one is tuned to some cable "McNews" telecast covering the Alaskan Governor as she *beamingly* makes a pronouncement years in the coming: "It gives me great pride to announce the opening of the Alaskan National Wildlife Refuge, ANWR, to oil exploration...."

If the message is lost on anyone in North America, it would be Carl and Angela who have migrated to the SUV's backseat and are presently engaged in some hasty but passionate, *fare-thee-well* lovemaking, the Governor's image little more than a blurry backdrop through the steamed-up windows. Almost drowned out by the rain beating down on the Navigator's roof metal, is the airport's P.A. system's taped warning: "The white parking area is for airport passenger drop-off only. Any unattended vehicle will be towed..." playing again and again and again, 24/7, to the point where it becomes an indistinguishable component of the airport soundscape.

Angela is atop Carl when it happens; a gentle but sudden lurching of the car, substantial enough to cause both to pause midstream, as it were.

Carl puts words to what both are wondering, "What the hell was that?"

But before Angela can figure it out, let alone answer, the SUV's front end begins tilting upwards in unison with the revving of a tow truck's diesel engine.

"Shit!" Angela shouts. Within seconds she's off Carl, buttoned up, and out of the car with a slam of the door.

Pulling himself upright, Carl wipes the condensation from the window. Looking out to the curb, he sees Angela, already tangled in heated argument with the tow truck driver and a policewoman.

"Why the hell're you towing me? I was just dropping someone off! Does this look like an unattended vehicle? Jesus, we were just looking for the airline tickets!..."

Carl can only shake his head and smile. The garish flat-screen then pulls his attention up to the now-clear image of the Governor, wrapping up her pronouncement:

"… as we take yet another bold step towards energy independence; all part of this administration's commitment to keep our nation strong in the face of adversity and free in the face of change." As the Governor then takes a pen from a gushing aide and signs the bill before her, the broadcast's camera cuts away to show the small audience of oil industry execs and workers assembled for the "photo op" on a pleasantly warm, blue day, out there on the north facing slope of tundra, their spattering applause just audible over the incessant whir of the Governor's helicopter's engines.

Hartsfield-Jackson International Airport

Carl moves along with the 554 other, mostly Asian, passengers passing through the gangway tunnel and into the China Airways A380. Still wet from the rain, still perspiring from the vaccine, still queasy from the night before, he hands his boarding pass to the flight attendant. She flashes a welcoming smile of perfectly bleached teeth and directs him — switching to equally perfect English — "First Class, up the stairway, sir. Enjoy your flight."

Surmounting the staircase, Carl finds himself somewhere in the middle of the vast double-decker plane. Looking both aft and stern, his disorientation brings a bemused smile to another flight attendant taking drink orders.

"May I help you locate your seat, sir?"

"Please," Carl concedes, showing the attendant his ticket.

"Row 47, seat 5; eleven rows up towards the front of the plane, sir," the attendant chirps, "May I get you a drink?"

"Just some — do you have grapefruit juice?"

"Of course. I'll get that for you."

"Thanks."

Carl makes his way to his empty seat assignment in the otherwise full compartment. But rather than taking his seat, he remains in the aisle, rechecking his boarding pass, confused.

Yet another flight attendant comes up to him, asking helpfully, "Something wrong, sir?"

"Yeah, is there another First Class section? I think maybe I'm supposed to be there."

The flight attendant checks Carl's boarding pass. "No, sir, this is your seat. May I get you something to drink?"

"But I'm supposed to be seated next to a business associate; a Dr. Jenna Williams."

The flight attendant glances at the eight year-old Chinese boy – ear buds reverberating audibly as he plays some electronic game – seated in the seat next to Carl's.

"Well, that's clearly not your business associate, now is it?" the flight attendant jokes. She then taps the boy's shoulder to get his attention. As the boy looks up at her, she speaks loudly to him in Mandarin: "May I check your boarding pass?"

The boy hands her his boarding pass.

"Row 47, seat 6. He's in the right seat," the attendant tells Carl, handing the pass back to the boy. "Why don't you go ahead and take your seat and I'll see if I can locate your associate. Dr. *Williams?*"

Carl nods. "Thank you."

Carl then takes his seat, smiling perfunctorily to the boy as he buckles in.

The boy beams back then asks Carl in stilted English, "White Devil?"

Carl isn't sure he heard the boy correctly, "Say what?"

"You White Devil, yes? Lady say I sit next to White Devil!"

"Oh, yeah? What lady was that?"

"Lady who trade me seats," he explains excitedly.

Carl stares at the boy for a beat, then stands right back up again, excusing himself from the boy with a cursory smile and a, "I'll be right back."

Carl descends the staircase into the vast, twelve-across economy class compartment, where seemingly half of Asia is currently trying to stuff oversized articles into the overhead compartments. Undeterred, Carl commences to squeeze and bump his way down one of the crowded aisles – no cheerful flight attendant around here to ask him if he needs help, or a drink, or both. Never having met Dr. Williams in person, he's going as much by the photographs he's seen of her in lecture brochures and journals and the Internet, as by the fact that there's a veritable dearth of African American women on the flight. In fact, there's just one. And there she is; shoehorned into an aisle seat in row ninety-one, a stack of journals on the tray in front of her.

At just a few years into her forties Dr. Jenna Williams hardly seems a candidate for retirement, yet that's her official status with the WHO. And, yes, as Stuart reported, she's attractive; but it's not the simplistic, easy-on-the-eye, magazine-covergirl, perfect-hair, glistening-skin, sex-kitten type attractiveness. Rather it's a much more rare and complex variety wherein confidence and intelligence are equal contributors, both of which ooze from an athletic, field-hardy figure. Sans make-up, sans frills, sans bling, she definitely connotes a low-maintenance, no-nonsense self-reliance as evidenced by her sensible shoes, sensible clothes, and sensible hair. In fact the only detectable accoutrement she appears to allow herself is the cheap, woven cotton, orange, yellow and green Rastafarian style "friendship" band tied to her left wrist.

Carl stands in the aisle beside her, nonchalantly moving his perusal from her Rasta wristband to the stack of journals she's studying, in an attempt to see if they are indeed science journals in an attempt to determine if she is indeed the world-renown epidemiologist with whom he's supposed to be seated. But, perhaps sensing his loitering presence, she speaks to him without looking up.

"I'll have a beer, please."

Carl smiles at her mistake. "Dr. Williams…"

She looks up, over her reading glasses, at him, expressionless.

Carl extends his hand. "I'm Carl; Dr, Carl Sims of the CDC."

"And just how does that preclude you from getting me a beer?" she asks, pointedly and without so much as a smile, and definitely not taking his offered handshake.

Carl is taken aback. Not quite sure what to do or say, he begins looking about for a flight attendant.

"Dr. Sims…"

Carl turns back towards her. "Yes?"

"I'm messin' with you."

"Oh."

"And I'll be messin' with you morning, noon, and night, so you'd best get used to it."

"I see. Well, nevertheless, I'm pleased to meet you," Carl smiles, extending his hand again.

"And field epidemiologists don't shake hands."

Carl retracts his hand again, embarrassed by his faux pas.

"And this particular one *would* like a beer, Chiang Tao if they have it," she adds, returning her attention to her journal and flipping a page.

Yet again, Carl finds himself jousted off balance by Jenna's conversation skills, or lack thereof. He's not sure if she's kidding; that's the problem. She's either overly wry or overly humorless altogether, but, for now, he's not sure which.

About then the airline's P.A. system comes on — *Please make sure your seat is in the upright position and turn off any electronic devices at this time* — repeating the message in Mandarin.

"I was told we had a lot to go over before we get to Shanghai."

"Asahi, if they don't."

"Dr. Williams,"

"Dr. Williams was my dad," she replies, growing exasperated, "My name's Jenna."

"Jenna —"

"Shanghai, yes, lots to do; what about it?" she mutters, flipping more pages.

"Well, I guess I'm just wondering — seeing how we have so much to go over — why you gave up your seat up in First Class to that kid."

"Why?" she laughs, scoffing. "How 'bout because in sixteen hours I will have forgotten all about those extra sixteen millimeters of leg room and that freshly-baked chocolate chip cookie, whereas he will remember it all until his dying breath. And on that you can bet yo' ass."

Carl stares at her — as she pulls off the cap of a yellow marker with her teeth and highlights a paragraph she's reading — knowing she's right.

"Flight attendants, please prepare the cabin for take-off," the P.A. system announces, prompting a nearby flight attendant to accost Carl in the most gentle manner possible: "Please, sir, time to return to your seat."

Carl stalls, clearly hesitant about returning to his assigned First Class seat.

Seated beside Jenna is a Chinese girl, all of ten, who stares at Carl, seemingly aware of his ambivalence. She holds up her boarding pass stub, sheepishly offering it towards him with a hopeful, toothy smile.

"Sir, we trade — yes?" she asks, ever so politely, as members of her family, seated around her, seem embarrassed by her forwardness.

By the looks and age of the girl, Carl surmises she's probably a sibling of the boy with whom Jenna swapped seats, which is probably where she got the crazy idea.

Carl shakes his head, chuckling dismissively, "I don't think so."

The girl's face falls, hopes dashed. The girl's mother quietly but sternly scolds the girl's audacity in a Wu dialect.

Without looking up from her journal, Jenna flips a page, purposely loudly enough to convey her disapproval of Carl's lack of generosity. And Carl gets it, feeling the intended wave of shame wash over him.

"Alright. Here," he capitulates, offering his boarding pass to the girl.

The girl pops out of her seat like some giddy game show contestant. After quickly snatching the boarding pass from Carl's hand and throwing him hers, she begins hugging and kissing family members like she's never going to see them again.

Carl shakes his head, smiling though not particularly happy about being guilt-tripped into his random act of kindness. Feeling entitled by his sacrifice, he vies – it's the very least Jenna could do, after all – for her aisle seat, telling her to, "Scoot over."

"Ain't gonna happen," Jenna scoffs, not even looking up.

Caving yet again, Carl swings his satchel from his shoulder, squeezes gruffly past Jenna's legs, and plops into the snug seat beside her. He glances up a last time to the Chinese girl, giddily touching the last few hands of family members as she bounces away up the staircase towards First Class.

"Feels good, doesn't it?" Jenna asks.

Carl tries to stretch out his legs, but can't. "I'll let you know in sixteen hours."

* * *

Somewhere within the deep-dark recesses of Carl's sleeping mind a recurring nightmare is playing out in the form of a grainy video. This is how the images of the event always come to Carl for that was his initial and only experience of it; a few seconds of some unedited, hand-held, amateur video that came anonymously in the mail. This happened back when Carl was maybe six. Carl's mother was watching the video in secret, tears streaming down her cheeks. In fact, it was her audible sobs which first drew Carl from his bedroom and into the home office where she was watching it on the family's one and only, seldom-watched, small television. It's the fragments of the event that haunt him; the brown paper wrapping the VHS tape had arrived in, torn up by his mom, colorful stamps from some far off and foreign land there on the floor beside her feet when Carl snuck up from behind. And why did she slap him and yell at him through her tears? Surely she loved him, and what had he done wrong other than to merely follow her sobs into the room. So, why the beating? Misdirected anger? Misdirected frustration? Misdirected schadenfreude? And then there's the video image itself; of some rally of sorts on some outdoor stage in some small, dust-dry, third world village. Who were those agitated masses in attendance? Were they Africans? Were they Arabs? Were they Asians? Were they South Americans? The anonymous but certainly terrified camera operator jerked about too quickly to know for sure. In fact, the only ethnically identifiable person in the video was that of the lone white male, in his fifties maybe, up there on the stage, trying to quell the incipient uprising with a loudspeaker. He had two aides with him, but they were quickly dragged off and presumably beaten. But it was the banner, strung up across the back of the stage behind the white man, that explained the event — that demystified and certainly personalized it — for Carl. The banner depicted a stick-figured family of two parents holding hands with two children, superimposed over a photograph of the Earth. And around the Earth ran a slogan printed out in English and another language:

Just two children. Just two billion. We can live with that, Yes, it was this banner that clarified the whole surreal flurry of video imagery for Carl; the banner that was too clearly visible once the white man was similarly dragged from off the stage and down into the angry mob, never to be seen nor heard from nor wrestled with nor played catch or soccer or basketball or Frisbee with ever again. Fortunately or not the video did not have audio — at least no helpful audio — just the staticy electronic blasts from the bullhorn, undecipherable, and the ardent but futile pleas and screams of the unseen camera operator, followed by scuffling sounds, followed by a loud cracking sound, followed by the silence marking the end of the recording.

And that pretty much is how the nightmare always plays out for Carl, sometimes chopped up and rearranged but otherwise pretty much the same.

The airline's P.A. system seeps through, now playing its Mandarin recorded message first, followed by the English version: "Please return your seat to its upright position and store your tray…." The announcement awakens Carl from his nightmare and transitions him to an equally disorienting state of consciousness, made so by the incessant din of the jet's engines, the subtle reduction of gravity as the plane begins its final descent, and by the alien chirps and clucks of half a dozen different Asian dialects all around him. Though chilled and trembling slightly, beads of perspiration nevertheless dot his forehead.

Jenna closes her journal, swigs down the last ounces of another beer, dutifully stows her tray up, then stands announcing: "I'm gonna hit the little girls' room before we land." She then takes a concerned notice of Carl, as he wraps his blanket more tightly around him. "You alright? You look sick."

Carl shakes his head. "I'm fine."

"You sure? You look sick."

"I'm *fine*."

"No matter, if you're not sick now you soon will be."

Carl looks at Jenna, a little puzzled by her prognostication.

Jenna explains with a smirk as she turns to leave, "Everyone's sick over here. You'll fit right in," before walking off up the aisle.

Carl drops his attention to the stack of journals on Jenna's seat. He picks one off the top and begins flipping through it, quickly finding it to contain the same, old epidemiological stats any student in this field has read over and over again: Infection percentages, mutation rates, weather correlations, herd immunization figures, hemagglutinin-neuraminidase combinations, ad nauseum. Carl drops the journal back into Jenna's seat with a bored, "Influenza — whoop-tee-do."

Carl then notices Jenna's weathered leather handbag sitting — rather carelessly, he thinks — fallen open on the floor. And he's about to look away when a glimpse — just a corner — of her olive green French passport snags his notice.

French? Huh, now what would a born and raised American be doing with a French passport? wonders Carl. Curiosity piqued, he looks nonchalantly about to make sure no one is watching, then casually slides the passport from the satchel. Flipping the pages he finds customs stampings from over four dozen countries in just the last year alone.

"Girl gets around!" Carl mutters, impressed. Turning to the very last stamped page he finds a U.S. Customs stamp: Port of Entry: Fairbanks, Alaska,

the momentum of folly

11 January 2010. "Winter in Alaska, how pleasant," he quips for his own amusement, before closing the passport and slipping it back into her satchel.

And he would probably have left it at that had he not noticed a manila envelope stamped, *Classified*. Noticing the envelope's seal was already broken Carl glances nonchalantly about again, and certainly up the aisle towards the *little girls' room*, then, all clear, similarly slides the envelope from the handbag. Unraveling the string looped around the button clasps, he opens the envelope and pulls from it four, black and white, eight-by-ten inch aerial photographs, presumably taken by a Russian satellite judging by the abstruse Cyrillic captions printed across the bottoms. Each photo seems to be of the same thing – some sizeable swath of some anonymous snowfield – each subsequent print a squared magnification of the preceding one. The first is of a frozen, south-by-southwest facing bay, with the actual focal point being some kilometers inland of the coast. The next is a closer detail of that focal point, showing what appear to be the skeletal remains of a small, long-abandoned settlement. The next photograph narrows the focus to a region not more than an acre in area, and located just north of the ghost town's limits. In that this area appears to be bordered by what looks like weathered fencing, Carl is led to the assumption this must have served as the town's corral or vegetable farm – the fence serving either to keep domesticated animals in or wild animals out. But this assumption holds only until Carl pulls up the fourth and last photograph; this one zooming in on the exact center of the fenced-in region down to a rectangular patch of undisturbed snow measuring – if the numbers on the photograph's legend are to be interpreted as metric standard – ten by twenty-five meters. And, still, this area would be unremarkable if not for the two, tall crucifixes – perhaps constructed of whale jaw bones, judging by their weather-bleached whiteness and natural curvature – which, along with some other obvious headstones protruding from the snow, suggests now the enclosed area is actually some type of graveyard. The long, north-stretching shadows cast by the crucifixes testify to a crisp and sunny day though, again, the only details Carl can know for sure are of the esoteric numeric nature; specifically 13:24:54, 19/05/2007, and 168°33" x 67°08" – whatever they might mean.

The plane begins to bank into its final approach. Similarly Carl can see Jenna, some twenty rows away, bumping and excusing her way back down the aisle and towards her seat. Normally such photos would make for a pleasant conversation but the delicate matter of their classified status makes Carl conclude that maybe he shouldn't mention to Jenna that he looked them over: if she wants to show them to him, fine, let her, but until that time he should just keep mum about it. Operating under that plan, Carl slips the photos back into their envelope, restrings the clasps, slides all of it back into her satchel while pretending to tie his shoes, then sits back upright again. To complete the ruse he pretends to have been all along gazing raptly – across a couple of the Chinese girl's still snoozing family members – out one of the plane's port windows to the glaring, polluted, endless sprawl of greater Shanghai. But after a few moments of this he barely notices that he *is* gazing raptly out to the polluted, glaring Shanghai sprawl – *endless*.

Carl pushes a luggage cart stacked with his and Jenna's bags and equipment from the crowded terminal lobby, through the automatic doors, and out to the more crowded Arrival curb. It's hard to know which is more overwhelming; moving from the dimly-lighted interior to the photon-saturated, eye-squeezing, hazy glare of the midday sun-less daylight, or the disorienting feeling of suddenly yanked from the relative order of the terminal and subsequently tossed on one's ass, so to speak, out into the utter chaos of the largest concentration of humans on the planet with all its intrinsic ear-piercing noise and, of course, lung-wrenching air pollution for which it has become infamous. "It's all good," a bumper sticker on a parked yet smoke-spewing taxicab explains to Carl as he pushes the cart past. And Carl is already shaking his head when the cabby, and dozens exactly like him, try to snag his business with the universal bark: "Taxi?' "Hotel, sir?" "Massage with happy ending?" Whether or not it is *all good* Carl will leave for the philosophers to sort out, all he can know for certain it that it is all the same anywhere he goes.

"White Devil, up here!" Jenna's unique sense of humor shouts down to him from the roof racks of an old, been-around-the-world-a-couple-times Landcruiser. She's up there – along with two Chinese WHO interns, a male and female both in their early twenties – already strapping equipment down for what looks to be a long, hard ride.

"Do you have to call me that?" Carl calls back.

Jenna grins wryly, then introduces the interns to him in Mandarin: "Wen and Tian, this is Carl. Carl, this is Tian and Wen." As they exchange handshakes and nods Jenna then translates into English for Carl's sake. "Wen and Tian are from the Shanghai office of the World Health Organization. Interns!"

"Cool, I finally get to work with people who makes less than I do. Do they speak any English?"

Wen, the male, hops off the truck and stands in front of Carl, "Fuckin' A, motherfucker. She-e-e-it, I be like, cracker-ass fluent. KnumI'msayin'?" Wen explains, following it up with knuckles, skin, a bro-shake, then a warm homie hug. "She-e-e-it, that's what I'm talkin' 'bout!"

Jenna shrugs, "He may have picked up a few words from me."

"Well, that and the fact I'm a diligent student of American haute couture – i.e., Rap."

"Fuckin' A," Carl responds, turning now towards Tian, the female. "And I suppose you – Tian was it? – I suppose you're just learning the language as well."

Tian pretends to hobble together a broken-English response, complete with repeated submissive bows: "Greetings to our simple-minded nation of peaceable peasants, White Satan. You want buy firecrackers, yes? Or cheap plastic crap maybe? We got lots cheap, plastic crap for you! Want see?"

Carl cuts Jenna a smirk.

After a boisterous laugh Jenna announces, "Alright, enough of the meet-n-greet crap, we've got us a virus to bag." She then settles into the Landcruiser's backseat, leaving the remainder of the packing to her minions. "Tian, where's my *medication*?"

"Right here, mama sun," Tian grunts as she lugs a battered white cooler with a red cross on it and wedges it amongst other hard-case gear in the back of the Landcruiser.

"Well, don't just chat about it: hit me on!"

"Yes, mama sun. Right away, mama sun. So sorry, mama sun," Tian smirks, opening the cooler to reveal the case of Chinese beer packed in ice. She pulls out a bottle and tosses it over the back seat to Jenna.

"Merci beau coot," Jenna responds, popping the bottle cap off with a couple of palm-smarting slaps, against the nearest metal door handle. She then takes a long, mind-numbing sip – *"Ahhh!"* – then settles into a reclined position across the backseat against some duffle bags, holding the cold bottle against her forehead, remarking: "Better than ibuprofen."

"So, you *are* French," Carl asks, settling into the front passenger seat.

"And we are talking about…?" Jenna asks, without opening her eyes, and in a tone just surly enough to let him know he is beginning to bug her.

"That *merci beau coot* shit."

"Oh, is that French?" Jenna asks, sarcastically.

"I was only wondering because your passport is."

Though her eyes are still closed, Jenna's face contorts with a hint of violation as she asks, "You went through my *stuff?*"

"Of course not. It just spilled out of your handbag thing on the plane." Carl invents, hesitating maybe a nanosecond too long, "I stuffed it back in."

However skeptical Jenna may be of Carl's excuse, she decides not to press the matter. "French, yes; I'm French," she says with a heavy sigh.

"But how's that? I mean, no accent or nothing: I always thought you were American."

"Suffice it to say, it's a long story about a short romance."

"So you weren't born in France?" Wen asks, sticking his upside-down head down through the open sunroof, as he ties down some luggage up there on the roof rack.

"Jesus, what is this; an interrogation?" Jenna snaps back up to Wen, managing to keep a hint of humor in her voice. "No, I wasn't born in France; merely married there."

Carl steals a glance at her hand – no ring – as she elaborates:

"I was born to a pair of passionate UC Berkeley paleontologists – very intentionally – right on the shores of Lake Victoria."

"*Very intentionally* because that's where the earliest evidence of homo sapiens were found?" Tian postulates.

"Yep. Right there beneath the welcoming shade of the Tree of Man. I *did* say they were passionate, didn't I?"

After maybe a moment's pause to reminisce about her parents, Jenna promptly changes the subject. She then pounds a fist against the Landcruiser's roof, shouting up through the sunroof to Wen.

"What the hell's taking so long, Wen?"

Wen tosses a net over the top of the luggage. "Almost there."

Tian climbs into the backseat opposite Jenna. "I'm ready."

the momentum of folly

After strapping the luggage net securely, Wen shouts, "Done!" then slides down through the sunroof and into the driver's seat.

"Let's roll, Kato," Jenna says, raising her beer in toast of the event, then sipping from it.

The Landcruiser's keys and ignition switch long missing, Wen "hotwires" it with the two wires hanging from under the dashboard. As the circuit is established allowing the electrons to flow from battery to starter motor, the engine sputters dutifully to life.

With a grinding of gears, Wen forces the manual transmission stick into first announcing, "We are, like, so-o-o outta here!" before punching the gas and steering the Landcruiser away from the curb.

"Fuckin' A," Jenna mutters, taking a long, thankful sip from her beer.

Some hours later the sun sits in a thick bed of haze on the horizon, looking more like an overripe persimmon than a dying star. *And far too easy to look at!* – that's what Carl is thinking as he stares wearily at it through the Landcruiser's windshield, his brain fried by the travel, the jet lag, the going away party, the vaccine overdose, the *et al.* Sleep; sleep is what he needs. About a week's worth would be nice. That and some exercise; endless hours of it. What he wouldn't give for a sweaty pick-up game of hoops right about now. As the Landcruiser nudges, stop-and-go, along through the almost hopeless gridlock of traffic, Carl finds himself searching the concrete jungle for a basketball hoop – either bolted to a building or, God forbid, freestanding – but the challenge seems to be of the needle in a haystack magnitude. Or some soccer; he hasn't played soccer in a while. But there seems to be no fossil remains of leisure left in this city; it all having been architected-over in the name of space efficiency. Why squander the real estate on a two-dimensional sports court when a seventy-story building is so much more productive? Build, build, build. Up, up, up. Down, down, down. Out, out, out. Money, money, money....

"Are we going to stop for the night?" Tian asks, timidly admitting even she is becoming weary of her hometown traffic.

"If we stop we only have to hop right back into it come morning," Jenna explains.

"The damage is greatest as done by the drip that is steady. Isn't that right, Dr. Williams?" Wen proselytizes.

Jenna winches at the garbled maxim, "Good said, student of language English."

"Yessiree, the journey of ten thousand kilometers begins at the beginning of the first millimeter." Wen turns towards Carl to add, "Confucius say."

Carl studies Wen's face, wondering if he's kidding.

Wen eventually smiles.

He *is* kidding. There's hope.

"Jesus, welcome to China," Jenna laments as she looks out at the gridlock. "Wen, is there any other road out of town?"

"This isn't so bad. I think we beat the rush," Wen calls back.

"Beat the rush," Jenna sighs. "You know, once upon a time, and not all that long ago, it didn't take all day just to get out of Shanghai. Once upon a time there were actually distinct villages here separated by, believe it or not, *wilderness*. Now look at it." Jenna alludes to the endless sprawl in every direction. "China, 1.3 billion and still growing in spite of its one-child policy, new world leader in CO_2 output, 1,000 new cars thrown onto the streets of Shanghai every day, consumer of more than forty percent of the world's coal, and building new coal-powered plants at a rate of one every twelve days. And then there's India; 1.2 billion and growing much faster than China due to no such family planning or restraint or foresight whatsoever, and increasing their fossil fuel consumption just as quickly. Hell, t'was a time the human population of the entire world was only one billion. Anyone care to guess when that was?"

"Uh, when sweet baby Jesus was born. No, sweet baby Mohammed. *Sweet baby Krishna!*" Wen blurts.

"Sweet baby someone anyway," Tian quips facetiously.

"Blasphemer, out with your tongue!" Wen scolds back at her with a sarcastic glower in the rear view mirror.

"Out with your *brain*."

"Well, good guesses all, but nowhere close." Jenna says. She then swings the question to Carl, now reclined in his seat — eyes closed and head pillowed by a somewhat giving daypack — desperately trying to get some sleep. "Carl knows. Tell 'em, Carl."

Carl answers without opening his eyes, "Sweet baby *Darwin*."

Jenna smiles and nods. "And what year might that have been?"

"1805."

"Yup, a mere two hundred years ago. And when did we hit two billion?"
"1928."
"Three billion?"
"1961."
"Four billion?"
"1974."
Tian and Wen are already looking at Carl with amazement.
"Five?"
"1987."
"And six?"
"July ninth, 1999."
"How do you know all that?" Tian has to ask.
Carl shrugs, still not even opening his eyes.
Tian turns to Jenna, "How's he know that?"
"Robert Sims; either of you ever heard of him?"
Tian shakes her head.
"Who?" Wen asks through the mirror.
"Dr. Robert Sims; one of the world's foremost environmental scientists. Founded *Just Two!* – an organization which attempted to spread population awareness worldwide and get everyone to adopt a voluntary two-child limit through a global billboard campaign. Very ambitious. Suffice it to say, he was Carl's father." Jenna then begins counting by fives fairly quickly, "*Five, ten, fifteen, twenty...* – c'mon, everyone!"

"Everyone what?" Tian asks.

"Count by fives! *Twenty-five, thirty, thirty-five...*"

Eventually Tian and Wen join in, "*Forty, forty-five, fifty...*"

"That's how Carl's father would start population discussions at schools; have all the kids count like that then tell them, *Okay, now keep that up for the rest of your life and you'll just barely keep pace the human population growth.*"

As Wen and Tian reel from the quickly adding numbers, Jenna takes another sip of her beer, before adding, "Very effective, I thought. But that's just me."

"What happened to *Just Two!*?" Wen asks.

Jenna shrugs, "It sputtered and died, like all good things."

"What happened to Carl's father?" Tian asks.

Before Jenna can answer. Carl blurts a pat answer meant to quell the discussion, "Sputtered and died."

Jenna honors Carl's decision to spare Tian and Wen the details of his father's demise. Instead she pulls another beer from her cooler and resumes her rant:

"Ah, but here's the cheery news: the world's population is currently zipping past 6.9 billion and heaping on a million more every four days, which shakes out to some eighty million, or a new Germany, each and every year, or an additional billion — nearly an India or China — every fourteen years or so."

Wen utters the dread felt by all, "That's crazy!"

Jenna nods as she pops open her beer, "And yet will we ever hear a peep out of any of the world's political or religious leaders or major media outlets that maybe, just maybe we shouldn't be spitting out as many kids as we can? *Heaven forbid!*"

"Why's that?"

"Because they're all fucking spineless," she begins, pausing only to take a sip of beer as if to reload. "They're afraid to offend anyone; afraid to dissuade any potential voter or over-breeding flock members, afraid of being labeled a pessimist by acknowledging the obvious fact that we're on a short path to global suicide, or afraid of being accused of hampering the economy — *It's the economy, Stupid.* No, excuse me, but you're wrong; *It's the environment, Stupid!* The environment is all that ultimately fucking matters and *it* is being trampled by too many fucking people!"

Jenna raises her beer in a sardonic toast, "So, a toast; a toast to *the momentum of folly.* Party on!" She then takes a long, anesthetizing swig.

Jenna's diatribe leaves a reeling silence in its wake. Tian and Wen dare not say or ask a thing more. Even Carl is speechless; surprised and even taken aback by Jenna's utter disdain for the species to which she had committed her life and talent to serving. In the darkness of the Landcruiser's cab, as they bump and squeak onwards into an uncertain night, he surreptitiously observes her; the scowl on her face, the frustration, the fixed resolve.

As if feeling his scrutiny, she turns towards him, engaging his stare with an even more critical one of her own; her eyes seemingly challenging him, seemingly asking: Are you up for this? Are you aware of what's at stake? Are you capable of transcending such trite notions as *Right* and *Wrong?* Are you man enough? Are you *human* enough?

Guangdong, China

It's morning again. Dawn. Just another day on Earth. The Landcruiser is stopped on the shoulder of a refreshingly un-trafficked, rural road. Carl is now sitting in the driver's seat, gazing out into the foggy mist obscuring the countryside. Some fifty meters away there's a silhouette of a farmer driving an ox-pulled cart. Due to the thick nature of mist the oxen, cart and farmer appear to be floating past, but Carl assumes they must be riding along some raised levee; there being so few miracles these days, even in Asia.

In one side of the backseat: Tian sleeps, curled up in an impossibly compact fetal ball — *How can she sleep like that?!* On the other side Jenna studies a map, aided by reading glasses and a headlamp. The fog-muffled pops of an approaching two-stroke, headlight-less motorbike are heard long before it is seen — *pop-pop-pop-pop...*. As it passes, Carl notices it transports what looks to be an entire family — father, mother, and three soiled children — all either barefoot or sporting plastic sandals, all expressionless, most somehow spawned in spite of China's one-child policy, all seemingly immune to the morning chill and the incipient day of toil, having been steeped in adversity since birth. And just as the Doppler effect is causing the motorcycle's engine *pop-pops* to drop in pitch as it passes, its handlebars nearly clip Wen, as he stands out behind the Landcruiser pouring gasoline from a five-gallon jerry can into its tank.

Wen shouts after the already vanished motorbike, "Shit! Buy a headlight, dickface!"

"What?" Carl calls back, unaware of Wen's brush with death.

"That dipwad nearly took my ass out. Hate that random shit."

The gas can emptied, Wen replaces the cap then calls up to Carl, "Try it now."

Carl pumps the gas pedal a few times then touches the two ignition wires together. And though there are sparks, and though the starter and battery seem to be doing their best, the engine doesn't turn over.

the momentum of folly

Wen shouts up again to Carl as he straps the empty jerry can to the back of the Landcruiser, "Might take a few tries before the gas works its way up to the carburetor."

Carl pumps the pedal as he touches the ignition wires again… still nothing.

"Might have to replace the fuel filter. Think there's a spare in the toolbox," Wen adds, ever the optimist, as he comes up to the driver's window.

Carl tries hotwiring it again — still no go — with the starter motor now beginning to groan as the battery's charge is gradually depleted.

Wen sniffs the air, "I don't even smell gas. Is the choke out?"

"What the hell's a choke?"

"Damn; you invent the automobile then forget how you did it: there's America's problems in a nutshell," Wen quips as he reaches in and pulls the choke lever out. "Now try it."

Carl touches the wires together again, the battery barely able to do its part. He pumps at the accelerator furiously.

"Stop pumping; don't wanna be flooding it now."

"How am I gonna flood it when no gas is getting there?"

"It's like overfeeding a starving kid. Ever done that? It's heartbreaking, man."

"Maybe we should let it rest."

"Rest? It's a *machine*; machines don't need rest."

Carl touches the wires together yet again, the battery hurling its last few electrons through the copper at the starter and causing it to turn. Sensing hope, Wen reaches in through the window again and delicately slides the choke lever back in, all very intuitively, and soon the engine coughs and sputters to life.

"Yeah, baby! See, no problem."

Carl rolls his eyes.

Wen opens the driver side door, telling Carl, "Slide over."

"But you drove all night."

"Which is why we're still alive. Slide over."

Carl begrudgingly capitulates.

"Besides, we need a gas station and you wouldn't know what to look for out here in the boondocks. They could be doubling as a bakery or barbershop or endangered species aphrodisiac emporium or all three; never know."

Wen releases the parking brake and gets the Landcruiser moving down the muddy, unimproved road again. "What the hell's a *boondock*, anyway?"

"It's a pier thingy where they, like, you know, dock boons," Carl invents, as he buckles into his seat.

Wen thinks about it, then turns back to Carl, "Now you're fucking with me," Wen is saying, just as he hits a giant pothole.

"Sure glad *you're* driving; I might've missed that one," Carl quips.

"Exactly," Wen replies.

The jolt awakens Tian. She rubs her eyes and stretches, then gazes out into the misty dawn, asking of no one in particular, "How much further?"

"I'm guessing about an hour," Jenna says, herself yanked unwillingly back to the task at hand.

"I have a dumb question," Tian begins to ask before being cut off by Wen.

"Now, now, there are no dumb questions; just dumb people. Isn't that right, Dr. Jenna?" Wen cracks sarcastically from the front seat.

"Shut up."

"Make me."

Jenna cuts through the quibbling with a hint of impatience. "What's the question?"

"Are viruses living organisms?"

"Yes!" "No," Wen and Carl answer simultaneously.

"Right," Jenna says.

"Who?" Wen asks.

"Both of you."

"How can we both be right?"

Jenna shrugs, "Just are."

As Wen and Carl exchange a dissatisfied glance, Tian adds: "I asked my biochem professor if viruses were alive and he couldn't really answer either."

"Yeah, well, what is life?" Jenna answers cryptically.

"Yeah, that's what I'm talkin' about!" Wen shouts with inscrutable glee. He turns then to Carl, "No beatin' about the brush with Dr. Jenna! Ever worked with her before?"

Carl shakes his head.

"If there's an opportunity to *meta* the *micro*, she's on it like flies on shit!"

the momentum of folly

Jenna dutifully ignores Wen to turn back to Tian. "If you're asking if viruses, like bacteria, are cells, or if they multiply by dividing, or if they use oxygen or eat or have anything resembling a metabolism, the answer is *no*."

Carl turns towards Wen, shooting him a *told you* glance.

Jenna continues, "But if you're defining life as the ability to replicate or to act in one's own best interest or to invade and conquer, then, *yes*, viruses are very much alive."

And now Wen turns to Carl, cutting him a *told you* glance of his own.

But Jenna is only getting started, "Then again, maybe the question should be rephrased: Are we *alive*? —"

"Hah! — here we go!" Wen says, facetiously warning the others of Jenna's incipient philosophizing.

"...Or, is there even such thing as life? Or is everything reducible to molecular level chemical reactions following the path of least resistance? Is then *consciousness* merely the result of the oxidation of carbon and hydrogen and the other atoms that together comprise our endorphins and neurotransmitters, or the cytosine, thymine, adenine, and guanine bases from which our DNA and RNA are created? Can life really be defined as anything more than chemical entropy? For that matter, is water — merely by virtue of its ability to evaporate or sublimate or similarly change states — or a fire—by virtue of its natural exothermic inclination to convert organic cellulose to carbon and CO_2 — are they also to be considered to be living organisms merely because they *change*? See? — 'tis a slippery slope, this attempt to define life."

"By that reasoning, there would be no such thing as free will," Carl opines, "insofar as every thought and, thus, decision is merely the result of chemical entropy."

"So it would seem," Jenna concurs.

"I read somewhere that humans possess a sliver of free will," Tian adds.

"A *sliver*?" Jenna repeats, rolling the theory about.

"Yeah. What do you think was meant by that?"

Jenna doesn't respond — other than a single, ponderous *"Interesting"* — nor would it be within her character to, at least not until she's completely mulled the theory over.

Some hours later raindrops begin to splatter against the windshield. Carl, now driving, turns on the wipers, which only seem to smear into squeaky arcs the bug parts splattered there the night before. He squints through the smear out into the brightening morning, the fog beginning to tear to reveal a higher layer of dark and portentous clouds.

"This rain isn't going to help matters," he tells Tian, now sitting "shotgun" beside him.

"Why's that?" she asks.

"Influenza doesn't spread well under wet conditions."

"Really? I thought the rain marked the beginning of flu season."

Carl shakes his head. "In some tropical areas that can be the case, but in more temperate climes – Europe, North and South America – the virus, quite counter-intuitively, travels best in low humidity; at the start of winter or early spring, when it's cold but drier. Precipitation literally knocks the virus out of the air; the less than ideal conditions resulting in lowered infection rates."

"So what do we do?"

"We persevere," Jenna blurts from her seat, even though – with eyes closed and legs reclined – she appears to be sleeping. "The bug's still out there, it'll just be a little harder to find."

Carl then directs Tian's attention outside to a passing rice paddy.

"There it is."

"There's what?"

Carl points towards a farmer, knee-deep in water, planting rice seedlings as a duck and pig forage on either side of him.

"The golden triangle of influenza."

Tian turns back to Carl, clearly puzzled, "What d'ya mean?"

"Ever wonder why virologists from the world over come here each year?"

"To China?"

Carl nods, "Particularly to the rice paddies of Guangdong Province."

Beginning to understand, Tian turns back towards the farmer and his animal entourage.

"Humans, pigs, and ducks?"

"The aforementioned triangle."

"Influenza thrives in birds, I know that much. So, what happens next; the ducks defecate in the water passing the virus on to the farmers?"

"Actually to the pigs which, of course, also live in close proximity with the farmers."

the momentum of folly

"So we get it from the pigs?"

"Usually. It's an easier jump since we share similar host proteins with swine that interact with the viral hemagglutinin and neuraminidase proteins; hence the 2009 season's Swine flu pandemic. We *can* catch influenza directly from birds but it's rare."

"Just from ducks?"

"Oh no; ducks, chickens, turkeys – pretty much all domestic fowl. Wild birds are natural hosts to all the known subtypes of influenza A but, unlike domesticated birds, usually don't get sick from them. Similarly dogs, horses even – probably most if not all mammals – can host certain strains, but it's because of our aforementioned relations with swine proteins that make us particularly susceptible to inter-species jumps from pigs."

"So I suppose every inter-specie jump causes subtle mutations in the virus."

"Every such jump *hones* the mutations into ever more successful ones. But the actual mutating happens within each and every infected cell – swine, fowl, or human. And because influenza, unlike most viruses, is made of highly mutable RNA instead of the more stable DNA, there can be, like, 10,000 different viruses bursting out of each."

"Ten thousand different strains from each of millions upon millions of infected cells?" Tian asks, reeling. "That's trillions of new strains, for which we have absolutely no antibodies!"

Carl scales back her math a bit. "Well, most of the mutations happen in non-gene coding regions. So, maybe not *trillions* of new strains, but a butt-load for sure."

"And it all starts right here in Guangdong."

Carl nods, "Some ninety-six percent of all new strains anyway."

Tian turns her amazement back to the passing farmer and his animals.

"The golden triangle of influenza."

Old Senate Building. Washington, D.C.

———

Dr. Hiro Nakayama looks all of his sixty-one years, and then some. He slides his thick bifocals back up his nose and leans towards the three microphones set on the polished wooden dais before him. As he resumes speaking his amplified voice echoes back at him, reverberating throughout the vacuous chamber of the United States Old Senate Building.

"… Global consumption of oil, coal, and natural gas is currently five times what it was in 1950, resulting in a twenty-one percent rise in atmospheric carbon dioxide – CO_2 – levels over that same time period. In order to search for a time when human activity had no effect, or only a negligible effect, on greenhouse gas concentrations, we would have to go back some two and a half centuries to the beginnings of our Industrial Revolution – the period when we really began exploiting the vast amounts of energy stored in fossil fuels. Since then CO_2 levels – a direct byproduct of the burning of fossil fuels – has jumped from 280 parts per million to its present 387 parts per million, adding an approximate two ppm per year. This 36% increase is the primary reason why average global temperature has risen 1° Fahrenheit over the past century. Some skeptics – here in this room even – point to last winter's record snowfall here in the Capital as proof that global warming isn't real, and famously built an igloo which they dedicated to Al Gore in an attempt to make their point. But the fact of the matter is the record snowfall is direct evidence of warming, insofar as the increase surface temperatures has caused a 4% increase in water vapor levels over the ocean just since 1970. More moisture, more precipitation; hence the record snowfall. This rise in average global surface temperature is unequivocal. The probability that this was caused by natural processes alone is less than 5%. This is the conclusion reached, after two decades of research by over 1,100 contributors, by the International Panel on Climate Change in its Fourth Assessment Report, released in 2007.

the momentum of folly

"Although there are predictable natural cycles – known as the Milankovitch cycles – that effect changes in the Earth's temperature and, hence, its greenhouse gas concentrations – among these: the 100,000-year Earth Orbit cycle, from circular to elliptical and back to circular again, bringing us varying distances from the Sun; also the 41,000-year Earth Tilt Cycle; and the 11,000-year Earth Wobble Cycle; not to mention the almost negligible eleven-year solar magnetic activity cycle – all of these, though significant in their impact on historic warming trends and ice ages, still have never brought atmospheric CO_2 levels to within 70% of what they are today; at least not at any time over the past 650,000 years as determined by data collected from Arctic ice core samples. These unprecedented CO_2 levels explain why eleven of the twelve warmest years - *eleven of the twelve warmest years ever recorded in at least the last 115,000 years* – have occurred just since 1996.

"This rise in the average global surface temperature has caused the world's sea levels to rise twenty centimeters during just the last century. Now, one degree Fahrenheit and twenty centimeters doesn't sound like a lot, but it has been calculated that an increase of just one degree Fahrenheit *more* will cause widespread drought in some areas and flooding in others, increased acidification of the oceans and the subsequent bleaching of coral reefs, further erosion and flooding of coastlines and large population displacements as ocean levels continue to rise, and significant reduction in natural snowpack and glacial reservoirs threatening the freshwater needs of hundreds of millions of people. And that's with an increase of just one degree.

"However, at current emissions output – both here and abroad – atmospheric CO_2 levels will likely top 800 ppm by 2100, or more than *twice* its current concentrations, or nearly three times what it's ever been over the past 650,000 years. This would cause the average global surface temperature to spike upwards of 9° Fahrenheit. In case you did not hear me: that's one degree over the course of the last century, *nine* degrees over the course of the next. That's if we stay the course, business as usual. That's if we do nothing.

"Now, as you are all no doubt well aware, The Copenhagen Climate Conference was an attempt to ratify reductions in greenhouse gas emissions. Targets varied from nation to nation; with over a hundred of the 192 nations present proposing a 45% reduction from 1990 levels to be met by 2050, in order to keep the average temperature increase to under 1.5°C by 2100. The European

Union proposed a noble 20 to 30% reduction on their own emissions by 2030, whereas the United States offered up only a 14 to 17% reduction from 2005 levels, and China, regrettably, would not commit to any reductions whatsoever. In the end the Accord was neither accepted nor rejected, but rather merely "noted;" presumably so the façade of something accomplished could be maintained.

"As frustrating as this insouciance was from an environmental perspective, it may ultimately prove to be a good thing that nothing was signed. I say this is because the Accord was already a weak compromise, with absolutely no "teeth" for enforcement and no timetable for execution. Had the U.S. and China and India and everyone else signed the treaty it would have been too easy to declare the Summit a victory — as China did nonetheless — and return to essentially business as usual. For even if those proposed 20% E.U. reductions had been adopted worldwide the sad fact of the matter is that atmospheric CO_2 levels would still top 770 ppm by the end of this century, causing global surface temperatures rise some five to six degrees, thus killing off any remaining coral reefs, thawing any remaining permafrost thereby releasing even more carbon and methane into the atmosphere, and triggering the extinction of an estimated 40% of our planet's plant and animal species, all within the coming century. And that's the case if we had signed on to the treaty."

Dr. Nakayama pauses to take a sip of his glass of water. Despite having recited these statistics in public many times before, they never fail to make him tremble. And of all his speeches this is arguably the single most important, so he wants desperately for his message to be clear, to be concise and, most of all, to be objective.

The members of Congress are reasonably intelligent people; no need for theatrics. Just give them the facts and they'll do what is necessary in order to avert global catastrophe — to do what is right. After all, it's only logical that what's in the best interest of all of humanity should also be in the best interest of the American people. And what's in the best interest of the American people; why, it's only logical that that is the goal of the Congress. Right?

That's what he had assured himself beforehand, in his own private pep talk. Nevertheless, it's a dire picture he's painting for them and he knows it. He also knows, deep down, that none of these people, no matter how concerned, no matter how powerful, can change anything. Senators, at best, can only look ahead six years. The President and his administration can only project four years. And members of the House of Representatives only two years. And by the fact they each and all must generate vast sums of campaign contributions just to get or stay in office, rendering each and all of them beholden to industries and corporations whose concerns about the future does not extend further into the future than the next quarterly profit statement; well, suffice it to say, Dr. Nakayama knows Congress is essentially powerless. Compounding that inconvenient matter, Dr. Nakayama also knows that unless some drastic voluntary reduction in global greenhouse gas emissions is adopted *immediately* by *all* nations, or unless something nearly cataclysmic happens *involuntarily* to cut anthropogenic greenhouse gas emissions – life on Earth will be changed forever. But he also knows this isn't likely to happen if left in the hands of the politicos. The situation is, in fact, utterly hopeless. We're past the tipping point. Life on Earth will soon be a living Hell. It's the momentum of folly thing. He's a scientist; he knows this to be true, and yet he continues; he'll try anyway. He'll do his damnedest to roll that stone back up that mountain. He'll hit his head against that wall yet again, only to have some coward with a website, funded by the coal, gas, oil, utilities, auto, you-name-it industries, spew out disinformation refuting his meticulous research. Then, citing those "studies," those predictable members of Congress in the pockets of Big Energy will censor Dr. Nakayama's report; just the way they did Dr. James Hansen's – twenty-five year research climatologist with NASA and Head of their Goddard Institute of Space Studies – back in 2006 when he attempted to make public his team's assessment that human activity was, "with 99.99% certainty," influencing global warming. Yes, they'll try to reduce Dr. Nakayama's testimony here today as mere opinion or, worse, a "hoax" all so that Big Energy can push ahead with new explorations, for which they will again receive billions in tax breaks in spite of their hundreds of billions in record profits; 'cause that's how the wheels between the government and big business are greased; that's how consent is manufactured, that's how spin is spun in a "free" society.

"Extrapolating current warming trends into the coming century we estimate much – as much as sixty percent – of the Antarctic ice shelf will melt. The Northern ice cap is expected to completely thaw – completely thaw – by 2040 or even sooner. Add to this the melting of the glaciers of Greenland and we may experience a rise in the mean ocean levels of as much as seven meters, thereby inundating several island nations and displacing as much as a third of the world's people including, for instance, Bangladesh and Holland. Insofar as the polar caps act to reflect solar radiation – not to mention acting as the Earth's air conditioners, if you will – their shrinking will only exacerbate the warming trend, resulting in an ever-accelerated rise in surface and atmospheric temperatures, with no end in sight.

'In conclusion….' When Dr. Nakayama says *In conclusion*, he can hear his Japanese accent, and though there was a time, not long ago, that this would embarrass him, it doesn't anymore. It doesn't because the data he's providing is just too important. It also doesn't embarrass him because, truth be told, he's just too damn angry now; angry at the world's governments for having not imposed greenhouse gas emission limits long ago, angry at corporate greed for intentionally obfuscating the facts about global warming – or timber stands or fish stocks or fresh water supplies or what have you – just so they can stuff a few more bucks into their pockets before the ship sinks; and, of course, he's angry at people for breeding irresponsibly. Nope; he's not embarrassed by his accent anymore: now he's just embarrassed to be human. And so he repeats himself:

"… *In conclusion*, I, along with most scientists in this field, have concluded that atmospheric CO_2 levels *must* be brought down to below 350 parts per million. We feel this is both economically feasible and environmentally *vital* in order to maintain life as we know it. In order to get there it is imperative that all nations – and especially China, the largest CO_2 producer; and India, the potentially largest producer; and the U.S., the biggest per capita producer; and the European Union, close behind – it is imperative that *all* nations commit to a much more stringent CO_2 reduction schedule than was "noted" by the Copenhagen Accord. Specifically, we are calling for a 45% reduction from 1990 levels to be met by 2030, and this coupled with strict compliance, verification, and enforcement. For unless such a commitment is made we see little hope of humanity surviving in any enviable manner beyond the next century. Thank you."

Upon finishing, Dr. Nakayama musters a frail smile as he gazes out to the Senate chamber, its one hundred seats ninety-two percent empty. Exacerbating matters, the only senators present are either reading some other pending legislation, conferring with aides, or unabashedly sleeping – but not a one, it seems, is paying attention.

the momentum of folly

As the futility of his efforts become apparent to him, Dr. Nakayama takes a deep breath and sighs. Then, as he begins to step away from the podium, he accidentally turns directly towards the unmanned, fixed C-SPAN 2 camera. But, rather than feeling suddenly self-conscious by the mishap and bowing all Japanese-like and quickly turning away, he decides instead to just continue to stare at the camera. He even takes off his glasses; seemingly peering – sans emotion and for a good half a minute at least – straight into the camera and through its unfathomably deep lens in order to take his appeal to the people – the little people, the *real* people– watching from the other side.

On that other side – the other side of the planet, as it happens – Dr. Nakayama's face, albeit pixilated and popping with static, is seen on the screen of Jenna's laptop computer, the C-SPAN 2 logo branded across the bottom of the live feed.

"Yeah, baby; gas station at twelve o'clock," Wen blurts out from the driver's seat as they pull into a small, rural town. He then turns to Carl, just awakening from a nap in the backseat. "Tell me you wouldn't've driven right past it."

Carl looks about, "I *still* don't see it."

"That's because you're looking for gas pumps and logos and shit; you've got to move beyond that. You've got to wrap your head around the fact that petrol is served up here in rusty 55-gallon barrels and plastic milk jugs," Wen jokes as he pulls up to the mom 'n' pop-ish looking storefront and parks the Landcruiser.

"Plastic milk jugs?" Carl asks incredulously, not sure whether to believe Wen.

"Yep," Tian testifies, from her shotgun seat and studying a map.

Carl shakes his head. "That's messed up."

"That's China; the mystical land of nuclear waste dumped into water wells, coal power generating plants in the middle of cities, and burning rivers," Tian laments.

Jenna takes a last look at her laptop's screen – a last look at Dr. Nakayama, now gathering up his papers and exiting the Senate testimony dais – then closes it. After staring off in space for a moment, she looks around then asks, "So, where are we?"

"The end of the road," Tian says, folding away the map with palpable frustration. "And you may take that any way you like."

Jenna climbs out of the Landcruiser to stretch out her weary traveler bones and look around. The others take this as a cue to do the same.

Wen heads for the store. "I'll see if I can find the proprietor. Would you prefer a robust Iraqi crude or a light, sweet Darfurian?"

Jenna calls after him, "Just ask 'em if they have a garage we can rent for the next week or so."

"For the 'Cruiser?"

"Yeah. Tell 'em we'll pay extra if nobody drives it or moves into it."

"Okay-doke."

"Tian?"

"Yes, Dr. Jenna?"

"How about checking to see if the local Club Med has any vacancies," Jenna says facetiously.

"May I assume anything with a roof will suffice?" Tian asks already heading off in search of accommodations.

Jenna nods, "A roof would be nice."

Carl has made his way up a slight rise behind the store offering a view of the village's freshwater port. There, on a red dirt knoll, he begins his regular stretching regimen – knee rolls, one side then the other, quadriceps, inner thighs, then hamstrings, etc. – as he gazes out over the wide, filthy river, rolling so slowly it's difficult to tell which direction it is flowing. As he moves from one rote position to the next he takes note of: fishermen tossing nets into the river from wobbly skiffs, an open sewage culvert oozing untreated waste directly into the river, children swimming naked and playing a game of tag while laughing so hard they nearly drown; all this as well as the aforementioned foreboding commingling of pigs, chickens and ducks.

"Lovely, isn't it?" Jenna quips, as she comes up to Carl, unnoticed from behind.

"*Primitive* is what I was thinking."

"More like post-apocalyptical."

Carl moves the conversation to the business at hand, "So, what should we be looking for; hacking coughs, runny noses, sneezing – the usual?"

"More than likely that phase has come and gone, if it was here at all."

"So, just set up shop and start collecting nose and throat swabs, and buy blood samples from anyone testing positive?"

the momentum of folly

Jenna watches as half a dozen piglets chase after a six year-old girl – their dirty-faced shepherd – tapping a stick. She shakes her head, "No need to spook 'em just yet. First we'll just test the pigs and ducks for antigens."

"I'll start unpacking," Carl says, turning back for the Landcruiser.

Jenna nods, "Right."

Before Carl heads off, he nods towards a trio of pregnant mothers, chirping amongst themselves as they stroller, push or drag one or two or even three children apiece. "What's up with all the kids?" Carl asks Jenna.

"What d'ya mean?"

"China's famed one-child policy; thought they were strict about that."

Jenna shrugs. "The law varies from province to province. Some allow a second child if the first dies or, worse, happens to be born a girl. Some just impose a fine for subsequent births."

"Meaning families can buy their way around the law."

"Yep. Or sometimes, particularly out here in the sticks, the law is just ignored."

"Well, so much for hope, eh?" Carl says, shaking his head as he walks away.

Jenna pauses, watching as Carl heads back down towards the Landcruiser. She then returns her attention to the posse of women and offspring, muttering Carl's words to herself so softly it registers as something between a thought and a sigh, "So much for hope."

It's a school house this time – not a church, not a post office, not a quasi medical clinic, not a pig sty – just some small, low, four-roomed, concrete and corrugated tin school house our influenza recon team has taken over; rented for a few hours or days or whatever it takes in order to search for something microscopic. The two long lines of Chinese villagers don't really know what the team has come in search of, all they know is that there's promise of a few yuans if they allow these foreigners in white lab coats draw a few drops of blood from their chickens, ducks, and pigs. A win-win obviously.

At the door Tian hands out three yuans – in new, crisp one and a two-yuan paper denominations – to each entering, critter-carrying villager. She then directs them to Wen, who marks each animal with an indelible purple ink, then divides the customers based on whether they carry swine or fowl, sending the former into the queue bound towards Jenna, and the latter into a queue bound towards Carl.

Wen goes to mark a new duck but finds traces of ink – despite an obvious attempt to pluck the stained feathers – already there. Not sure what to do, Wen calls out to Jenna, unworried that the middle-aged woman who owns the duck, or any of the other villagers for that matter, will understand any of their conversation: "Hey, Dr. Jenna, we got us a repeat offender here. What should I do?"

Jenna sits cross-legged on the floor drawing blood from a piglet. She answers without hesitation: "Boot her out on her ass."

"But it only costs us, like, what, thirty-five cents?" Tian asks, pleadingly.

"Which is like a gazillion dollars to these people. Nope, don't want to be starting them down that slippery-slope to a life of crime. Next thing you know they'll be opening sweatshops and selling sequined jeans to The Gap; don't need that hanging over our karma."

Wen turns back to the woman, explaining in Cantonese she'll have to leave the building. For a cheater she musters an admirable defense – pleading eyes, children to feed, drunken no-good-for-nothing husband, the whole bit – all to which Wen apologetically shakes his head as he turns her towards the door.

For Jenna, the incident brings to mind an anecdote of a flu recon past: "This one time, back before we got smart and started marking the animals, we were out in Bumfuck, Egypt – come to think of it, I think it *was* somewhere in Egypt – anyway, this woman comes through with her sick-ass chicken and, I swear, I couldn't draw a drop of blood from it. Not a damn drop! It was probably that poor bird's twentieth time through the line," she says, laughing so infectiously some of villagers can't help but join in. Settling down, Jenna wipes the tears of laughter from her eyes with her shoulder sleeves, adding: "Lost all faith in humanity right then and there."

Looking up, Jenna notices Tian and Wen are laughing as well, but not Carl. Quite to the contrary, Carl takes each new bird handed him, quickly and perfunctorily draws a sample, then shoves it back at the owner, sans any acknowledgment.

Jenna hands the pig back to its farmer owner, thanks the old man in Cantonese, then calls out to Carl. "Hey, White Devil, it won't kill you to thank them, you know."

Carl doesn't even dignify her comment with a reply. Still looking pale, sweaty, sickly, he draws blood from the next duck then hands it back.

"At least he's efficient," Wen quips.

Jenna nods, "Like workin' with a damned robot."

Blood cells under high magnification come into focus. It's the evening now in the same four-roomed schoolhouse as Carl stares down through the lens of a florescent microscope checking for anomalies that would be brought instantly to his attention from the fluorescent stain he adds to each sample. Seems like half his life already has been spent bent over one of these damned microscopes. He pulls out the slide, files it under the "normal" category, stains the next blood sample, smears it over a glass slide, sandwiches it between another slide, inserts it beneath the microscope's big, bad eye, focuses it again... more cells — healthy, thriving red blood cells.

"There's nothing here," he calls out, without even looking up.

Nearby, Jenna sits stuffed in a child's way-too-tiny school desk, making her look like some African American version of Snow White, willingly held hostage in the cramped domicile of the Seven Dwarfs. An ELISA field test kit is set on the desktop providing her with an orderly array of serum spun down from the blood samples drawn today. She is searching for a ubiquitous presence of antibodies throughout the serum samples which would alert her to an epidemic infection — any infection would show up — but, so far, she has stumbled upon nothing more than one might have to call *normal*.

"Here either," she calls out in reply.

"Which is good, right?" Tian asks as she takes away the ELISA tray just tested and hands Jenna a new one.

"She's right: you guys sound almost bummed that you haven't found any flu virus. What's up with that?" Wen calls out from across the room, where he sweats over a manual centrifuge he's hand-cranking in order to separate the samples' red blood cells from the clear, yellowish serum.

"What's up with that second batch of sera?" Jenna responds, deflecting his question.

"I'm workin' on it. I'm workin' on it!"

Jenna tests the next tray — "Negative" — then hands it back to Tian asking, "How much of the blood have we tested?"

With a quick glance, Tian compares the stacks of tested trays to the stack of untested ones estimating, "Well over half of the first batch."

"So, roughly one-third of all the samples from both swine and fowl and still nothing..." Jenna mutters, guesstimating — with the benefit of her years of fieldwork – the likelihood of finding any indication of influenza based on the samples tested thus far.

"Alright. Forget it. This is a dead end," she sighs, pushing the tray away.

Her judgment call brings all activity to a halt.

"So, what now?" Tian asks.

"Time to find a new village?" Wen follows.

"I reckon," Jenna replies, standing now and stretching out her cramped limbs.

"How about one with electricity this time?"

"What, you no like workout?" Jenna jokes sarcastically, pinching Wen's thin bicep. "No wonder you've got those spindly arms."

"Hey, these are the mighty arms of a scientist!" he jokes back, flexing his muscles.

As the others laugh at Wen's antics Jenna unwraps a new hypodermic needle.

The only one not laughing is Carl; clearly not amused. "Let me check that last tray," he says, extending his hand towards Jenna.

Mindlessly holding the hypodermic needle between her fingers, cigarette-like, she picks up the ELISA tray just tested and, with the same hand, passes it across to Carl as she continues her sarcastic ribbing of Wen, "It must be comforting to know you'll always have that career in bodybuilding to fall back on in case science doesn't work out."

"Yes, very comforting," Wen confirms.

As Carl, not quite looking either, goes to grab the tray from Jenna, the tip of the hypodermic sticks him between his fingers. "Fuck!" he blurts, more angered by the jabbing than the subsequent crashing of the tray of samples to the floor.

"Oops," Jenna responds, somewhat apologetically. "Sorry."

Carl glares at her.

"Relax, Carl, it was a clean needle. See? – I just unwrapped it."

Despite her showing him the wrapper, Carl's anger is not allayed.

"Jesus, Carl, chill already. It was clean. Besides, there're no viruses here!"

"I'll try to *chill* if you try to be a little more careful."

"*Oooh* – high drama!" Jenna replies, with high sarcasm.

Just then the team's satellite cellphone rings, prompting Jenna to extemporize as she reaches for it, "It's probably Carl's lawyer."

the momentum of folly

Jenna picks up the phone and answers, "Jenna Williams.... Shit. Okay. Where?... No, but we can get there. We're actually done here. When was it detected?... Alright, we're on it."

Jenna closes up the cellphone, pauses to ponder the ramifications for a moment, then turns to her team, uttering in portentous understatement: "We've got us a hot one."

* * *

It's hard to believe there are still late 1950's vintage Helio Courier planes in operation anywhere in the world but — due only to the fact that the CIA's Air America employed then discarded an undisclosed number of them in this region during the covert stages leading up to the Vietnam War — there are, and one of them — fitted up with floats — is ferrying Tian, Wen, Jenna, and Carl a few thousand meters above a carpet of olive-green rainforest. Jenna sits up front alongside the Chinese pilot, a map open across her lap. She shouts over the single-engine din something in Cantonese to the pilot, who nods back. She then turns in her seat to shout, over the second row of seats where Tian and Wen play a computer game on one of their cell phones, to the cramped, not-really-meant-for-passengers, back row where Carl naps, stretched out over gear cases and duffle bags, "Ever been to Laos?"

Carl shakes his head.

Jenna shouts again as she points down, "The Mekong."

Carl turns his attention out the window and down to the ribbon of emerald green river snaking through the jungle. Logically he knows that within an hour they'll be down there, but for now — separated by the Plexiglas window and the plane's rattle and hum — it feels like some phony museum exhibit trying but failing to depict another world.

The Helio Courier floatplane is in one of those steep, banking turns charter pilots do just to distinguish themselves from the overly-regulated passenger pilots or their underly-experienced amateur brethren. It's a ninety-degree banking turn that has adrenalin pouring into Carl's synaptic clefts, thus brewing up a hot pot of fear up there in his cortex as his face stares straight down the wing as it's tip seems to brush the treetops. *Note to self: Never fly with a pilot who believes in reincarnation.*

And the floatplane is still in that ninety-degree pitched turn as the scenery out Carl's window changes from jungle blur to the emerald-green waters of the Mekong in a blink of an eye. And in that blink, Carl's eyes lock with those of an equally surprised woman of about his age moving a primitive skiff up the river with a long bamboo pole. And in that instant that their eyes engage – that mutual opening of their respective *windows of the soul* – the acknowledgement is passed that: *We could mate. We really could. We both want it.* It's what biology demands even if societal dogma, familial complications, and sundry jealousies prohibit it. To breed. To carry forth the seed. To mix and mutate and tumble the double helix of our subtly distinguishable strands of deoxyribonucleic and ribonucleic acids; it's hopelessly complex yet at the same time basic but it's what the survival of the species relies upon, what it demands. And suddenly, inexplicably, a soundtrack usurps Carl's inner voice; it's Barry White and he's singing, *Let's get it on!...*

But that aforementioned blink passes, and with it that aforementioned potential mate of a woman, and soon the plane's steeply banking turn is flattened into an arrow-straight approach, pontoons soon slapping against the tiniest of waves, and the subsequent dragging force of the heavier medium shoving everyone forward against the seat or dashboard in front of them. *Seatbelts? We don't need no stinkin' seatbelts.* This is the Third World, and welcome to it.

In the hectic chaos of the First World time skips ever forward, but here in the sweltering jungle it bends and stretches and overlaps. That's how balance is maintained; the conservation of the fourth dimension. That's why it can be so surreally discombobulating when a Third Worlder is suddenly plopped into the First World or vice versa. Carl is feeling it now as he lets his fingers drag through the barely cool water of the Mekong, as the barely-floating, motorized skiff Tian had negotiated pushes the team upriver – or is it downriver, or does it matter? Certainly it doesn't matter to Carl; not the way he feels. He's Conrad puttering into the heart of darkness, that's all he knows for sure. And what about that captain standing in the stern of the boat; eyes clenched into slits, batik headband and sarong, Olde English 800 T-shirt, barefooted, hand-rolled cigarette in sunburned lips; is that the same guy as piloted their plane, or the woman with whom Carl shared that adulterous glance from the window? Or just one of those anonymous but handy doppelgangers that show up from time to time in the service of Destiny? It really doesn't matter. *Nothing matters* — that's the hypothesis Carl has come to, not so much out of crystalline epiphany as out of a gradual beating down of the ego until nothing is left, not even a hand able to lift a white rag of surrender. *Nothing matters*, which of course translates in modern parlance to *fuck it*. Carl closes his stinging eyes, head pounding — *fuck it*.

As the skiff rounds a bend in the river the din of heavy machinery pulls Carl's attention towards a hillside undergoing clear-cut deforestation. With chainsaws and bulldozers and even an enslaved elephant or two, what isn't being filleted into lumber is burned in smoldering slag piles, converting lush rainforest to barren grazing land, and later to squalid megaslum, and tucking a tidy profit away in the process. *Slash and burn*; a dying art for sure.

Carl turns his troubled glance back towards the boat's stern to where Jenna sits — reclined against some rice sacks, feet up on her ever-close-at-hand "first aid" cooler, her expression unreadable beneath her Cal Bears baseball cap and one-year-out-of-fashion sunglasses, that ever-present "cold one" in hand. Watching the same slash and burn spectacle, she takes an anesthetizing sip from her beer then by chance turns towards Carl. After their wordless exchange, she opens her cooler, pulls out another ice-cold bottle, and tosses it to him. Carl catches it, twists off the cap, and takes in a long, cool, quenching, mind-numbing swig, thinking to himself — *Now it makes perfect sense why she keeps this stuff in the first aid cooler* — before returning to the mindless distraction of watching his fingers drag through the water again.

The Doppelganger at the helm blurts out something in some choppy dialect. Though his words may be indecipherable to Carl his anxiety his apparent. Wen nods to the Doppelganger then turns to translate for Jenna and Carl, "Border."

At a border crossing — presumably dividing Cambodia from Laos and consisting of little more than a flagged rope slung across the river, and a bamboo guardhouse set out on a rickety dock — a pair of young guards with old guns order the skiff over to them in order to conduct the *de rigor* border crossing. The Doppelganger complies, and soon the skiff is parked at the dock.

"I'll handle this," Wen tells Jenna, Tian, and Carl. "Give me your passports." Then, with the team's documents in hand, Wen climbs from the skiff onto the dock and begins the negotiations.

As Wen explains their expedition to the pimply-faced teenage guards, Carl leans in to Jenna to whisper, "Are they Cambodian or Laotian?"

Jenna shrugs, "Laotian I suppose, not that it matters," already pulling out nigh-worthless paper currency from her money belt.

Carl watches her, confused. "What do you mean?"

"It's just a run-of-the-mill, turd-world, shake-down. These guys' senior officers probably embezzled their meager pay so this is the only way they make any money."

Wen righteously argues with the guards, pointing to the team's documents, showing them passports and visa stamps, showing them the medical equipment. But the guards — one in particular, the other seeming as if he's just learning this art — remains recalcitrant. The Doppelganger, bowing and pressing his hands together in the universal gesture of submission, begins pleading with the slightly more senior of the two guards. This only seems to anger the guard, who shouts back at him angrily something to the effect of *Shut up!* But as the Doppelganger persists — no doubt hoping it will increase his expeditionary guide fees — the fed-up more-senior guard nods to his protégé. Heeding the order, the protégé gives the Doppelganger a brisk crack in the forehead with the butt of his rifle, sending the Doppelganger tumbling backwards into the skiff. Tian gasps and rushes to the Doppelganger's aid, nursing the already swelling and bleeding lump. The younger recruit shouts at Tian to move away from the Doppelganger, conveying what she doesn't understand by cocking and aiming his rifle at the Doppelganger. Frightened, she scoots away from him, fearing that shots are about to be fired.

The senior guard then pulls out his pistol and shouts some order to the Doppelganger who apparently heeds by climbing out of the skiff, overboard and into the waist-deep water, and, with head bowing and hands still pressed together pleadingly, commences a back-peddling, wading retreat towards his Cambodian homeland. Then, just to be sadistic, the senior guard fires off two shots, one on either side of the Doppelganger, just to underscore the point that he *could* kill him if he wanted — it was within his power — if he wasn't such a nice guy. Cowering, the Doppelganger continues bowing and retreating all the way to shore and then some. Then, surmising he's probably out of their range, he turns and begins to run off into the safety of the obscuring jungle. *Ah, to live to see another day!*

Almost as soon as the guard holsters his pistol and the threat subsides, Wen resumes arguing the team's case.

"Forget it, Wen," Jenna says, pushing past him. "These morons speak only one language." Jenna then steps into the faces of both guards and begins shouting down at them like some angry mom, first in Cantonese, then French, then whatever bits of Vietnamese she can regurgitate, all the while crumpling and tossing yuans in their faces. Perhaps sufficiently insulted, or perhaps the wheels of migration sufficiently greased, the senior-most guard eventually nods to his protégé to return the papers to Wen. He then turns for the guard hut, pausing only to reach down into Jenna's "first aid" cooler and pluck two ice-cold bottles, then heads off, allowing the mosquito netted hut door to fall closed behind him.

"Motherfucker!" Jenna seethes aside to Carl. "The only reason I'm going to let him get away with that bullshit is that I'm overly rational."

"Yeah, that's what strikes me about you," Carl smirks back.

"It's true. And I'm not particularly proud of it."

The protégé guard shoulders his rifle, raises the counter-balanced gate, then waves them through the checkpoint.

Wen steps to the helm of the skiff, pull-starts the smoky, two-stroke motor, then pilots the skiff towards deeper waters. As they pull away from the dock, the senior guard calls facetiously out to them from the guardhouse, perhaps the one English phrase he knows, "Have a nice day!"

Jenna flips them the finger, which only cause both guards to laugh.

Jenna shakes her head angrily then reaches into the cooler for another pair of beers. Tossing one to Carl, she asks him facetiously, "You're a G-man, can't you call in an air strike or something?"

Carl catches the bottle and pops it open on the skiff's gunwale. "Consider it done."

Tian, not quite sure they're only joking, turns a troubled glance towards Wen.

Wen laughs and shakes his head.

It's that time-slip thing again. If there's a chronological progression, if it's the same day just hours later, it doesn't feel like it – it could as easily be some hours earlier, or so it seems. Presently, at this point in time, Tian is up in the bow reading, Wen sleeps, Carl stands at the helm, one hand on the long throttle/rudder pole, squinting ever upstream, and Jenna is the one, sitting in the stern near Carl, allowing her fingers to drag mindlessly through the barely translucent green, soft, almost lanolin, water. Then, as if out of nowhere, she laughs to herself.

Puzzled, Carl studies her for a while, then asks, "Those jerks at the border?"

Jenna shakes her head, still smiling at her abstruse recollection.

"What?" Carl presses, having to almost shout over the noise of the tiny outboard motor.

"Snowball fights with my stupid, little brother growing up. He had the arm, of course – jock – but I'd always cream his ass."

"How's that?"

"I had this method – *le Method*, I called it – you know, tossing two snowballs simultaneously; one kind of lobbed up there to distract him, then the second fired under radar. The ol' one-two. Worked every time. Used to piss the hell out of him."

As Jenna laughs again at the memory, Carl looks about at the steamy jungle on either side of them. Puzzled anew he has to ask, "What made you think about snowball fights out here?"

Jenna thinks about it, then shrugs and shakes her head. "Dunno."

Too enervated by the sweltering humidity to press the matter, Carl lifts his attention back upstream. From around another bend in the river something captures his gaze, something that looks like it doesn't quite belong.

Jenna follows his squint upstream to where the twisted and burned carcass of what was once a sturdy, mach-two-capable, F4 "Phantom" jet hangs in a tree.

"Your Vietnam War era tax dollars at work," she surmises, staring now down to her handheld G.P.S. device. "I think we're close. There should be a village a couple clicks in-country from here, river right." She scans the riverbank for a suitable landing, then points, "Park it on that sandbar right over there. Maybe we can hide the S.S. Minnow here in the brush so it doesn't get ripped off."

Carl nods, turning the skiff towards the sandbar and cutting the engine.

the momentum of folly

Wearing backpacks weighted down with their tightly-packed biosafety level three suits and the minimum compliment of equipment necessary to conduct a mobile viral assessment, the foursome wends its way through the jungle, single file along a well-worn path; Wen leading, then Tian, then Carl, then Jenna, consulting the G.P.S.

"There's a clearing up ahead," Wen calls back, adding, "Yeah, village too."

"Must be it," Jenna calls back, tucking away the device.

Wen pauses instinctively behind the last cover of brush at the periphery of the clearing. The others pull up on either side of him in order to peruse the situation before jumping in.

The village, too small to warrant a name, consists of some forty bamboo huts elevated on frail stilts two meters or so above the flood plain prone ground. Ducks wander about foraging for bugs. Hogs graze on whatever waste, table or human, is dropped through the floors of the huts. Smoke from cook fires emanate from many of the huts, as do the sounds of deep, hacking coughs.

"Tuberculosis?" Tian asks.

Jenna shakes her head, then directs their attention towards a dying pig, front legs buckled beneath him, rear legs clawing at the earth trying to push itself forward, eyes wide and frightened. "TB wouldn't be affecting the pigs."

"Pneumonia?" Wen asks.

"That'd be my guess. Pneumococcus, likely."

"So that means it's bacterial?"

Carl shakes his head. "Not necessarily."

Jenna elaborates: "The virus lays waste to the immune systems leaving the body defenseless against any subsequent viral or bacterial infection that comes along, pneumococcus being one of the most common and lethal."

A slight breeze rakes through the trees and causes Wen — first him, then the others — to catch a whiff of something awful. "Jesus, something died!"

Troubled by the mounting symptoms, Jenna slings off her backpack. "We better suit up."

Minutes later the team is about halfway from the edge of the clearing to the village, with each member enveloped head to toe in a white, moisture-proof, vapor-tight, rip-stop biosafety level 3 field suit, air provided via an elaborate, battery-powered filtering system designed to keep every known pathogen — bacterial or viral – out. But despite all the high-tech engineering that went into the relatively lightweight armor, there's no getting around the fact that anyone wearing such a suit looks unflatteringly hokey. Spandex might look cooler, but it wouldn't keep the bugs out. So, as it is, the team looks more like a pack of astronauts from some way under-budgeted science fiction flick from the sixties than a team of cutting edge virologists/epidemiologists. But such is fashion in the service of function.

Jenna is up ahead of the others by a good twenty meters. Carl walks with Wen. Tian lags behind, a bit overwhelmed by what they are encountering, this being her first time in a "hot zone." En route they pass dozens of corpses, some respectfully, obviously the earliest of the victims, laid out and shrouded with rice cloth, others, the more recent and more plentiful, hastily tossed into heaps.

"Lot of corpses for a tiny village," Wen tells Carl.

Carl nods, "A lot of corpses for a *big* village. A lot for even *Shanghai.*"

Carl pauses to peel back one shroud to take a look at the body beneath; an otherwise healthy-appearing woman, maybe in her late twenties, exhibiting no obvious symptoms of trauma or suffering. Wen steps up beside Carl to look at her.

"Hemorrhagic fever? Dengue?"

Carl shakes his head. "No indication of bleed-outs or pox. Just some slight discoloration: note the bluish lips and fingertips."

"Cyanosis?" Wen asks, incredulously.

Carl nods then sketches out the probable course of the disease with his gloved index finger down the dead woman's neck and into her chest. "That's essentially how viral pneumonia plays out; the immune system chases the virus down into the lower respiratory track, all the way into the epithelial cells of the alveoli, the deepest, darkest otherwise most sterile recesses of the lungs. Then it floods the bronchial trees with a veritable cytokine storm of every kind of white blood cells, antibodies, enzymes, and toxins it's got. The lungs then fill with collagen, fibrin, various cell debris, proteins, and whatnot until there's simply no room for air anymore. The actual condition is called ARDS."

"Acute Respiratory Distress Syndrome?" Wen asks.

"Exactly. The heart's right ventricle, here," Carl is pointing again, "try as it might, simply cannot pump the fluids from the lungs. So either her heart failed, or, because of lung congestion, she couldn't get enough oxygen into her blood, no matter how fast she breathed, then just died of fish-out-of-water-esque exhaustion."

"So she essentially drowned."

Carl nods, "Suffocated in her own juices." Carl then notes the dead pigs stacked nearby. "And the fact that the pigs caught it is a strong indication it was brought on by flu."

Wen conducts a quick assessment of the corpses scattered all around them. "Five, maybe six dozen dead. Half the town might be here. I've never heard of influenza with that kind of mortality rate!"

"Except for H5N1."

"Bird Flu?" Wen asks skeptically. "But there's only been like a hundred reported cases of it in all the years it's been around."

Carl nods, "And over half of them died."

"But all very isolated; handfuls of people here and there, close-knit families mostly. The virus just hasn't shown itself capable of making the interspecies leap."

Carl nods, "Until now."

Wen stares at Carl, clearly troubled by the prospects.

"I'm just saying it's a possibility which we shouldn't overlook," Carl adds as he lays the shroud back over the woman's lifeless body. He then moves over to the next pile, removes the irreverent blue tarp covering it, then checks over the stack of other corpses, all seemingly those of young adults, an anomaly not lost on Wen:

"I would have expected to see a lot more corpses of infants and old people, but most of all these seem to be young adults – the strongest!"

Carl nods, "That's the cruel irony of particularly lethal strains of influenza; it's the ones with the healthiest immune system that are most likely to die."

"Carl," Jenna calls from up ahead.

Carl and Wen catch up to where Jenna is examining another corpse, that of a young boy.

"How old; four?" Carl asks, guessing the boy's age.

"If that," Jenna answers.

"Wen and I noticed most of the corpses seem to be of young adults."

"Most of the corpses you've *seen* you mean."

Carl and Wen are both a bit taken aback by Jenna's quick dismissal of their observation.

"I'm just saying—" Carl begins, until cut short by Jenna.

"Incomplete sampling can lead to misdiagnosis. Fieldwork can't be guesswork. Let's not draw any conclusions until we have all the facts."

"So, you don't want us telling you what we observed?" Carl says, a little peeved.

Jenna cuts Carl a look before replying, "Exactly. And I especially don't want you taking something I might say, however gruffly, personally. We're in a hot zone; I shouldn't have to handle you with kids' gloves! Got it?"

Carl and Jenna exchange a glare, with Carl eventually backing down.

"Got it."

"Thank you. Now give me a diagnosis here," she tells Carl, pointing down to the boy's lifeless body.

Capitulating, Carl places his gloved hands on the boy's chest, checking the ribs one at a time, the two mil of protective layers essentially dividing the world into separate existences; one safe for the moment, the other expired.

"No broken ribs. Sternum's in place."

"What's that mean?" Wen asks.

"Means he didn't cough to death like the others," Jenna explains.

"Reyes?" Carl hypothesizes.

Jenna nods.

Wen turns from Jenna to Carl for an explanation.

"Reyes Syndrome: cranium fills with fluid, compressing the brain stem and choking off all impulses to the heart and lungs, basically shutting them down."

"Doesn't sound like such a bad way to go."

"It's not," Jenna confirms, "for a virus."

Tian comes up cautiously, with obvious trepidations, from behind Carl to peek around his shoulder at the corpse of the little boy. Almost immediately upon seeing the boy's lifeless eyes she begins to hyperventilate, seemingly unable, for whatever reason, to take her eyes off those of the boy's.

Feeling her tightly clutching his arm, Carl turns towards her. "You alright, Tian?"

Gasping now, with eyes wide, she looks as if she's about to become nauseous.

"I think she's gonna hurl," Wen notes.

"She better not," Jenna states coolly.

the momentum of folly

Panicking, Tian tries to rip off her facemask. Wen and Carl immediately pull her hands away from her mask to prevent her from doing so. Carl then wraps his arms around her in a tight bear hug to keep her arms pinned down and out of self-inflicted danger, as both Jenna and he begin shouting orders at her.

"Don't you dare take that mask off! Hear me? Don't take it off!"

"Tian, relax. It's alright. It's alright. Deep, calm breaths. It's alright…."

Unable to suppress her nausea, Tian vomits in her facemask.

"She's gonna suffocate!" Wen says, worriedly.

"No, no; she's fine," Jenna assures him. "Been there. Done that."

After a couple nauseous episodes Tian, exhausted, is indeed able to calm down; her safety contained within her suit, as too her vomit.

"Are you okay?" Carl asks her.

She nods then, reeling at the stench with which she's trapped, mutters, "Gross!"

"No one twisted your arm to be here," Jenna tells her, unsympathetically.

"Hey, Dr. Williams, how 'bout cutting us a little slack here," Carl says, gently admonishing Jenna. To which Jenna rolls her eyes and sighs, before returning her focus to the corpse of the young boy, which she doesn't even bother recovering with its shroud before moving on to the next corpse stacked alongside him.

Carl turns back to Tian, giving her as reassuring a smile as he can muster under the circumstances.

"Hey, guys…" Wen says quietly, lassoing their attention as gently as possible.

Carl, Jenna, and Tian turn to find… a dozen or so surviving villagers – some coughing, all looking on pleadingly.

Jenna studies the villagers carefully. "They think we've come to help. They're not going to like it when they find out we're just after blood samples."

"We have needles and saline, right? We could pretend like we're administering vaccinations," Tian suggests.

Jenna turns towards Tian, impressed by her devious pluck. "Honey, you just might have a future in the bug biz yet!"

Tian flashes Jenna an embarrassed, puke-stained smile.

"How about you and Wen go grab our kits from the boat – maybe wash up while you're at it – while Carl and I devise a game plan."

Tian nods.

"We're outta here," Wen says, as he and Tian head back for the boat.

Jenna turns back towards the villagers, regarding them as she speaks aside to Carl: "Somewhere between giving phony shots and pretending to treat their sick, we're going to have to somehow convince them to let us take lung tissue samples from their deceased loved ones."

"What about cremating the bodies?" Carl asks.

"That too," Jenna confirms, sighing at the work that awaits them.

"Good times," Carl cracks, ever so wryly.

"Yeah. Good times."

Less than two hours later the team is back at the grind, their mobile viral recon shop set up in the largest of the stilt-elevated huts. Stacked orderly around them are all the requisite cases and items necessary for the well-equipped field lab; the dry ice coolers, sanitizing fluids, cameras, laptops, hand wipes, emergency chemical shower, injectors, hazardous waste depository, etc. And from one of the walls hang the vital charts to be filled out – the "spot map," "line listings" and "histograms" – all necessary in order to track the source and spread and epidemiology of the virus.

Still safely encapsulated within their biosafety suits, Carl, Wen, Jenna, and Tian respectively draw blood from the incoming queue of villagers, separate the sera from the blood samples with the hand-crank centrifuge, test the sera in the ELISA trays, and, yes, administer placebo inoculations.

Carl is in the process of trying to locate a vein in the withered arm of a very old woman. Once he does he sticks a needle in it. As her blood begins to fill the needle's cylinder, he inadvertently locks eyes with the old woman. He tries to coax a smile out of her with a feeble one of his own, but she isn't having it.

Jenna calls out from across the room, "Fortunately this town is fairly isolated. Maybe the virus hasn't traveled yet."

"Well, someone had to report the outbreak, right?" Wen asks.

"Good point."

"Who do you think did?" Tian asks.

"Reported it?" Jenna shrugs. "Someone who knew at least what an outbreak was and knew at least to call a doctor who knew to call the WHO."

"Who knew to call us," Wen surmises.

"That's how it works."

"Missionaries!" Tian blurts.

"Missionaries?"

"Yeah, they're about the only ones who bother making contact with remote villages."

"Bless their hearts," Jenna cracks.

"My parents were missionaries. They used to drag us to villages like this."

"Well, bless their hearts too."

"Whoever it was, they're gonna have to be tracked down. They could be carrying," Carl says.

With a sufficient quantity of blood drawn, Carl pulls the needle from the old woman's arm, sterilizes then bandages the puncture wound. As she rolls her sleeve back down she begins speaking insistently at him; her abstruse Laotian dialect sounding like the barking yaps of a small dog. Carl shakes his head to her, "I don't understand. No comprendo." But on she goes, louder and faster now until it seems as if she's railing at him.

Carl calls to Wen, "Is she mad at me?"

Wen shrugs, "Dunno. Probably. I understand this dialect about as well as you."

Carl tries to dismiss the old woman, "Ma'am, you go. Next!" But she won't have it; instead, his attempts to move her along only seem to make her more insistent, more demanding that he understand exactly what she is trying to convey to him. She points to herself, then to others from her village in the room: an old man, bent with antiquity but otherwise healthy; another old man, similarly ancient yet unaffected health-wise; and then, another elderly woman, this one helping her coughing, probably pneumonic, thirty year-old grandson. Still barking at him, the old woman now grabs Carl's hand and taps her own chest with it, then uses it to point, slowly and deliberately, back to each of the other very old folks she had already pointed out.

Carl turns back to the old woman, shrugs apologetically then tells her, "I'm sorry, I don't understand."

Exasperated with him, the old woman sighs audibly, shakes her head, then turns and walks away, flapping her arms in frustration and complaining aloud as she goes.

Carl turns back towards Wen for some sort of explanation of the old woman's antics, but only receives back a similarly confused shrug. Carl returns his attention to the next person in his queue; a teenage boy, seemingly healthy but for the tiny beads of perspiration clinging to his nose. Carl rolls the boy's sleeve up, sticks him with the needle and begins to draw his blood. As the cylinder fills, Carl's attention is snagged by the curiously unwarranted event of laughter, so out of place, erupting from across the hut. There, twin girls, six-ish, prove to be the source. They are standing with Jenna, all seemingly laughing over the fact that their pet pot-bellied pig's orange, yellow and green Rastafarian woven necklace matches their own Rasta style wristbands; which of course matches Jenna's – Carl recalls – though hers is hidden beneath her biosafety suit. Jenna is speaking with the twin girls in her very limited Laotian; laughing with them, as she scratches behind the pig's ears. And then, quite by accident, she happens to notice Carl is watching the exchange. Caught before she can construct an adequate subterfuge, her eyes involuntarily avert from his. Thus, in a wordless instance, suspicion is aroused. *But suspicion of what?* – that is what makes no sense to Carl.

Carl pulls the needle from the boy's arm, cleans the area of the skin, bandages it, smiles and nods to the boy, calls out, "Next," then glances back at Jenna as she hands the pig back over to the twin girls.

Five o'clock finds our team still outfitted in their biohazard suits but alone in the hut they've taken over in order to process the blood samples taken this afternoon. That Carl knows it is five o'clock comes from his habit of checking his cell phone's clock every few minutes, a habit he's grown too used to working in the CDC lab where five o'clock meant something. Back then it meant catching a ride back home with Angela in her Geo, and thereafter, who knew? But things have changed. Here and now, five o'clock only means the sun is still hanging high in the sweaty Southeast Asian sky with no end of the workday in sight. And where might Angela be at this moment? – Los Angeles, no doubt, learning the ropes of her new job at Aegis Pharmaceuticals. Making new friends. Carl glances at his cellphone again: 5:01. Old habits die slowly.

Tian sits cross-legged across from Carl at the low kitchen table where, perhaps just a day or two ago, the hut-owners might have been eating dinner. Where that family is now – fled town, hunkering down in some relative's hut, or stacked like cordwood in one of the corpse piles outside – is anyone's guess. All that can be stated for certain now is that their home is making for a pretty good ad hoc laboratory, and that their kitchen table is proving to be a suitable lab desk for Tian as she drips the centrifuged samples of the entire town's sera into the ELISA kit's ninety-six well plates, as Wen and Jenna hover over her shoulders, watching with keen interest as each new drop is tested to see if there's a change in color in the fluids. There isn't.

"No reaction," Tian tells them, as if they weren't aware of the same results.

"Have we tested everyone?" Jenna asks.

Wen nods, "Dead or alive."

"So what's that mean?" Tian asks, turning to Jenna.

"A new strain, right?" Wen hypothesizes.

"That or just not one of the more common ninety-six strains our kits are designed to test for," Jenna explains. "Carl, on the other hand, is comparing it to the CDC's database of every strain of influenza ever captured. He'll be able to tell us if it's a new one or not." She turns towards Carl, "So what say you, White Devil?"

Across the table, his Western legs folded uncomfortably beneath him, Carl peers into the infrared microscope, comparing the Laotian strain's stained cell slides to strains previously catalogued and held in the CDC database on his laptop computer. But as each new antibody tag reveals a different color he is forced to admit, "No matches."

"Does your database there include H5N1?" Wen asks.

"Yep. And I would've bet dimes to donuts that that's what this would turn out to be, but apparently not."

"Not what?" Tian asks.

"Not the dreaded Bird Flu," Wen answers.

The news cause troubled glances to bounce about the researchers. Jenna moves over to Carl, nudging him aside with a no-time-for-niceties, "Lemme see."

Carl abdicates the microscope to Jenna. As she settles in at the lenspiece he types a command on his computer that brings up onto the laptop screen what she is seeing through the microscope, then uses this as an opportunity to elaborate on the Bird Flu for Wen and Tian's benefit: "Basically, on top of the pyramid, there are three types of flu viruses; influenza A, B, & C. Influenza A are then classified by the two surface glycoproteins hemagglutinin and neuraminidase. Insofar as there are 16 known hemagglutinin proteins and nine known neuraminidase proteins they can combine to create all of our presently known 144 influenza subtypes."

"Not to be confused with the myriad different *strains* of influenza beyond that," Jenna cautions, without lifting her eyes from the microscope.

"That's right. Anyway, of these, only three main subtypes are known to infect both humans and birds – H5, H7, and H9 – and are thereby given the distinction *Avian* influenza. So, by partnering each of these with the nine different neuraminidase proteins, we get a grand total of 27 potential subtypes of Avian influenza."

"But the *biggie* – the one most dreaded – is the H5N1!" Wen interjects.

"Right, that's because it's long been feared that H5N1 – which packs the highest mortality rate of any known influenza – would eventually mutate to the point where it was readily capable of making the interspecies leap from birds to humans. I thought this might just be that historic moment, but apparently not."

"Well, I wouldn't rule it out just yet," Jenna adds, still peering into the microscope.

"Why not? All the tests came back negative," Carl asks, clearly taking umbrage in what he perceives as an attack on both technology and his own methodology.

"I'm not doubting your science, Carl. I'm just saying these tests aren't 100% conclusive; maybe the strain has mutated just enough so as not to be recognized, or maybe our sampling here today was bad – though I doubt that's the case –, or maybe whoever entered the H5N1 sample into the database, way back when, simply misclassified it. We don't know. Hell, I'm probably responsible for ten percent of those strains in there, and I'm certainly capable of a fuck-up now and then."

For some reason none of Jenna's explanations ring true with Carl, and nor with Wen now that the two of them have exchanged a doubtful glance across Jenna's back as she continues peering down at the virus through the microscope's eyepiece.

"Jesus, that was quick," she mutters, to no one in particular.

"What?" Wen asks.

"Just about every cell is infected," she remarks, a subtle sense of alarm apparent in spite of her attempt at scientific detachment.

Carl pulls up on his computer screen an archived picture of an influenza virus as photographed using electron microscopy. Then, pointing to the various parts of the virus, he explains the situation to Wen and Tian, "The hemagglutinin gene – this kind of spiky antler thing right here – it's what binds the virus to the cell's sialic acid receptors. Not long after the binding *absorption* happens at which point the cell is pretty much history. If for whatever reason the virus cannot penetrate the cell, the hemagglutinin can detach itself to allow it try to find a cell it *can* invade."

"Mind you not all viruses work this way," Jenna elaborates, still from the microscope. "This is somewhat of a unique ability of influenza. As is what it can do once it does invade a cell."

"What happens then?" Tian asks.

"Carl?" Jenna asks, deflecting the question.

Carl complies, "Most viruses merely fuse with the cell's membrane. Influenza, on the other hand, as well as some other viruses, penetrates the cell through what's called the clathrin-dependent endocytosis pathway."

"Is that what allows it to hide from the immune system?" Wen asks.

"Essentially. Therein, the acidic conditions found inside the cell's endosomes – cell subcompartments – cause the virus's membrane to dissolve enabling the virus's genes to insert themselves into the cell's chromosomes. These genes then impose themselves upon the cell's genome—"

"Body snatchers," Tian quips.

"Basically, yeah; insofar as this causes the infected cell to begin manufacturing *viral* proteins instead of its own."

"That's messed up," Wen declares, underscoring his gift for understatement.

"Yep," Carl confirms, then turns to Tian. "Then there's the RNA verses DNA matter that we talked about before."

Tian nods.

"What's that?" Wen asks.

After a *go-ahead* nod from Carl, Tian explains it for Wen, "Influenza, unlike the vast majority of viruses, encode their genes in the highly mutable RNA molecule rather than in the more stable DNA one. This means there can be hundreds of thousands of subtly different mutations of the virus present within a single cell by the time it is ready to explode."

"How long does that take; from absorption to explosion?" Wen asks.

"Only about ten hours, right?" Tian checks with Carl.

Carl nods, "And with so many mutations – *swarm mutation*, it's called – influenza has up to a million chances to expose the cell to the single most efficiently lethal strain it can come up with. And after that cell explodes all the other cells are infected and get up to a million chances to hone that lethal strain even further."

"So it's, like, always shape shifting," Wen posits.

"*Antigenic drift* it's called. There's antigenic *shift* as well, but that's far less frequent. HIV and Coronavirus – the common cold – are similarly dynamic since they too are RNA based. This is why all three are so difficult to vaccinate for; they're forever mutating."

"Which is why you guys have to come back to Guangdong each year; to hunt down the most prevalent and nasty mutation," Tian adds.

"Right. But the opposite is true for the much more stable DNA based viruses – say polio or smallpox – one vaccine can last generations because they mutate so slowly."

"All of which makes influenza the most highly evolved, potentially lethal virus of them all, in my humble opinion," Jenna interjects, adding a coda meant as a subtle, little dig at Carl, "And to think some virologists would rather study ebola."

"Have we come up with a morbidity rate?" Tian asks.

"Antigens are present in everyone we've tested; dead or alive."

"So *everyone's* got it?" Wen asks, incredulously.

Jenna nods, "Then again, a morbidity – who all has it – of 100% is not uncommon with influenza epidemics; it's very easy to catch and, hence, spread."

"What about a *mortality* rate?" Carl asks Wen.

"Until I get an exact census for the town, I can only guesstimate," Wen replies, "but upwards of thirty percent."

"*Way* upwards considering not everyone that is going to die has yet."

"And that's with the less-than-ideal warm and rainy conditions," Tian adds.

"So where would you put the number?" Wen asks, turning to Jenna.

Jenna shrugs, "Sixty, sixty-six percent?"

the momentum of folly

"Two out of three?" Wen asks incredulously, "Two out of three people here will die from this?"

Jenna confirms his assessment with a glum nod.

Wen reels, "Damn, not even H5N1 packs that kind of mortality rate. Those are numbers you might expect from Marburg or Ebola, not some little flu bug!" Wen reels.

"Little flu bugs can be just as nasty. Entire villages have been wiped out by little flu bugs. All it takes is the right mutation and no previous exposure."

"So we really could have an entirely new strain here?" Tian asks, worriedly.

Jenna nods, "That or an all-but-forgotten oldie but goodie."

"Either way this thing could spread like wildfire if it gets out!" Wen states, as the dire possibilities of their discovery dawns on him.

"Feels nice to be needed, doesn't it?" Jenna quips.

Suddenly from outside shouted orders are heard; first from one direction, then another, then another, causing all activity within the makeshift lab to grind to a halt. The team looks at one another worriedly.

"Sounds like the village is being surrounded," Wen notes.

"Which is hardly ever a good thing," Carl says, turning towards Jenna for some sort of explanation.

But before Jenna can answer to allay their concerns, the sounds of automatic "small arms" fire erupts in short bursts from all sides. The bursts are followed by screams, both of agony and remorse, and then more bursts of gunfire.

Carl scuttles to a nearby window and steals a peek outside. There he can see a pair of villagers – a woman and child judging by what fleeting glimpses he can catch of them – as they weave between other huts, until another burst of gunfire drops them in their tracks.

"Jesus," Carl mutters.

"What's going on?" Jenna asks in an urgent whisper.

"They're shooting everyone."

Jenna scoots herself over to the window beside Carl, trying to steal glimpses – in spite of their limited vantage point proffered by the hut and the awkwardness of the biosafety suit – of the terror taking place outside, and all while trying to keep her head low so not to become a target herself. One such glimpse reveals a trotting trio of, presumably, soldiers outfitted in camouflage fatigues and gas masks. One soldier points his pistol up towards a nearby hut. Another, armed with an M-60 and heeding the directive, riddles the thatched domicile with bullets, while the third sets it ablaze with a couple billowing plumes from a flamethrower. Jenna ducks her head back in below the window. With eyes wide and chest heaving, she is clearly worried yet still in control of her senses. Trusting no one more than herself, she takes quick assessment of the situation then issues the order, "Alright, leave everything."

"What about the serum?" Carl asks.

Jenna shakes her head, *"Everything!"*

Then, from below their own hut they hear voices. Tian begins to gasp until Jenna cuts her a quick and threatening *don't-you-dare!* glare. Another order is called out just beneath them, followed by the unmistakable sounds of small arms weaponry being locked and loaded.

All eyes are now on Jenna, the unequivocal boss. Sans hesitation she points across the hut's main room towards the floor-mounted, one-meter square, three-inches thick concrete cooking slab in the kitchen area, demonstrably mouthing, "There!"

Wasting no time, Wen, the closest, scurries on hands and knees towards the slab, followed in quick succession by Tian, Carl, and Jenna. Drawn to the noise of their transit, bullets, fired from at least one automatic weapon, begin ripping up through the hut's elevated floor, making chaff of the rice straw mats and feeble boards.

"Faster!" Jenna calls out, just loudly enough.

Reaching the hearth slab, Wen quickly sits on it, brushing aside the still hot cooking embers with his gloved hands. Within seconds Tian and Carl are on board as well and doing the same, followed soon thereafter by Jenna who basically throws herself into their midst. Crammed together on the too-small area, they clutch one another in an effort to minimize their exposure to the gunfire tearing up from below within the umbra of the protective slab. And the deafening barrage – consisting of both the short bursts from a smaller caliber assault rifle, and the more sustained blasts from one of an obviously larger caliber – seem to last an eternity, whereas, in reality, it's probably no more that ten or fifteen seconds' worth. Several of the shots – maybe five percent of the thousand-plus rounds fired – peck at the bottom of the slab but are unable to chip their way through, while the rest, the vast majority, rip through every square foot of floor space. And then, suddenly, silence as the gunfire is halted.

the momentum of folly

Unwilling to move, the team members bounce nervous glances about as they listen intently for any sounds from below. Soon they hear another order being shouted, this one oddly perfunctory in its tone.

Jenna turns towards Wen for an explanation, but – not understanding it – Wen can only shrug and shake his head. Then comes the unmistakable sounds of a flamethrower, followed by the crackling sounds of dry kindling being consumed in a sudden inferno, followed by the stench of both kerosene and burned rice straw wafting up through the tattered floor.

"We're on fire!" Tian says.

"*Sssh!*" Jenna says snaps back, instinctually comprehending the nature of their quandary; that they must risk burning alive while listening for the assault team's moving along before making their break. And that's exactly what each of them is doing, *listening*, when the last burst from the small caliber rifle, a clip's worth at best, comes ripping up at them again. Zeroed-in on where they have hunkered, most of the shots ricochet off the hearth's bottom. But one manages to tear through the arm of Carl's biosafety suit, fortunately only grazing his arm. He and Jenna exchange a look, each instantly cognizant of the possibility that his protection against the virus has been compromised.

Reacting immediately, Jenna sets out back across the ripped up floor.

"No!" Carl tries to order her – quietly, urgently – but to no avail.

Reaching the tattered daypack that doubles as their first aid kit and toolbox, Jenna quickly grabs it and beats a retreat back towards the relative safety of the hearth. And she's almost back when that voice from below spots her. Once again it shouts an order that is heeded with a maelstrom of gunfire; wildly spinning, barely aimed gunfire that seems only to have the bottom of the hut in its crosshairs. Smoke and chaff and noise choke the perforated room as Jenna scrambles back, hurling herself back on top of the others once again. Sans hesitation she opens the pack, pulls out a roll of duct tape, unfurls a few feet's worth, and quickly begins wrapping it around the tear in Carl's suit.

The voice from below, apparently convinced they've snuffed any life from this hut, then orders his minions away to the next hut. With the subsequent cessation of gunfire all that can be heard are the sounds of the broiler on high just beneath them as the engulfing fire switches fuels, from the kerosene starter to the bamboo and thatched straw.

"We can't stay here," Carl states, hinting for an evacuation.

"Obviously," Jenna retorts, ripping off the end of the duct tape and tossing the roll aside.

"So, how should we do this?" Wen asks.

"Well, it's actually quite simple," Jenna explains, her sarcasm biting through even here: "When I say *bolt*, we bolt. Got it? Try to use the smoke as cover."

Carl looks at her incredulously, "You act like you've done this before."

"Baby, I grew up in Oakland," she deadpans, while digging further into the daypack for something. Finding what she's been fishing for, a small hand mirror, she tosses the pack aside then extends the mirror a minimal distance down through one of the many holes in the floor of the hut. Using the mirror as some sort of upside-down periscope she maneuvers it to obtain a fair if shaky glimpse of what is transpiring outside. The M-60 can be heard ripping up another hut halfway across the village, followed soon thereafter by the *whooomph!* of the flamethrower. From another direction there's the more distant sounds of the lighter caliber assault rifles, along with the expected screams and pleas, followed by a couple efficient pops from a pistol.

All eyes are on Jenna as she finishes up her surveillance. "They seemed to have moved on. Everybody ready?"

"Do we have a plan?" Carl asks.

"What part of *getting the fuck outta here* don't you understand?"

"Just wondering if we should stick together —"

Wen shakes his head adamantly, "Too easy a target for automatic weapons."

"He's right," Jenna concurs.

"Fine, but how about a general direction?" Carl asks, "I assume we want to try to meet up afterwards."

"I admire your optimism," Jenna cracks wryly.

"You said to use the smoke as cover; how 'bout we follow it back into the jungle?" Tian suggests.

"Sounds like the best idea yet."

Just then one of hut's main support joist beams buckles causing the corner of the hut to drop nearly to the ground.

"Let's go!" Jenna barks, now pushing her team members towards the nearest gaping hole in the floor. *"Go! Go! Go!"*

the momentum of folly

Oddly, Carl drops through the hole in the floor with that old adage stuck in his head; *Out of the frying pan and into the fire.* He didn't dare say it up there in the hut, it just sounded too trite considering the seriousness of their situation, but that's what he was thinking the whole time. *Out of the frying pan and into the fire.* Strange how the mind can dally even when wired on adrenalin.

When Carl hits the ground he finds himself all alone. No sign of Tian and Wen who had presumably touched down before him. Nor of Jenna who was presumably to follow. This isn't wholly surprising considering the thick and obscuring smoke, and the roar of the fire just above him, and the roar of the other fires consuming the adjoining huts. It's all very chaotic. And, of course, handicapping it all is the fact that he's still enveloped in his airtight biosafety suit, which hampers the body's perception even under ideal conditions. And these were hardly ideal. Exasperating his visibility woes, soot was gathering on his suit's plastic visor. And when he attempted to wipe the soot away with his gloved hand it only smeared it around, thus exasperating those *visibility woes* even more. Then there was what was going on *inside* the visor; for it seems that having been roasting up there in the hut had caused him to sweat like he might after an hour of pick-up basketball on a muggy afternoon in summertime Atlanta. Bag all that sweat up in a moisture tight suit and you get condensation on the ol' windshield. Which Carl had big time, compromising his vision to a fraction of what it should be.

But his hearing was still working fine, and it was telling him the blazing hut looming just above was about to come crashing down on his pumpkin head. Ducking low beams, stumbling over burning debris, even the occasional body or three, Carl eventually makes his way to a relative clearing, but somewhere still within the village. There's an open well here, so maybe it's the town center, he surmises. He thinks to look skyward in an attempt to ascertain which direction the wind seems to be blowing, so to follow the smoke away per their well-thought-out escape plan. But what with all the problems he's having with his visor coupled with the fact that the intense heat rising from the burning town seems to be lifting the smoke in a swirling plume heading only upwards, Carl really has no idea about which direction he should run. He wishes he could just rip off his suit and take his chances with the virus. But what were those chances: one in three? Not good odds; that much he knew. Wouldn't be prudent, even under these conditions.

Suddenly someone is shouting something at him in some Asian dialect, and from very near by. He turns, but sees nothing. *Am I hallucinating?* – that's what he is wondering, until he hears it again. Squinting, straining to see through the smudge glare penetrating his visor, he gradually makes out two forms, dark and silhouetted against the backfires. As they step closer and the smoke lifts a bit he sees that one of them carries an AK-47 and the other the flamethrower. Both are outfitted in camouflaged chemical warfare suits. Through their gasmasks Carl thinks he sees Asian eyes, but isn't certain of it. Nor can he be sure of any rank or military affiliation whatsoever. Paramilitary? Mercenaries? – Carl hasn't a clue. The one, seemingly the officer of the two, shouts again at Carl, this time pointing to his hands. In response Carl shakes his head, trying to convey the universal *I don't understand* gesture. Turning towards one another they speak briefly amongst themselves. After the flamethrower guy shrugs, the "officer" reaches for his sidearm, a Vietnam War vintage Colt .45. Carl swallows hard, thinking to himself, *So, this is how it ends. All that, what? – effort, emotions, joy, pain, desire, suffering? – and this is all how it ends? Dissatisfying to say the least!* Carl wants to close his eyes, but the officer shouts at him again. Carl stares back, shrugging now. The officer turns the pistol around and, holding it by the barrel, hands it to Carl. Befuddled, Carl takes the pistol, trying to play it cool. The officer then points at a pigsty nearby and shouts what appear to be more orders; orders to kill everything therein, by Carl's crude interpretation of the officer's body language. Carl nods. The officer, growing impatient, shouts at Carl – *"Dah!"* – a single syllable which Carl translates as *Go!* Heeding the edict, Carl begins walking towards the pigsty. This seems to satisfy the officer and his subordinate, as the two then turn and begin trotting away. As they go, the officer guy points to a still-standing hut which the flamethrower guy promptly torches, and off into the smoke they vanish. Still confused but playing along, Carl trots away in the opposite direction, pumping off a few shots into the air for good measure as he goes.

    The flames prove to be a better indication of the prevailing winds than the direction of the meandering, indecisive smoke. So, against instinct, against better judgment, Carl aims his flight in the direction towards which the towering, leaping flames are leaning. It was all very counter-intuitive, this running in the direction of the flames. Probably not a gene that made it too far down the human DNA ladder before being burned into extinction, Carl was thinking as he weaved his way past collapsing structures and more scattered bodies, these all shot. How did he get here? It was all so very surreal. What were those few fateful decisions he had made that led him to this point in time? There was the one wherein he chose virology over becoming a doctor. Then there was that other fork in the road; the one foist upon him just a few months ago by Bronwyn back at the CDC. He had wanted to do Level Four & Five research – the "sexy" stuff – not this "boring" Level Two crap. Influenza recon: where's the excitement in that?

Just as Carl, still running, is beginning to sense he is nearing the town limits, two "Huey" helicopters swoop overhead, further obfuscating what was already a swirling chaos of smoke, soot, and dust. Carl never actually sees the helicopters – he only hears them, and maybe glimpses their hulking dark shadows – but as they move towards one distinct end of town – and hovered there, presumably to evacuate their goon squad assassins, it being "Miller Time" after all – Carl instinctually runs off in the exact opposite direction. A straw "coolie" hat, driven by the helicopter wind, tumbles past him: *Follow it!* – some little voice in his head shouts.

The smoke thins to mere wisps as Carl runs from out of the last of the burning structures. Up ahead of him await the hundred meters of open grazing land that rings the village then, beyond that, the welcoming jungle. Even through his soot-smeared visor Carl can make out another fleeing biosafety suit; white, like his. He chases after it, quickly gaining on it as it stumbles again and again. From up further ahead Carl can hear Wen shouting out: "Tian! Tian!" followed by something in Mandarin that feels like, *"This way! Hurry!"*

Tian is on her hands and knees, seemingly sobbing, when Carl reaches her. He calls out gently, "Tian, it's me, Carl. Let me help you."

Nearly as quickly as it takes Carl to say those words and place an encouraging hand on her shoulder, Tian is up and running again, instantly emboldened by just his presence. Soon they reach Wen, still in his biosafety suit as well, waiting just within the peripheral vegetation. He takes one of Tian's hands, urging her onward, "We have to keep moving."

"Where's Dr. Williams?" Carl asks him.

"Dunno. Where'd you get the gun?"

Carl looks down at his hand, surprised to discover he's still holding the pistol. Without answering, he tosses it into the thick of the jungle.

The revving helicopter engines turn Carl's attention back towards the village. As the Hueys lift into the sky, their door-mounted M-60s begin shooting down anything in the village or periphery below that might still be clinging to life. Wen shouts and points, "Here comes Dr. Jenna!"

Carl wipes his visor with his sleeve as best he can, and is still only barely able to see Dr. Williams running towards them, some thirty meters away, the daypack slung over one shoulder.

"Dr. Jenna, over here!" Wen shouts to her.

Upon reaching them Jenna doesn't even pause as she shouts, "Keep running! Keep running!"

With Jenna in the lead now, the team resumes their flight deeper into the thickening jungle.

"Can we take off the suits?" Wen calls out, no doubt feeling as encumbered by the bulky bag of sweat.

"Not yet. Wait until we're a kilometer in, at least!" Jenna shouts back, then thinks to ask, as if in an afterthought, "Everyone alright? Tian?"

Tian nods; things could be better but she's not complaining.

"Wen?"

"I'm good."

"Carl, how's the arm?"

"Good. I don't even think it's bleeding," Carl shouts back from the rear.

"Alright then, let's pick it up a bit. They're likely to be shooting at anything they can spot. Even a napalm strike wouldn't surprise me," Jenna shouts, now quickening their flight as she leads them, single-file, away and into the jungle.

After some ten minutes of what might have felt like an all out sprint to anyone not on steroids, Jenna rips off her facemask and slows to a trot, then a walk, then, at last, to a stop, telling the others, "Alright. Alright, that should do it."

The others similarly pull off their masks and coast to a stop; each sweaty, out of breath, and still terrified.

"Shouldn't we, like, change course?" Wen asks, worriedly.

Jenna, bent over and wheezing, shakes her head. "They weren't after us."

"They weren't?" Tian asks incredulously. "Sure felt like it."

"Who were they after then?" Wen asks.

Carl breaks it down for them: "The bug."

the momentum of folly

"The *bug*? The virus?" Tian asks.

Jenna, still bent over, hands on knees, spits then nods, "Fighting it the most efficacious way known to humankind."

"Oh, so those were the good guys!" Wen says sardonically.

"Yep, those were the good guys."

Something catches Carl's attention, some eighty meters away from where they all have paused. At first he's not certain it isn't a natural formation, though the straight-edged horizontal and vertical features suggest otherwise. As the others begin to remove their biosafety suits and continue trying to make sense of the violence just witnessed…

"I don't get it; were they *troops?*"

"That or mercenaries; I don't know."

"You've seen this sort of thing before?"

"No, never. I've only heard of it happening, particularly with Ebola in Africa, but I guess I never quite believed it."

"I don't get it; they just swoop in and *slaughter* everybody?"

"What's not to get? You saw that mortality rate; just imagine if that got out."

… Carl wanders towards the enigmatic formation, drawn thither by the same curiosity that killed the cat, and leaving behind Jenna as she attempts to put the attack in some sort of historical context for the others:

"In Africa they've been known to barricade the roads and trails leading into a hot zone, leaving the people stuck therein to die and killing those – with guns, rocks, spears, whatever – who try to escape. Sounds cruel but it's nipping the suffering in the bud."

"The ends justifying the means."

"Precisely. I just didn't know they still did that sort of thing.…"

Halfway to the structure, Carl can make out its *all but hidden* features, currently in the process of being reclaimed by the jungle. And closer still he begins to feel a sense of frightened exhilaration as the size of the structure becomes more apparent to him: it's at least forty meters long and fifteen wide and shaped like a greenhouse, but without the requisite glass walls and ceilings. That is perhaps what is most puzzling about it; its sheer enormity. Clearly it's not a hut like the structures in the village being reduced to ashes not two kilometers from here. Clearly this edifice had more forethought put in to it, making it seem like an institutional effort, whether governmental or religious. Carl rounds the nearest corner of the structure and – compounding his surprise – discovers it to be just one of four such buildings; three of which are identical and aligned maybe five meters apart, with each in similar states of decay. The fourth seems to be a centrally located building intended to somehow service the others, perhaps in the capacity of mess hall or worship center. Also, the surrounding area – though covered with vegetation now – attest to a concentrated effort to carve a settlement out of the wilds, with vestiges of levees and rectangular rice paddies all now just vague features to be re-imagined.

Carl moves to the nearest building. Reaching out with his still-gloved hand, he pulls aside the vines growing over what appear to be a window, and is surprised to find bamboo bars, horizontal and vertical, filling the space. Grabbing one such bar he gives it a shake. It holds. Putting more effort and both hands into it, he shakes it again. This time, owing to the decay, the bamboo bar breaks off in his hands. Taking the next logical step, Carl sticks his head through the aperture in an attempt to peer into the structure's dark interior.

"Careful," Jenna calls out from behind him, as she too is drawn by curiosity to the building. Soon she is at his side and peering into the same murky darkness. "You never know, it could be booby-trapped."

"D'ya think?"

"No, but that's how it always is in the movies, right? – that or there's some hunkered-down, loaded for bear, paranoid soldier in there who somehow didn't get word the war had ended. You know, that kind of thing."

"I thought it was a greenhouse at first but there's not enough light to grow anything, except maybe mushrooms."

"Corrugated tin roof; serious stuff. I doubt it's about mushrooms."

Jenna, liberated from her biosafety suit, begins kicking at the remaining window bars, determined to get inside.

"You don't seem too concerned about booby-traps now."

"I'm over it," Jenna confirms, as she continues busting down the bamboo bars.

Carl uses this opportunity to peel out of his suit. "How long do you think it's been abandoned?"

"A decade? A century? Hard to say," Jenna replies, grunting as she issues the last of maybe a dozen kicks at the bamboo bars, this one managing to break

the momentum of folly

through the last of them. She then puts one leg over the low windowsill and ducks inside. Carl follows her in, both of them pausing just inside to adjust to the dim light. As Carl's eyes adapt the first thing he notices is the raised, plank flooring.

"Wood planks, not bamboo. Milled even."

Jenna nods, "Definitely a government job. Had to bring the wood down the Mekong from the highlands."

"So why put a prison way out in the boonies here?"

"I'm guessing it's a work camp," Jenna says as she crosses the width of the room over to where shelves are built against the walls. There she brushes aside decades' worth of dust and cobwebs to get a better look at what is stacked on the shelves, commenting ominously, "But I could be wrong."

Carl leans in beside her to see what she has found; human skulls — scores, hundreds, thousands of them, maybe tens of thousands — each meticulously stacked and numbered, presumably for identification. Jenna gently picks up one and blows the dust from it.

"Epidemic?" Carl hypothesizes.

"Then what; cut off their heads and shoot 'em just to be orderly?" Jenna says, sarcastically, turning the skull around so Carl can see the bullet hole in the back of it.

"Okay, maybe not."

Carl takes a 360° look around the room to see if all the shelves similarly contain rows of skulls. They do, prompting Carl to posit another theory: "Khmer Rouge?"

Jenna nods, "Ostensibly." She replaces the first skull back onto the shelf and picks up another, this one obviously that of a young child, three, maybe four years old. As she examines it, she elaborates, "Pol Pot was one fastidious motherfucker. Targeted the intelligentsia first. After that it was easy. 1.7 million in all. They've found complexes like this all over Cambodia and Laos; reckon just not this one."

After the objectively scientific part of her examination, Jenna turns the skull so to stare straight into its hollow eye sockets; which she does for several seconds, seemingly mesmerized by it, seemingly sans emotions.

Watching her frozen there, transfixed, for what seems to him a disturbingly protracted time, Carl grows concerned, "Dr. Williams?"

Carl's verbal nudge pops Jenna out of her entrancement. She opens her eyes wide and takes a deep breath, but her attempt to appear unaffected by the child's skull and its premature fate, is belied by the tears welling in her eyes. Placing the skull back in its dusty divot on the shelf, she says, "Let's get the fuck out of here."

Dark clouds drag their heavy bellies across the higher ridges, obscuring them, probably already raining — up there in the highlands — but not yet down here in the barely rolling hills of the jungle floor. Not yet, but soon.

The recon team continues single-file through the dense undergrowth, still purposely avoiding using a trail, still purposely moving as directly away from the eradicated village as they can employing their vague sense of direction-by-committee. Exhausted by what has been the quintessential *long day*, each generally keeps whatever thoughts they might have to his or herself. Wen is up ahead, ripping and trampling a path through the brush and vines with both arms. Tian follows on his heels, carrying both of their tattered biosafety suits, like footballs, wadded in each arm. Some meters behind them follow Carl then Jenna. Jenna carries both their suits in the daypack, while Carl does their ripping and trampling.

Without turning, Carl voices what he's been pondering ever since she first muttered it, "*Ostensibly?*"

"That's right," Jenna replies, barely taking any time to pick up their interrupted conversation.

"How so?"

Jenna shakes her head. "Oh, you don't want to get me started."

Oh, but he *does*. "If it wasn't the Khmer Rouge who killed those people, who was it?" he presses.

"You mean, *what* was it?"

"What do you mean? — *What*," Carl repeats, perplexed.

"Nobody ever wants to talk about the impetus of genocide. Ever notice that? It's, like, taboo. Much easier just to declare the perpetrators *evil* and leave it at that."

"But you have your doubts."

"Don't misunderstand me: what Pol Pot did back there was horribly and unequivocally wrong, but something brought him to it. Do you think he or whoever anguished about killing that kid? I do. I certainly do. I mean, I'm sure he was no saint, but to write him off as merely evil or insane is naïve, and probably even dangerous."

"And Hitler?" Carl suggests, gently encouraging her to elaborate.

And she does, a palpable rant now evident in her voice. "Hitler, Stalin, the Hutus and Tutsis, the Chinese in Tibet, Indonesians in Timor, Serbs in Kosovo, Dayaks in Borneo, Shiites and Sunnis, the Jangaweed in Darfur slaughtering Sudanese *as we speak*, what's transpiring in the Congo *as we speak*; what they all did was/is unspeakably atrocious, but that doesn't change the fact that something led them to believe they had no choice. We're all human. We're all capable of this. People are not innately *evil*. People are innately *fearful*. People are innately *protective*."

"Your aforementioned *what*, as in what causes genocide."

Jenna nods as she pauses to squint up at the floral canopy and feel for rain, "And it's bound to get a whole lot worse before it gets any better. A hard rain's gonna fall."

She then calls up ahead, "Wen, which way's the boat?"

Wen pauses and turns, "What?"

Exasperated, Jenna re-submits the question in Mandarin.

Wen checks his compass, then points in nearly the opposite direction they are presently moving, "Back that a-way."

Jenna sighs heavily, then looks around. "It's getting dark. Alright, we'll sleep it off here. Wen, Tian, how 'bout making us some cushy mats out of whatever you people used to make them out of, while Carl and I go look for water."

"Cushy mats, got it," Wen replies, too wasted to add the salute.

Jenna begins down towards a subtle ravine, beckoning the stationary Carl – "Are you coming?" – as she brushes past him.

Understanding that hers was not so much a question as an edict, Carl takes a deep, sighing breath, then follows after her.

Time; where does it go? Minutes later Carl finds himself trudging along a few steps behind Jenna down the gently sloping topography, hopefully towards a stream or other freshwater source. But this isn't what he's thinking about. He's thinking about what Stuart had said about Dr. Williams back in their house: *I'd follow that ass through the Valley of the Shadow of Death, and with a smile on my face!* And how did Stuart know she'd be wearing tight khaki jungle shorts? – damn prescient of him.

Carl feels the first few drops of the imminent rain streak down his face and arms. Jenna must have felt some as well, because she's now walking with her eyes closed and her face tilted skywards – inhaling deeply, arms held out at her sides palms upwards – relishing the prospect of a cleansing downpour. Her better judgment usurped by Nature's intoxicating allure, she steps out of her shoes. *Sensible shoes,* Carl admires, as he walks past them, *sensible but now apparently discarded.*

"Carl?"

"Yeah?"

"Take off your shoes," she says softly, without turning towards him.

Carl hesitates, "Do you really think that's a good idea?"

"I do."

"Staph, jungle rot…"

"Surely you've learned by now not to argue with me."

Carl begrudgingly obeys. Standing, flamingo-like, first on one hopping leg then the other, Carl pulls off his hiking shoes and socks, tucking the latter into the former and prudently carrying them along by his fingers, as he continues with his feeble excuses, "… hantavirus, malaria…."

But if Jenna is even listening, nothing in her expression or pace – relaxed but steadily onward – is evidence of it.

Carl steps carefully along the jungle floor, waiting for something to jab up through the soles of his feet, or to step on a python or some three-pound spider. But nothing like that happens. Instead, the leaf-covered soil is cool and unbelievably soft – welcoming. As Carl is watching his toes gently depress the padded carpet with each new step, he can't help but notice too Jenna's shirt, discarded there on the ground. Slightly shocked, he looks up in time to see her pull off her athletic jog bra – up and over her head – which also she drops by the wayside. Now it's just those aforementioned tight, khaki jungle shorts, leading him onward through that aforementioned Valley of the Shadow of Death, and soon she slips out of those.

"Now your clothes."

"C'mon, Dr. Williams," Carl protests, feebly.

"Where are you from, Carl?"

the momentum of folly

The change of tack disorients Carl. "Atlanta."

"I mean originally."

"Colorado. Up near Steamboat Springs."

"No – *originally*."

The question stumps Carl.

Knowing this, Jenna answers for him: "You're from the *jungle*, Carl. One exactly like this. We both are." She turns towards him, driving home her point with her atavistic nakedness.

"So, what's that got to do with taking off my clothes?"

She glares at him for a beat before snapping back, "Nothing. Nothing, Carl. Only that this will likely be the only fucking chance you'll ever get to experience what our ancestors experienced; walkin' through the East African jungle one rainy day when Njobo said, *Antelope went 'im this way*, and Dorf said, *No, me quite sure antelope went 'im that way*, and the two took their families and parted ways never to see each other again for another 70,000 years." Jenna pauses, still staring at him, then, "So, take off your clothes."

"I have a girlfriend, you know," Carl tries.

"And I've got a husband, *whoop-tee-do*. But d'ya know what? – life is short."

Fed up, Jenna turns and begins walking down towards the subtle babblings of a gently flowing stream, deeper into what is looking less like a jungle and more like a thoroughly wild garden.

And Carl watches her, barely aware he has removed his shirt and is working on his pants.

Above... the silhouettes of monkeys flutter through the upper canopy against a pale orange sky. The dissonant cries of parrots rend the otherwise tranquil mists. A spider puts aside its web weaving for a time to hunker down beneath a leaf for the incipient rain. A luminescent green boa slides, like liquidity itself, down the underside of a limb.

Below... dwarfed by Nature to the point of insignificance, a naked Carl is a top a naked Jenna. The barely audible rustling of leaves, a few grunts, a few groans, but nothing artificial. So why all the fuss? – just another pair of mammals doing the chore. Pleasure; just biology's ruse to keep reproduction going. Guilt, shame; maybe this is all that separates humans from the rest.

Beads of condensation from the mists gather on a tiny fig, joining one another, aggrandizing, slipping down the skin of the fruit to the very bottom. Once there, with nowhere to go, the drip dangles, growing to the point, some five millimeters in diameter, where the surface tension can no longer resist gravity's pull. And then it drops, plummeting more than forty meters from its origins way up in the high canopy. En route downward it changes shape, from teardrop, to spherical, then to a flattened blob as — slapped about by wind resistance — it obtains its terminal velocity of nine meters per second. As chance has it, the drops lands upon a broad-leafed rubber plant before reaching the jungle floor, and from there slides down the leaf's ravine-shaped spine until at last it drips again, less than a meter this time, into Carl's open and awaiting mouth.

Carl is lying, still naked, on his back on the soft ground. Dropping his attention from the leaf and the next drip gathering there, he gazes over to Jenna; lying on her side, presumably sleeping, a few meters away. She too is naked, but for that cheap Rasta friendship bracelet at which Carl is looking — pondering, puzzling over. Is that the laughter of those twin girls, probably dead by now, he is hearing; the ones with the similar bracelets, oh, and the pot-bellied pig with the similar necklace? *Rasta bracelets; what's up with that?* Carl is one of those people who frown when they are not able to figure something out, and that's what he's doing — frowning. But at least he's figured out it's not the girls' laughter he's hearing; sure, maybe it's what he's *imagining*, but it's not what he's actually *hearing*. What he's actually hearing turns out to be another mosquito, revving up its wings to take to flight from nearly the exact, still-itchy spot on his abdomen where that Mexican mosquito tanked up just a few days ago. This one, a Tiger Mosquito, is about four times the size of its North American cousin but keeps to the same modus operandi: bite, suck, leave, lay eggs, die. And, tanked up, that's just what this one does, with that same, annoying, 165 million years-old buzzing.

Clued in to the jungle timing — *part* of the jungle now — Carl closes his eyes, turns his face back skyward again, opens his mouth... and catches the next drop of water that falls from the rubber plant leaf.

Shanghai International Airport. Two days later.

Despite all the new steel and concrete and mirrored glass stretching to the sky, something about Shanghai International makes it feel like just another Third World airport, but on growth hormones. Perhaps it's the overworked, underpaid ground crew and terminal employees, putting in fifteen-hour days only to try to sleep it off in their shoebox-sized, shared apartments before having to don their uncomfortable suits and First World smiles again way too early the next morning. Perhaps it's the gaping lapses of security and the pretense of customer service. Or perhaps it's the *Is this all there is?* malaise chipping away at the big promise of the Cultural Revolution, felt by all but the few sitting on the pantheon of power. Some societies have to believe in the *carrot* of Heaven and the *stick* of Hell to survive. Some have to believe in the joy and self-fulfillment guaranteed by capitalism to all those who are willing to just get off their asses; *Work hard, happiness is just within reach!* Other societies get by on plain old oppression. While still others rally behind *Le Revolucîon!* – no matter how long ago *Le Revolucîon* was. Modern China seems to be an amalgamation of all of these diverse paths to happiness. But when will it change; not just for China, but for all humanity? What will keep humans caring for one another, growing food and teaching kids and hauling bedpans for strangers, once the fear of God and false fulfillments of materialism and threat of death and suffering and the phony goal of freedom are finally transcended? Is there a point to this? Is there a goal in human evolution? Is there a pre-destined, ideal, ultimate terminus?

These are the thoughts oozing through Carl's mind as he leans, delirious and sweating again, on the team's cart of luggage and crates and whatnot out on the tarmac at the "Special Cargo" check-in area. *Special* – that word gives him something to ponder over as he gazes out through the wobbling heat mirage hugging the tarmac; gazing mindlessly out at plump aircraft the size of ships coming and going through the smoggy haze to all points on the over-heated globe. *Special* – and now, perseverating over the word, it quickly decomposes to meaninglessness as, somewhere behind him, Tian and Wen can be heard chatting in Mandarin as they unload the last of the team's equipment from the Landcruiser, separating the CDC's stuff from the WHO's and stacking them onto separate piles. Up ahead, Jenna stands at the Special Cargo check-in window, exchanging documents and questions and explanations with the airport Customs employee therein. But it's all a surreal blur to Carl; the way he feels, it's all so pointless.

Jenna turns and walks back towards him. As she folds away the documents and lifts her attention to Carl's face, her expression becomes one of concern.

"You okay?" she asks, walking up to him.

"I'm fine," Carl assures her.

"You look like shit."

"Thank you, but I'm fine."

Unconvinced but changing subjects, she calls out to Tian and Wen.

"How're we coming along?"

Tian slams shut the Landcruiser's tailgate, "We're done."

"Good. C'mere a minute."

After Wen stacks the last crate on the CDC pile he tosses a big-brotherly arm over Tian's shoulders and walks her over to where Carl and Jenna wait.

Jenna takes a breath to begin her farewell address.

"Alright, first item of business: I'll be filing a report as soon as I get back to Geneva. And I assume, after getting my report, they'll be wanting to speak with each of you as well."

"On the outbreak or the massacre?" Tian asks.

"Both, I'm sure. So, it wouldn't hurt to jot down every detail of what you saw, especially since this process could take months – don't want to forget anything – and be prepared to be called in to give a formal deposition. Got it?"

Tian and Wen nod.

"Questions?"

They shake their heads.

"Okay, I'm not good at goodbyes, especially teary ones. So let's get this over with," Jenna says, spreading her arms to embrace Tian. "Don't worry, these things always get better."

After Jenna releases Tian, she turns to Wen. Similarly Tian moves on to Carl.

"Well, in spite of everything, it was nice working with you," Tian says.

"Likewise," Carl replies, not too good at goodbyes himself.

"Do you think I'll have to tell them about barfing in my suit?"

Carl smiles and shakes his head. "But you can if you want."

Tian flashes a grateful smile up to Carl, then hugs him again, tightly.

"Alright, alright, enough already. It's my turn!" Wen teases, pulling Tian away from Carl, and hugging him himself.

"Take care, bro," Wen tells Carl, patting his back.

"You too. And keep an eye out for this bug. If it escaped it's gonna hit the ground running, and governments are notoriously slow to react," Carl tells him.

"Will do," Wen assures him.

Pulling apart, they smile at one another.

"Boom, there it is," Wen says, wrapping his arm back around Tian's shoulders and turning her away, she waving her final farewell blindly to Jenna and Carl as she and Wen walk back towards the Landcruiser.

"China will be in good hands," Jenna says, watching Wen and Tian walk off.

"Yeah, someday," Carl comments, closing the lid on the empty, stainless steel briefcase meant to carry samples of the influenza serum back to the CDC.

Jenna watches him latch the case.

"Do you think you'll get in trouble?"

"Whatever for?" he scoffs, "just for returning empty-handed from possibly the most lethal flu outbreak of the last ninety years, or maybe ever? Who could get upset with me for that?" As if to underscore his sarcasm, he angrily tosses the case onto his pile of luggage.

"You might explain they were shooting at you."

"What's that expression? Excuses are like assholes; everybody's got one."

Jenna smiles. "I think you're being a little hard on yourself."

"Yeah? What about you? Won't anyone back at the WHO be upset about your coming back empty-handed?"

"You're forgetting; I'm retired."

"So, what was this about? – just a hobby?"

Jenna smiles at Carl, seemingly studying him again but saying nothing. After what amounts to an unnervingly protracted beat she pulls off her daypack and, unzipping it, pulls out two cylindrical, milled-aluminum canisters. She then holds up both, one in each hand, as if for him to choose either one.

Bewildered, Carl takes one and begins to unscrew its lid.

"Careful," Jenna warns with understated calm.

Carl pauses then, heeding the suggestion, gently unscrews the lid. Once opened, he sets the lid down then carefully slides from the canister a small rack securely holding three sealed, glass vials, each approximately two-thirds filled with a reddish-yellow fluid recognizable to any seasoned virologist as blood serum. Carl looks up at Jenna.

"The Laotian strain?"

Jenna nods.

"You actually thought to grab some?" Carl asks, incredulous.

"Wouldn't've left there without it."

From some forty meters away, Wen honks the Landcruiser's horn as he and Tian drive off, waving. Carl looks from them back to Jenna.

"Do they know?"

Jenna shakes her head. "I figured it might be safer for them if they didn't, as I don't know who exactly they report to."

Her reasoning sound, Carl nods.

"So," Jenna begins, mustering a rare smile, "cheer up; you won't be returning empty-handed after all."

Carl stares at her, her smiling face now every bit as disorienting as the bustling airport and sprawling metropolis that envelops them.

The Chinese Special Customs Agent looks over the three vials securely racked within Carl's stainless steel CDC attaché case, as well as what only seems to be a cursory glance down the DHL courier forms.

"Centers for Disease Control, Atlanta, Georgia," Carl tells him.

To which the agent nods a begrudged, *Okay*, then hands an electronic clipboard across the counter for Carl to sign, which Carl does and hands back, after which time the agent returns Carl's passport and documents, after which time Carl locks the case, after which time the agent applies security seals and biohazard labels to the case, then tosses it on the conveyor behind him.

"Thanks," Carl tells him.

To which the Special Customs Agent nods perfunctorily, motioning impatiently for Jenna's documentation and similar steel attaché case. Jenna sets her case on the counter, opens it, and spins it towards the agent, telling him, "World Health Organization, Geneva, Switzerland."

As the agent inspects the case and documents, Jenna turns towards Carl, noting sardonically, "I always loved that."

"Loved what?"

"You risk your life for these people and then they act like they're doing you a favor by letting you put your itsy bitsy box on an airplane," Jenna smirks, regarding the Customs agent.

Carl stares at her, taken aback she would dare say such a thing within earshot of the very person she is criticizing, of the very person upon which the safe passage of her ever so important cargo relies. Then again, she's right.

"Okay," the agent blurts, similarly tossing Jenna's case on the conveyor behind him before pulling down the steel shutter of his Special Cargo Counter window – closed.

Jenna and Carl turn and begin walking away from the counter, now burdened with only their carry-on daypack and laptop case respectively.

"So, how long 'till your flight?" she asks.

"Like five hours. Why?"

"I'd like to show you something."

Jenna and Carl climb out of a taxi and into a sea of pedestrians, somewhere in the heart of downtown Shanghai. As Jenna pays the cabby Carl looks about, gawking up at the towering skyscrapers in all directions.

"This feels about as far from Nature as one can get," he tells her, having to shout over the mid-morning din as they join the urgent flow of ant-like, gotta-be-somewhere pedestrian traffic.

Jenna nods, "Slow-cooked frog."

Carl isn't sure he heard her right.

"What?"

"Slow-cooked frog: ever heard of it?" she repeats.

"That's not what we're having for lunch, is it?"

Jenna smiles and shakes her head.

"They say if you toss a frog into a pot of boiling water it'll have the sense to jump right out. But if you put it into a pot of *cool* water, which you then slowly heat to a boil, the frog will cook to death without ever noticing the increasingly intolerable conditions."

"I don't suppose you're implying anything allegorical in that," Carl quips facetiously.

After a perfunctory smirk in response, Jenna pulls their forward progress to a complete stop near a five-way roundabout intersection. She then turns towards Carl, just standing there as the clone-like river of Shanghai-ites bump and bustle past. Carl is feeling uncomfortably self-conscious; both from being, yet again, the focus of Jenna's inscrutable stare, but now also from being an obvious obstacle in the foot traffic – one of the two rocks in the otherwise free-flowing stream of humans.

"What?" he asks, wondering if Jenna's stopping was arbitrary or intentional.

Jenna widens her smirk then nods in a direction directly behind Carl's back. Following her nod, he turns about, seeing nothing at first other than just another wide and busy street, back-dropped by a wall of skyscrapers and yet another one under construction.

But then he sees *it*. *It* is a mere billboard painted on the brick wall of the soon-to-be-demolished, three-story building currently all but hidden beneath the scaffolding and steel girder frame of a newer, bigger building being erected in the obsolete building's place. And though *it* is mere billboard the very sight of it stabs Carl through the heart. Though chipped and faded, the simple, grade school children's artwork and text – printed both in Mandarin and English – are still visible, and its message still all too clear:

"For them. For us. For it." – it says across the top of the three-panel display, with a kids-created crayon drawing of some elephants, tigers, frogs, and polar bears, under the first "For them" section; a similarly cartoonish depiction of a two-child family under the "For us" panel; and a nearly round, blue, green, and white reproduction of the Earth under the "For it" part. Then, below the art-work, the caption: *"Just two kids. Just two billion. We can live with that."*

"Recognize it?" Jenna asks.

"Of course," Carl replies glumly.

"Thought you might like to see it, you know, before it's demolished."

"Thanks," Carl says, not meaning it.

"I thought you might be, I don't know, proud; it being your father's legacy and all."

Carl shakes his head bitterly, "What can be said about someone whose greatest achievement is a billboard?"

"I would have to say that depends on the intent. If it's to sell cigarettes or light beer, not a lot. But if it's a self-less attempt to save humanity from trampling itself into oblivion, I'd say that's something of a triumph."

"Generous praise, don't you think?"

Jenna levels a stare at him. "Don't you think you're selling your father short?"

"Not really, considering I was part of that family he virtually abandoned when he set out to foist his two-child campaign upon the world."

"You sound resentful."

"I *am* resentful."

Jenna hesitates, debating whether to tell him more. Then – perhaps deciding it would help him, or perhaps deciding *what the hell* – she begins to fill in the story:

"Carl, I was here with your father when he and a group of school children painted this billboard. Possibly you weren't aware of what your father was doing at the time, especially considering you were hardly in grade school yourself, but I was a high school exchange student here at the time, and I was very impressed by his efforts."

Carl is seething; Jenna's revelation coming as more of a personal intrusion into a painful memory than a healing insight.

"I was also here when he came back and put up that," Jenna says, now turning 120° and directing Carl's attention to the digital LED numerical display installed above the entry of the Hard Rock Café restaurant located across one of the other streets terminating into the intersection.

"What's that?" Carl asks, spitefully.

"Thought you'd recognize it: it's a Population Clock. There's a handful of them scattered around the world; universities, museums, Hard Rock Cafés, etc. There's one near the concert hall in Stockholm where they hand out the Nobel Prizes. That's the one that first caught my eye."

"Six billion, eight hundred and eighty-six million, nine hundred and thirteen thousand, four hundred and something," Carl reads from the red LED display, unable to cite the number precisely insofar as the last couple digits – particularly the ones column – are a whirling blur of changing lights.

the momentum of folly

"Current World Population; that's what those Chinese characters under the display say. Two-point-nine births per second, nearly two-thirds of them malnourished and miserable from day one."

Jenna turns from the Population Clock to Carl again. "It was your father's goal to put up one of these in every city and village so that people the world 'round could get a sense of the mathematics of our population explosion in order to begin to grasp the dire consequences of it all."

"The momentum of folly."

Jenna nods, "As he referred to it — yes.

"Well, if that was his goal he obviously failed."

"Maybe he didn't succeed, but that was hardly his fault."

Carl takes a big breath, and releases a heavy, moving-on sigh.

"So, is this why you dragged me here?"

Jenna glares at him, growing weary of Carl's resentment of his father.

"Yes, Carl, that's why I dragged you here."

From the perspective of oblivious passersby, it's just another Chinese taxi pulling up to the Departures curb at bustling Shanghai Airport. And, emerging from the back seat, just another pair of sojourners from continents far away; one, an attractive black woman, the other, a sicker-than-shit gringo.

Jenna watches as Carl slides out of the cab into the harsh sunlight, squinting, perspiring — again, still.

"Okay, *Godspeed*, as they say. This bug'll be knocking on America-the-beautiful's door before you know it."

Carl begins to nod, but is cut short by a sneeze, prompting Jenna to feel his forehead then look at him with concern.

"If you're worried about the Laotian strain, I didn't catch it," he tries to assure her.

Jenna looks at her watch, "That was forty hours ago… you shouldn't be showing any symptoms yet even if you had caught it."

"I *didn't!*" Carl states obstinately, slinging his laptop case strap over his shoulder.

Jenna nods, opting not to argue with him. "How many layovers are you looking at between here and Atlanta?"

"Just one big overnighter in Anchorage."

"Well, do yourself a favor and pop for a hotel. You need some rest to give your immune system a chance to recover. Preferably some place quiet; away from the airport."

"Any recommendations?"

Jenna shakes her head. "Sorry. Never been there."

"Never been? – to Anchorage or Alaska?" Carl asks, a little confused.

Jenna hesitates. "Either."

"What about those two weeks last winter?"

Jenna is clearly caught off her guard by the question. For the first time in her life, she's speechless.

"There was a stamp in your passport," Carl explains, innocently enough, and certainly without any hint of suspicion.

"You went through my stuff?" she asks, suddenly accusatorily.

"Just your passport. On the flight over, you dropped it when you went to the bathroom."

And just like that, Carl finds himself again the focal point of her searing glare.

"I'm sorry, but I don't get what the big, fuckin' deal is: Your daypack thing was open and spilling its guts out on the floor, and, *yes*, I picked up your open passport, then stuffed it back in your pack knowing that's what I would have *appreciated* your doing for me. And, *yes* – guilty as charged – I happened to glance at the page that happened to have that Alaskan port-of-entry Customs stamp. Jesus, I know you're bad at goodbyes but this is ridiculous!"

Jenna's wrath eases some. She musters a conciliatory, "Sorry," then extends her elbow for the virologists' handshake.

Carl considers the elbow touch momentarily, but instead kisses Jenna full on the lips; a kiss that lasts considerably longer than mere friends might exchange, but considerably shorter than that of genuine, passionate lovers.

When she pulls away – and of course it would be her – both are left not quite knowing what to think or feel about anything, and there is certainly nothing in either's inscrutable stare to guide the other.

And so, after a protracted, wordless exchange, Carl turns and walks away towards the airport check-in building.

And Jenna stands there watching, trembling ever so slightly.

University of Melbourne, Australia.

Some two hundred graduate students sit in the darkness of the ultra modern multi-media hall, listening in rapt silence to a lecture accompanying the Power Point presentation they are watching. Though the course title sounds rather tedious – Political Economics of Natural Resources – the horrorstruck look on each student's face suggests the subject matter today is anything but boring.

On the gigantic screen high-definition, motion, aerial shots of smog-choked Mexico City – endless and sprawling – are being shown. Off to one side and dwarfed by the projection, visiting professor, Dr. Fernando Perez, sixty-three, delivers his matter-of-fact lecture in flawless English, colored by a Columbian accent.

"2003 marked the first time in history in which the number of people living in urban areas surpassed that of those living in rural ones, as society continues to transition from an agrarian to an industrial-based economy."

He pauses to keep his lecture paced to the images being projected.

"Greater Mexico City, currently at 29 million and growing by fourteen hundred per day, most of this influx coming from failing farm communities. Whereas global *rural* growth is expected to peak around 2020 at 3.3 billion, 99.5% percent of humanity's final buildup will be concentrated in existing cities, and most of this, sadly, in slums."

The screen cuts from Mexico's slums to Manila's, then to Jakarta's, then to Dhaka's, then to Karachi's, as Dr. Perez continues with his narration.

"Karachi, Pakistan; world's second largest city now with over thirteen million just within its city limits and a population density of 3,612 per square kilometer, it throws six hundred new cars on its already traffic-clogged streets every day.

"Not to bore you with the good ol' days, but back in 1948 – about when I was that proverbial twinkle in my genetically-gifted parents' eyes – there were only eighty-six cities with populations of one million or more. By 2020 there

the momentum of folly

will be over six hundred. This rampant growth has given rise to the phenomenon of the *megaslum;* where basic infrastructure – sewage, running water, electricity, policing, etc. – have either never existed or now lay in utter decay."

The projection cuts to a listing helicopter shot skimming over the rooftops and squalor and smoldering wreckage of some vast, seemingly endless African slum, as Dr. Perez elaborates: "Lagos, Nigeria; just sixty years ago a bustling yet functional city of 290,000, now growing at nearly that much – 275,000 – per annum to the point where greater Lagos is now Earth's largest contiguous urban sprawl, home to an estimated eight to nine million just within its metropolitan area and countless millions more spilling out beyond its official city limits."

The screen now shows street-level, hand-held shots of Bombay, India, as Dr. Perez continues: "Greater Bombay, Mumbai: thirty-three million. One toilet per five hundred inhabitants. *Hey, Baba, how's it going in there? You almost done?* Overall, India's water demands are now twice what its aquifers can sustain, portent of a massive famine, and this in a country where already half of its children are malnourished and another eighteen million are born each year."

The projection now displays aerial footage of Kabul, N'Djamena, Addis Ababa as Dr. Perez drives home his point: "In Afghanistan, 98.5 percent of its urban populace live in slums. In Chad, 99.1 percent. In Ethiopia 99.4 percent. And, like most slum dwellers, many of these people – and please remember they *are* people, crying, laughing, *wanting-better-for-their-children* people – more often than not they live in the toxic shadows of railroads, refineries, coal-powered electricity generators, dumps, and chemical plants."

And now newsreel footage of genocide in the Republic of Congo fills the screen, serving as generic backdrop to the visiting professor's commentary: "An annual growth rate of a mere two to three percent causes a nation's population to climb twenty-fold in a century. Whereas a banker might term that *compounded interest*, we in the urban planning biz call it *compounded suffering*. In all of the world's 194 nations only fourteen have stabilized populations. Of the remaining 180 at least seventeen – termed "failed nations" – are in a current state of collapse with all of the others following hot on their heels."

Dr. Perez concludes his sobering lecture as more footage of human squalor and suffering alights the projection screen, this time represented by the inhabitants of Cairo's sprawling public landfill, who live within its vast mountains of waste.

"Cairo's public dumps; though rarely touted in travel brochures is actually much, much bigger than the pyramids – visible from space even – and home to millions of Egypt's most destitute. Some of its children are born, raised and die here without ever even seeing the city to which their slum, their world, is inextricably conjoined."

As the camera slowly zooms in, the screen begins to tighten in on a quartet of prepubescent children sifting through the heaps of trash for anything they might be able to recycle and resell – scraps of copper wire, bottles, used hypodermic needles. With sunken, brown eyes they stare at the camera as they continue with their diurnal toils, the screen ever tightening on their expressionless faces.

"Most of the world's children no longer go to school. Illiteracy – like malnutrition, infant mortality and infectious diseases – are all on the rise. It is said that if you want a peek into the future of humanity – into the lives of your *own* children and grandchildren – you need to look no further than at any of today's megaslums."

Somewhere over the North Pacific Ocean

A tray of warm, freshly baked chocolate chip cookies is pulled from a small convective oven. The "baker" – an Air China flight attendant – then carries the tray from the galley of the aging 747, through a divider curtain, and into the First Class section, doling them out to any passenger who might desire one. She then pauses in the aisle beside seat 3B and asks with a wry grin: "Would you like a warm, chocolate chip cookie, *Dr. Sims?*"

"Two, please," a beaming eight year-old Pakistani girl replies, nodding shyly.

The flight attendant spatulas the requested cookies onto a small plate and sets it before the girl, smiles, then moves on down the aisle. "Cookie?..."

Meanwhile, downstairs in the jumbo jet's "Last Class" section, Carl sits crammed into a window seat amongst a pack of raucous Pakistani kids, no doubt less fortunate siblings or cousins of the polite cookie-eater upstairs. Sure, he's pale, clammy, sweaty, baggy-eyed, sneezy, coughy – all that – but that's just what one might expect him to be considering all that he's been through this past week – having been dragged through Asia's rectum and all, figuratively speaking. Nonetheless, despite all the distractions both internal and external, he is focused on the task at hand; which in this case is the streaming-live-video-Internet conversation he's having with his housemate Stuart, who is seen on the screen of Carl's laptop shoveling yet another heaping spoonful of cereal into his mouth as he carries on with his end of the chat from the kitchen of their bungalow back in Atlanta.

"So, in spite of the stamp in her passport thing, what makes you think Dr. Jenna was lying about having never been to Alaska?" Stuart is asking, while pulverizing the cereal with the same mouth.

"Do you have to talk with your mouth full?" Carl asks, with disgust.

Stuart nods. "Multi-tasking," he replies, muffled and with food spilling out.

Carl rolls his eyes, then muses over Stu's question: "What makes me think she was lying?... she had that look on her face."

"That look on her face," Stuart repeats skeptically.

"Yeah, you know, that *look*."

"Right. Okay, seeing how I'm your roomie and all, ergo, required to take your side on everything except rent and refrigerator disputes, let us suppose for the time being that you *are* right about her lying. Okay? So, now the question becomes *why?*" Stuart pretends to ponder the question for a second or two, then, "*Ding!* – I have the answer."

"What is it?" Carl asks, seeming to barely notice the laughing Pakistani kid climbing over his seat to chase after her squealing little brother.

"Simple: she went there to cheat on her husband."

"She's not that kind of girl," Carl tries, hesitating just enough to make Stuart skeptical.

"Uh-huh, now *you've* got that look on your face!"

"C'mon, Stu, help me out here."

"Okay, okay," Stuart capitulates, scooping in another spoonful of cereal to help him think. "Starting with what we know: she's an epidemiologist, right? – so, maybe, just maybe, she went up to Alaska to research an outbreak. How's that for help?"

"Was there one?"

"One what?"

"An outbreak, moron."

"Oh, I'm the moron? Oh, but wait, stop the presses: who is that on the other end of the computer screen asking our aforementioned *moron* for help; oh, none other than *über* moron Dr. Carl Sims!" Stuart snaps back.

"This is your idea of *help?*"

"You know what your problem is, Carl? – you lack focus. You're like those Pakistani kids climbing all over you; you're too easily distracted. You've got to learn to... what were be talking about?"

Carl sighs and rolls his eyes.

"And to answer your question: *No.*"

"No, what?"

"*No*, there haven't been any outbreaks up there in Alaska!" Stuart replies, now feigning exasperation. "At least not recently; you know, not since the Spanish Flu."

Carl pauses. "The Spanish Flu hit up there?"

"*Duh* – big time! Wiped out entire Eskimo, Inuit, whathaveyou, villages. Seventy percent mortality rates some places."

"Seventy? Why so high?"

Stuart empties the last of the box of cereal into his bowl. "Dude, you're out of cereal. Mind picking some up on your way home? Damn heartless of you, when you think of it; leaving your crippled roommate home alone, cupboards bare and all. Pray to God I have enough pot and bong water to see me through these lean times," Stuart adds, reaching across the kitchen table for his bong.

"Uh, need I remind you the Internet passes, like, right through the NSA?" Carl says, urging his roommate to use a little more discretion.

"Dude, you're right. My bad. How 'bout we use code words? Instead of *pot* we'll say *Al Qaeda*. And instead of *bong*, let's see... oh, how 'bout *dirty bomb*? Kinda rhymes." Stuart takes a hit off the bong, seemingly not too troubled by the prospect of domestic spying, then adds, "Oh, and handles; let's see, I'll be *Holy Jihad*, and you be *Pig-faced Capitalistic Swine*. Okay-doke? By the way, you'll have to clean this *dirty bomb* when you get home, *Pig-faced Capitalistic Swine*. And I hope you scored some *Al Qaeda* while you were in Asia, you know, for the *Holy Jihad*, wink-wink."

Carl sighs, exasperated, then tries to steer the conversation back onto the tracks. "My question is: why was the mortality rate so high up there when it was only, like, less than one-percent throughout the rest of the world?"

Stuart exhales. "What the fuck are you talkin' about?"

"Alaska. The Spanish Flu pandemic..."

"Oh, right. Simple – actually there's a couple of theories – one of the more plausible being that a significantly-less-lethal-strain of H1N1 swept across most of the rest of the world in the *spring* of 1918, and subsequently gave all those people significant immunity to the subtly-different-but-vastly-more-lethal-mutation of the strain that ripped through later that *fall*. Sadly however, that immunizing strain skipped over some of the more remote Eskimo communities and other isolated villages around the world."

Carl nods, understanding. "Leaving those Eskimos with no immunities against the lethal strain that followed a few months later."

"Learn you fast, Pig-Faced Capitalistic Swine. Holy Jihad shall reward you with dirty bomb upon your return – if you catch my drift, wink-wink."

"What's the other theory?"

the momentum of folly

Stuart shrugs, "I don't like it as much, but basically is postulates that the strain that hit up yonder there was just nastier; by a factor of, like, seventy-times."

"That must've been one hell of a die-off."

"Yeah. Could you imagine having a *girlfriend* that was seventy times nastier?" Stuart asks, drifting again. "Oh, there was another theory — may have even been Dr. Jenna's — that theorized — 'cause that's what theories do, right? — that theorized it may not have been the Spanish Flu at all that slammed into those Eskimo villages, but rather some other, much more lethal, subtype that was circulating, though not nearly as widely, at the same time."

"Avian?"

"That was her contention, but it didn't seem plausible to me."

"Why not?"

"For fucksake, moron; think about it: it's not like Eskimos waddle around their rice paddies with their ducks and chickens in tow!"

"You're saying they don't have much in the way of domesticated fowl. So, what about migratory birds?"

"In November? — that's when the pandemic slammed into the Arctic, you know. By then any bird worth its feathers would be far south of there sipping a Mai Tai!"

"The birds could've left it behind to fester and mutate in —" Carl replies, struggling to make sense of the mystery.

"In what? — it's not like they have much in the way of a pork industry either."

"They have sled dogs; which they *sleep* with, right?" Carl says, his hypothesis beginning to gain momentum the more he thinks outside the box of normal epidemiology.

"*Canine* influenza?"

"It exists. And what do Eskimos eat, particularly in the winter? Whale blubber? Seals? Walrus?"

"Spam?"

"The point is she may have stumbled upon an entirely new *golden triangle* of influenza antigenic drift or antigenic shift mutation mechanisms!"

"Yeah, but the *likelihood* is she *didn't*. And the *fact* is, we just don't know."

Aware that Stuart is probably right, Carl changes the subject: "So, what did they do with the bodies?"

"Mass graves, dude. When peeps are droppin' that fast that's about all you can do; dig a big hole and toss 'em in."

Carl is nodding to the theory conjured by Stuart when he suddenly remembers the Russian satellite photographs of just such a mass grave site that Jenna had in that brown paper envelope marked, *Classified*.

"She had satellite photos of a cemetery," Carl tells Stuart, as he tries to figure it out.

"Who did?"

"Dr. Williams."

"She did? Was it an *Eskimo* cemetery?"

"I'm not sure, but it was all covered with snow. Oh, and it had crosses – you know, *crucifixes* – that looked like they might've been made of whale jawbones."

"So, was it a mass grave for sure? Could you see any corpses?"

Carl shakes his head, "It was all undisturbed snow. God, I wish I could remember the coordinates; they we're stamped right on the photographs!"

"If you saw it, it means it's still in your brain somewhere. Maybe have one of those Pakistani kids hypnotize you," Stuart teases.

"I wonder why she didn't talk about them; I mean, it's not like there weren't plenty of opportunities."

"Who?"

Carl groans, exasperated. "Tell you what: when I say *she* or *her* how about you just assume that's our little code word for Dr. Jenna Williams, alright? – especially seeing how that's the only she or her we're talking about."

"Unless of course the topic happens to drift to your knocked-up ex-girlfriend, now tramping around as personal *bee-atch* to the CEO of Aegis Pharmaceuticals."

Carl glares at Stuart through the computer.

"Oops, tender subject matter. Sorry, dude," Stuart apologizes, taking another bong hit, adding, as he tries to hold in the burning smoke, "That's just the latest rumor going 'round the shop… Probably not true…. Maybe I shouldn't've said anything."

"Have you heard from her?"

"Dr. Jenna?"

"No, Angela."

"Hah! – *see?*" Stuart says, victoriously as he releases the smoke.

"Fuck you."

"Hey, I've got an idea: how 'bout we change the subject? As in, how 'bout them Red Sox?!"

"Bronwyn was right; you *are* a dickhead."

"Naw, I'm serious: 1918; the Red Sox, World War I, the Spanish Flu – what a year. By the way, you know the Spanish Flu didn't start in Spain, right? It started in Iowa, or Kansas or something. It was just that the Wilson administration had a propaganda/censorship effort in effect that prohibited mention of the outbreak in the papers. Wanted to keep people focused on the war effort. Wasn't until the pandemic spread to Spain that it got wide press; hence, the Spanish Flu misnomer. One Congressman got sentenced to twenty years in prison merely for opposing the war. Geez, those were the days, my friend. My great grandma still talks about it like it was yesterday; she caught the Spanish flu."

"So, how'd she fair with the 2009 H1N1 pandemic?"

"No sweat. She, like just about every other ninety-somethin' year-old, still theoretically carried the antibodies, so she didn't even bother to get a vaccination. I urged her to – explaining how even within the H1N1 subtype, strains can vary and all – but she said, *Fuck that, shit!*"

"She said that, huh?" Carl asks skeptically.

"Verbatim. She's part sailor," Stuart avers, before recalling: "Bronwyn called me a *dickhead*?"

But before Carl can confess he only made up the dickhead aspersion in order to get back at Stuart, his brain is hijacked by the recollection of another incident from the Laotian village; namely, the incident of the *very* old lady, shouting at him in her abstruse dialect while emphatically pointing to all the other *very* old villagers – all exhibiting no signs of infection.

"Shit," Carl mutters to himself.

"*Shit*? – as in shit-*head*? Now I'm confused: did she call me *shithead* or *dickhead*? Big difference, you know. Shithead I could live with."

Carl stares blankly from the screen, pondering matters of much more gravity.

"Carl? Roomie? You okay?" Stuart asks, troubled by his roommate's sudden catatonia. "You've got that stupid, vegetative, nothing-goin'-on-upstairs look on your face; not that that's all that unusual for you –"

"The outbreak in Laos; I think it could be the same strain that struck those Eskimo villages way back when!"

Now Stuart is the one taken aback. "You tested it against HINI, right?"

"I did."

"And?"

"Negative."

"What about for H5NI?"

"Same."

"Well, then we do indeed have a mystery."

Carl racks his brain, trying to connect the dots. "Her theory about another virus, or maybe even a co-morbidity of it with Spanish flu, seems like the only explanation for why the old people of the Laotian village were unaffected. Also –" Carl pauses as he recalls Jenna's lashing response to hearing his and Wen's report regarding the village corpses. "It was weird; we were trying to tell her that the preponderance of the corpses we had come across seemed to be of young adults. I mean, we were just expressing our surprise, and she, like, got all up in my grill about it."

"Young adults; that's not good. Did you guys calculate a mortality rate?"

"She also seemed almost determined that my not being able to identify the virus against any in our database – that it had to be a mistake."

"Well, isn't that curious?" Stuart wryly understates. "And what did you say the mortality rate was?"

"Sixty, sixty-six-ish percent."

"*Two-thirds?* – Jesus, that's higher than either HINI or H5NI on their best days! If this motherfucker gets out –"

Another mental flashback – this one of the Laotian twin girls with their pot-bellied pig all with their matching Rasta bands – gives Carl cause to interrupt Stuart with another stark revelation: "They planted it."

"Planted what?" Stuart asks, trying to follow Carl's rapid flow of circumstantial assumptions.

"The virus – whatever it is. They deliberately caused the Laotian outbreak."

"You mean you *think* they did."

"No, they *definitely* did."

Stuart pulls back, visibly skeptical. "Professor-Dr.-Jenna-foxy-WHO-tight-khaki-jungle-shorts-foxy-Nobel-Laureate-foxy-Williams?" he asks, with a purposely incredulous tone.

Carl nods.

"Uh, okay. And you mentioned *they*; as in, she was not in this alone. So, like, who's *they?*"

"I don't know."

Stuart doesn't even try to hide his skepticism, "I see; you don't know *who* deliberately planted the virus to cause the outbreak of untold suffering, except that Dr. Jenna Williams, one of the foremost humanitarian altruists of our time was involved."

"Yeah."

Stuart rolls his eyes. "Okay, skipping over the *who* and *how*: any idea *why* they would do such a thing?"

Carl is shaking his head, racking his brain, but then he remembers Jenna taking him out of their way to see the Population Clock mounted above the entrance to the Hard Rock Café in Shanghai – its LED display a whirling blur of red numbers. And he can still recall her words, *"There's one around the corner from the Nobel building in Oslo, Norway. That's the one that first caught my eye."*

Carl's epiphany causes him to begin trembling.

Noticing the change, Stuart becomes concerned. "You alright, dude? You don't look so good, not that you looked so good before –"

"I know exactly why they did it."

"O-kay, well, like, hit me on."

Carl shakes his head, "Not now."

"Not now? Jesus, Carl. You know, postulating that *they* purposely set off an epidemic is a pretty heavy accusation; so why won't you at least tell me *why* you think they did it?"

"It's, I don't know, kind of hard to explain."

"Hard to explain," Stuart repeats, taking offense to Carl's excuse.

"I'm only beginning to understand it myself."

"You know, you can go to hell. And by the way, you're lookin' sicker than shit. Are you sure there's no chance you caught this bug?"

"Yes, I'm –" Carl begins, until now recalling Jenna's *accidental* sticking him with the needle in China, and her casual, *"Oops."* But this image is followed quickly by another; of the bullet ripping through the arm of his biosafety suit in Laos, which Jenna subsequently risked her life – scrambling across the burning, bullet-riddled hut to fetch her roll of duct tape to repair his suit – seemingly all in an attempt to *prevent* him from becoming infected. The juxtaposition of contrary images and motives perplexes Carl. He blanches, shaking his head in denial.

Sensing Carl's ambivalence, Stuart leans towards the camera mounted on his computer screen in order to convey the seriousness of the situation to Carl. "Jesus. Carl; not to belabor the obvious, you know, but seeing how you're on a crowded jet and all – recirculating air, doorknobs, *blah, blah, blah...*"

Carl stares back at Stuart's face on the computer screen, his confidence that he's disease-free quickly eroding.

"Carl, you know what you have to do, right?" Stuart is asking, nudging.

Carl can feel a wave of anxiety wash through him; he's never felt as uncertain of something in his life, and yet he's shaking his head even as the implications of his denial fester. "I'm not going to have them quarantine this flight."

"Why the hell not?"

"We don't even know for sure if I have it."

"Which is exactly *why* you quarantine it!"

"But I shouldn't be symptomatic yet; it hasn't even been three days."

"Three days? What the fuck, dude? Seventy-two hours is just a rule of thumb. Influenza can begin presenting itself in as little as twenty-four hours! Who the hell told you three days?"

Closing his eyes, Carl can still feel Jenna's hand on his forehead, feeling for a temperature.

"Carl, listen to me, alright? One hundred million people last time; that was the toll the Spanish Flu inflicted. And that was with a *one* percent mortality rate, not *sixty-six!* And it was also long before we had jumbo jets and other mass transit efficiently zipping it to every corner of the world. "

"It just doesn't make any sense that she would infect me."

"But her doing in an entire village *does?*" Stuart counters.

"But she –" Carl begins to say.

"What? – fucked you?"

"I was going to say *risked her life.*"

"But she fucked you too, didn't she?"

Carl looks at his hands, shaking. He glances about the cabin at his fellow passengers – the Pakistani toddler crawling after his sippy-cup under Carl's seat

— nervously trying not to admit that more than two-thirds of them could be dead by week's end because of him.

"Damn it! Look, Carl, there's a simple solution here: in seventy-two hours everyone on that plane will either be symptomatic or not. *Then* we'll know for sure. Do you hear me? Carl?"

From Stuart's perspective, Carl is looking almost catatonic again, or, at very least, not like someone who should be entrusted with a life or death decision, especially one involving his own liberty.

"Alright, fuck it, I'm calling the CDC in Anchorage!"

"Stuart, no."

"*No?* Fuck you, you brain-dead moron; I'm calling 'em," Stuart says defiantly, adding, "And this is what *you're* going to do: you're gonna send me a blood sample A-fuckin'-S- fuckin'-A- fuckin'-P so I can check it against the Laotian strain you couriered back. You did ship it separately, right?" Stuart asks cautiously.

Carl nods.

"Least you did something fucking right." Stuart checks his watch, "Let's see, you'll be touching down in about seven hours; that should give them fair enough warning." Stuart turns back to Carl, "Until then try not to sneeze on anybody, got it?"

Again, capitulating, Carl nods.

Stuart smiles reassuringly, adding "Good. So, like, have a nice quarantine, dude," before flashes a peace sign and ending the transmission.

Carl stares at his blank laptop screen, reeling. Reclaiming his senses, he removes his headset and takes a pensive look around the cabin to his four hundred-plus co-passengers; potential plague carriers all, whose only mistake was in being on the same flight. Feeling a sneeze coming on, Carl hastily pulls a vomit bag from the seat pouch in front of him, fumbling with it as he tries to open it. Then, just managing to get the bag's open end over his nose and mouth, he sneezes explosively into it, filling the bag tightly with his exhalation. He then pulls the bag carefully from his face — some snot and saliva clinging to both — and quickly and meticulously closes and seals it. Feeling a stare, Carl glances over to the five-year old Pakistani kid sitting next to him; who is staring with quiet befuddlement at the weird white man who sneezes into barf bags.

And Carl wants to smile reassuringly to the boy... but can't.

Alaska International Airport, Anchorage

There's only the faintest hint of the nascent dawn out on the eastern horizon as the China Airlines 747 touches down on Runway Fourteen, destroying what had been a veritable picture of tranquility – of idle flocks of gulls and geese and a lone and hungry bald eagle up on the approach light scaffolds – all now shattered by the otherworldly intrusion of running lights and strobes and headlights and tire smoke and squeals and hydraulics and dropping of the engine cowlings and subsequent air-breaking. After the hulking plane finally slows to a crawl, it turns – as if instinctually – towards the main terminal but then stops in its tracks, seeming to hesitate there for a protracted amount of time before turning another one hundred and twenty degrees and beginning a slow, uncertain taxiing out towards the dark, seldom-used, far western end of Runway Six.

From within the plane Carl presses his face to the window, straining to see up the runway. But from his limited vantage point he can only just barely see the lighted quarantine area, hastily set up out on the loneliest corner of the airport out against the edge of the Cook Inlet, the absolute furthest point of airport property from the terminal and people in general.

Despite the flight attendants' specific orders to the contrary – "Please remain in your seats with your seatbelts fastened…" – most all the passengers are unbuckled and up and pulling their carry-ons from the overhead compartments in that futile effort to be among the first off the plane. But Carl knows better. He knows they'll be lucky to be allowed to de-board, or see the sky, or breath fresh air at all for at least seventy-two hours. In fact, he knows it will probably be more like a *week* as he's done airplane quarantine training drills many times before. Why, he's even organized such drills as the representative CDC "expert" tasked with training local emergency responders – airport security, TSA, police, fire department, DHS, etc. – on how to handle such situations. Yes, he's an expert on such matters, so all the emergency trucks and vehicles rushing past the taxiing plane – hyper-vigilant lights and sirens ablaze and ablare, and EMT personnel therein, fumbling with their biohazard suits – none of it surprises him..

Quite antithetical to the behavior of his fellow passengers, Carl takes a sip from his water bottle and settles even deeper into his seat. Gazing at his own reflection in the plane's window, he wipes the visible beads of sweat from his brow with his sleeve, then catches himself muttering aloud, as if to someone else: *Doesn't make sense she would infect me; she risked her life!...*

Out beyond his reflection in the window, portable construction lights and thrown-up cyclone fencing appear to slide past as the plane taxis into the quarantine area. Craning back towards the rear of the plane, Carl notices security personnel outfitted in biohazard suits closing a gate in the temporary fencing just after the plane enters. And, shortly thereafter, the plane comes to a final and jarring halt, parking in a vast and garish pool of portable floodlights.

Once again the plane's PA system barks information – something about a temporary quarantine, and about telephones that will be provided, and some obligatory apology for the inconvenience, and some vague explanation about how this is only a precaution, *blah, blah, blah* – which all the tortured, bleary-eyed passengers of course ignore. If they had listened to the announcement they would know their efforts to de-board were futile and would return to their seats. But of course they didn't, so as a result they bump and push forward, annoying one another with over-stuffed carry-ons, only to pack up like half-witted cattle before the sealed exits. *"Ladies and gentlemen, please return to your seats!"* – all for naught.

Carl looks up over some thirty rows seats towards the exit ahead of him. There he can just barely make out the frantic scene taking place: a six-pack of biohazard-suited EMT personnel enters the plane and barks something unintelligible through gas masks to the now very worried-looking flight attendants, some of whom have taken to clutching clean hand towels to their mouths and noses. Craning about to look behind him back down another couple rows of seats, Carl can see a similarly confused and frantic incursion is happening there at the rear exit. Settling back in his seat, Carl ponders the situation for a beat: sure, he could endure the quarantine, and probably even should, but then again that morsel of logic – *It doesn't make sense; she risked her life!*– underscored by the fact it was *her* who initiated their lovemaking.

"Screw this," Carl mutters to himself. Then — and perhaps utilizing the reptilian part of the brain that's proven so adept at *fight or flight* situations over the millennia — he nonchalantly stands, snags his carry-on satchel from the overhead bin, then sits back down again. Next he pulls from the satchel his navy blue windbreaker, with CDC written in bright yellow lettering across the back and, making sure no one is paying attention, casually dons it.

Up ahead the six-pack of biohazard-suited EMTs has split in half, with three of them now working their way down each aisle. Glancing towards the rear of the passenger compartment, Carl can see that the other team of EMTs has done the same. Assuming both teams are on the hunt for him, Carl finds himself looking about for something else to abet his escape. Above him he notices the console storing the emergency oxygen units. Glancing slyly about to make sure again no one is watching, Carl reaches up, opens the unit, and yanks out its oxygen facemask. Keeping his head low, Carl dons the facemask, takes a here-goes-nothing breath, then stands. Swinging his satchel over his shoulder, he immediately adopts an authoritative air then begins pushing his way past his fumbling co-passengers, barking out through his facemask such vagaries as: "Stand aside... Please return to your seats... Make way... Comin' through..."

Carl saves his most authoritative posturing for the three EMTs. Encountering them midway up the aisle, he flashes them his CDC photo I.D. and promptly barks to them: "We've secured the stern, why don't you three check the upper deck. The docket says he should be in First Class."

Successfully duped, the three EMTs nod and promptly begin ascending the spiral staircase for the First Class section, permitting Carl free access to the exit.

Carl de-boards the 747 down a staircase gangway. Looking out to the quarantine area he sees the passengers being directed towards any of five inflatable, 100-person capacity mobile barracks by oxygen-masked DHS agents. With these armed agents being the only thing standing between him and the gate, Carl extemporizes yet another flurry of commands knowing — as a G-man himself — how unquestioningly and, ergo, *good* they are at taking orders:

"Don't unload the upper deck until I get back with more inflatables," Carl tells them as he climbs onto an empty electric light luggage cart parked near them.

But one of the DHS agents speaks up: "But we already have enough beds for all four hundred, fifty-five."

"Beds are one thing; *space* is another; last thing we want to do is to overcrowd them. Don't need another Fort Dixon," Carl explains cryptically, finalizing the ruse with a salute. He then turns the electric cart towards the already opening gate. Passing through the gate, he shouts out more orders to the two biohazard-suited National Guardsmen posted there — "Nobody comes within a hundred meters of the containment area without a mask, nobody enters without a bio-suit, and nobody *but nobody* leaves! Got it?"

"Yes, sir!" the Guardsmen reply, snapping off crisp salutes.

And Carl returns a salute to them as well before driving away, out of the quarantine area and down the deserted runway, off into the nascent dawn.

The Allosphere. Museum of Natural History, Santa Barbara, California

---

As the name implies the Allosphere is spherical; some ten meters in diameter. It's innovation was the anticipatable evolution of the very first Kinetoscope – a "peep show" type box into which a single person at a time leaned their head and viewed a short film loop – invented by one of Thomas Edison's assistants, W.K.L. Dickson, way back in 1893. The technical wonder of the Kinetoscope was soon usurped by the first *projected* motion picture, invented by the Lumiére Brothers, Louis and Auguste, in 1895. But the art form would not rest there. Along with such "bells & whistles" as sound, color, 3-D, and, of course, Odorama, the motion picture stretched itself from the early three-by-two aspect ratio to the wider screen Panavision. The Imax theatre experience was the logical next generation along this theme of expansion, as was the 360° Movie, as was the Allosphere. What the Allosphere did that was innovative to the motion picture technology was to bring this ever-wider-screen trend to its logical terminus by completely enveloping the viewer within the projected image. This was accomplished through the use of fourteen individual projectors shooting off in all directions, projecting their precise, contiguously interlocking images onto the interior of the sphere. At first pioneers of the Allosphere tried using standard "silver" screen material, but this was found to be way too reflective, causing the sphere to become flooded with trapped light which washed out the other projections until the overall effect was akin to trying to watch a drive-in movie during the day. Too much light. To solve this problem, the Allosphere's screen is made from a metal screen mesh, just porous enough to allow sand, but nothing much larger, to pass through. The room beyond the sphere has to be painted a flat black to create a non-reflective void from which no light can bounce back. And out there, mounted on the frameworks holding together the sphere, are 470 tiny speakers that conjoin to provide an all-enveloping sound sensation to compliment the all-enveloping visual experience. Of course in order to take this all

the momentum of folly

in one has to somehow get to the center of the sphere and, ideally, hover there without blocking any of the projections. This is somewhat inelegantly handled by the skewering of the sphere at its equator with a narrow metal grate catwalk onto which some twenty audience members can be crammed at a time. The result, though maybe less than perfect, is enormously impressive nonetheless. But the evolution of the Allosphere has not stopped there, especially now that three-dimensional visuals and computer-generated images are being added to the mix, along with variable temperature and humidity effects, and even man-made wind – from gentle breezes to howling gusts – blowing through the structure. Hence, short of anti-gravity and utter sensory deprivation, the Allosphere has all but perfected the virtual reality experience, and thereby pushed the envelope on the state of the art of cinema.

Dr. Alyesha Singh first experienced the Allosphere when she traveled from her native University of Mumbai, India to take up the Graduate Dean chair in the Marine Sciences Department at the University of California, Santa Barbara. On most days parking is easily found in the lot adjacent the Marine Science buildings, which is on the part of the campus that juts out into the Pacific; hence the moniker, "Campus Point." But on days when the swells are coming in just right – say, at twelve to fourteen feet, out of the west-northwest at 295° on twenty-one second intervals – on such "epic" days surfers will gladly risk the $40 ticket or yet another arrest warrant in order to park at the Marine Sciences lot. Thus it was that on one such day Dr. Singh found herself having to park in the lot servicing the Kavli Institute of Theoretical Physics, and muster the three-kilometer trek across campus lugging along her laptop and an armful of books. But her effort was not without the silver lining of passing her through the hitherto unexplored Media Arts and Technology building and, as luck would have it, just when they were hosting the inaugural grand unveiling of the Allosphere. A sucker – like every academician – for cubes of cheese served on toothpicks and cheap wine out of plastic cups, Dr. Singh set down her load for a bit and took in the Allosphere demonstration. There, standing on the catwalk with a dozen or so others, she first experienced a very realistic, live-action production of a simple walk along the beach replete with the cries and visuals of seagulls passing overhead and the crashing of waves from any number of directions. After five minutes of that she and the other viewers donned hokey pairs of 3-D glasses and then experienced a three-dimensional virtual reality ride through the tucks and folds and synaptic clefts of an actual brain scan.

At the time Alyesha was searching for a gimmick that might hold grade school kids' gnat-like attention spans for long enough to teach them about humanity's impact on the oceans. And thus it was almost a classic case of *Providence* that she stumbled upon the Allosphere or, arguably even that, just two years later, due to California's $42 billion budget deficit, the UC's funding was trimmed ten percent and the Allosphere project had to be nipped in the bud and hocked. Luckily, Alyesha had the gumption to approach a local billionaire philanthropist woman and asked her, even before they exchanged hellos, if she would purchase the Allosphere and donate it to the Museum of Natural History so that she, Dr. Singh, could create a community outreach program for public school kids in order to teach them about ocean science. *"You could use the tax deduction, am I right?"*

Cut to two years later and here stands Dr. Alyesha Singh, Distinguished Chair, Visiting Professor, Dean, et al, in her floral-print sari amidst twenty, 3-D glasses-sporting fourth-graders standing on the catwalk grate here in the center of the relocated Allosphere. The show today is all her creation; basically it's an inside-out view of a transparent Earth, with the enthralled audience there on catwalk gazing out from the core to the multiple layers representing: the oceans and all their sea life and the proliferation of oxygen-depleted dead zones, subterranean crude oil deposits and fresh water aquifers, farm and grazing and urban and toxic wasteland sprawl and the inversely proportional declines of wildlife and natural habitat, the polar ice caps and waning glaciers, shrinking forests and waxing deserts, the opening and closing of the ozone holes, as well as numeric footnotes tracking parts per million concentrations of various pollutants, carbon dioxide, nitrogen oxide, methane, and water vapor, atmospheric and oceanic temperatures and ph levels, increases in hurricane and typhoon frequency and magnitude, rising ocean levels, and, of course, human population. All in all it's a tool to convey the impact human enterprise is having on the natural world in a way both comprehensible and engaging to all, but especially to kids.

The Allosphere now has the class of fourth-graders enveloped in a virtual aquarium. Using a wireless remote Alyesha zooms in and navigates the class towards a giant turtle, filmed from below as it swims in the South China Sea off the coast of Thailand.

"The Green Sea Turtle, once common in the Atlantic, Pacific, and Indian oceans, is now expected to become extinct in our lifetime and only because it has the misfortune of making a nice soup. In all, each of the large ocean predators species has seen its numbers plummet ninety percent or more in just the last fifty years…."

Alyesha now envelops the class in a litany of endangered species shown in their natural habitats, wiping from one to the next as she names them off:

"…This includes sharks, swordfish, tuna, halibut, cod, flounder, and even skates, all thanks to the efficiency of drift net fishing and sonar and our insatiable and growing appetite. Lower on the food chain…"

Alyesha now *swims* the audience through schools of sardines and krill, submerged penguin flocks, and even pods of whales, as she continues her narration:

"Krill stocks – the diet of arctic creatures from penguins to whales – have diminished eighty percent in just the last thirty years due to global warming. The same foe has put both the walrus and polar bear on the endangered species list due to the rapid loss of arctic ice…."

The underwater camera now shows walruses rooting with their tusks for clams through the rocky ocean bottom, then follows a polar bear and cub swimming and swimming and swimming through open ocean in seemingly futile search of a chunk of ice onto which to claw their way upon. This scene crossfades to one of stark contrast: life-less oceans with bottoms thick with dead crab and fish carcasses, bleached coral reefs and rotting phytoplankton….

"As if rising sea levels, over-fishing, and the fact of the oceans are become ever more acidic due to their absorption of ever increasing levels of CO_2; as if all those weren't already enough, we have yet another unfortunate phenomenon taking place – that of vast hypoxic and anoxic zones – also known as "dead zones." These dead zones, some larger than states, are low-oxygen pockets doubling in both numbers *and* area every decade or so. And we find they are occurring primarily in regions which were once among the most productive fisheries in the world. Now, due to a triple-whammy combination of global warming, over-fishing and human effluent, these nutrient-rich regions are becoming choked with rotting *phytoplankton* – an algae that smaller fish feed off before the bigger fish gobble them up and so on. But now that fish stocks are so much lower and the amount of phytoplankton so much higher, instead of being eaten the phytoplankton simply rots and dies. The chemical process of this rotting sucks all the oxygen from the water, after which time the phytoplankton then settles like a blanket of white mud on the ocean floor."

The projection then dissolves from the life-less ocean floor and bleached reefs, to shots of savannah scenes around the world showing the mentioned creatures as she continues:

"Moving inland now, Bali and Javan Tigers, Barbary and Cape Lions, all hunted into extinction by people fancying themselves as sportsmen. Rhinoceros – African White and Black, Indian and Sumatran – have seen their populations reduced to under two thousand due to poaching that continues even today, all because their horn is mistakenly believed to be an aphrodisiac, which I'll leave to your parents to explain. Similarly, poachers are to blame for the imminent demise of all wild tigers, which numbered over 100,000 just twenty years ago, now number just 3,200 by the most recent count. Same is true for elephants, walrus, and sperm whales, this time because of mankind's inexplicable lust for ivory...."

And now the screen dissolves to a jungle setting – showing Paradise parrots, Silverback gorillas, Spix's macaws, impalas, pandas, hippopotamuses, koalas, chimps, manatees, Birdwing butterflies, and on and on – as she now focuses on the root cause of the problem:

"In a nutshell, the problem has to do with the fact that it takes 5.4 acres of land to support the average human; 17.8 acres for Europeans, 23.5 for North Americans. Hence, as our global population continues to explode, thousands of animal species – in fact, an average of three per day – will be driven into extinction as we usurp their habitat in order to feed and house ourselves. So, unless something drastic is done to reverse this trend, all these species I've shown you here today will become extinct within your lifetime. And, as the old saying goes, *extinction is forever.*"

As the screens within the Allosphere return to the inside-out shot of a vibrant, living Earth, a fourth-grade boy raises his hand.

"Yes?" Dr. Singh says, calling on the boy.

"So, like, what's going to happen?" the boy asks, clearly shaken.

Dr. Singh pauses, wondering how one is to explain to a ten year-old that all hell is about to break loose. What exactly is her responsibility here? Should she be perfectly forthright and tell this little boy that he and his classmates here will be amongst the only generation of humans to experience an extinction event?

the momentum of folly

That's the truth: is that what she, as an educator, should tell him? And, if so, how is she to describe or prepare this child for the unprecedented war and famine and suffering he will almost certainly experience? As a scientist, as a parent, how does one stare into this innocent child's eyes and tell him he is going to witness horrors on a scale unimaginable by any generation of humans before?

Dr. Singh realizes she has taken too long to respond to the boy's question; she can see it now in the suddenly terrified countenances on the rest of the class, in the angered glowers of the parents who have volunteered to escort the class on this educative, supposedly fun, field trip, in the embarrassed teacher's furrowed brow. Yes, verily, Dr. Alyesha Singh has taken way too long, and so she does what anyone who finds themselves caught in such a predicament should do; she musters a smile and, as simply and as pleasantly and as *convincingly* as possible, tells the little boy: "Everything's going to be just fine."

"Really?"

After another thoughtful pause, Dr. Singh nods then confidently if cryptically replies, "Yes, *really.*"

Alaska International Airport, Anchorage

The long, arctic days this time of year barely seem to end before they begin anew, even though the sun seems content to doodle for hours behind yonder ridgeline before mustering the responsibility to finally rise and shine. And why should it? After all, it's not even four a.m. Anchorage will be asleep for the next several hours still, so what's the rush? Just because the horizon is waxing to a pale yellow and the chirps of unseen birds can be heard over the distant whines of airliner engines, that's no reason to get up, is it?

Due to the still pre-workday hour this private part of the airport – contiguous to yet miles from its commercial wing – has the feel of a deserted ghost town. Apart from the crow pulling fast food wrappers out of a trashcan, there's no sign of life around here, not even on the electric luggage cart Carl *borrowed* to aid his escape from the quarantine area maybe an hour ago now. The cart is presently parked out in the open amongst the private hangers and bush pilot shacks, near a Fed-Ex drop-off box and a more-spacious-than-usual, wheelchair-accessible, rarely-if-ever-serviced, plastic "port-a-potty" restroom.

Not that anyone is likely within a mile of here, Carl has nonetheless locked himself inside the aforementioned port-a-potty. Distraught, shaky, bleary-eyed, sweaty, pale, sleepy, restless, you name it, he hovers over the stinky toilet with his sleeve rolled up, his arm strapped junkie-style, and a hypodermic needle stuck into it. Anyone who happened into the stall here would certainly misinterpret his actions, for, despite what it might look like, he's not shooting up; rather, he is merely drawing a sample of his own blood. Once the needle's vacutainer vial has filled with a reasonable amount of blood, he slides it from his vein. He then grabs a Fed Ex envelope and opens it hastily, but then hesitates. It's not the *"Do not ship liquids, blood or fluids in this package"* warning on the envelope that gives him pause, instead it's the bar code printed there used for tracking the package's route. Carl considers the tracking bar code for long enough to weigh the consequences – both for and against – of continuing with his plan. Deciding to proceed he drops the vacutainer vile into the envelope and seals it, then discards the hypodermic needle down into the toilet, where it plops upon the piled island of excrement surrounded by a blue "sea" of deodorizing chemicals therein. He then pulls a pen from shirt pocket and tries his best, under the circumstances – foot up on the toilet, using his thigh to write against – to legibly address the envelope to his and Stuart's 1414 Peach Lane bungalow back in Atlanta.

That done, Carl turns in the stall and contemplates the filthy, mechanic grease-stained sink. There's a pedal on the floor. He pumps it bringing a trickle of water to the sink faucet. Someone has left a can of Borax powdered soap on the sink. *This'll work.* The mind; oh, how it wanders. Even under critical circumstances such as these Carl finds his brain repeating that old *You know you're a redneck if...* joke. How did it go? *You know you're a redneck if you marvel over how gas stations can keep their bathrooms so clean.* Something like that. Funny how it's still funny, even if it doesn't bring a smile to his face. After washing the blood from his arms and the sleep from his eyes, and trying in vain to find paper towels in the empty dispenser before resorting to drying his hands on his pants, Carl finds himself taking the first hard look at himself in a mirror in more than a week. And it's probably for the better that it's one of those stainless steel mirrors, so obscured beneath rival gang tags that he can barely see his sorry reflection, let alone recognize it. But there it is, staring back at him with some sense of purpose, however wavering. *Gang tags in a filthy, stinky port-a-potty?* – the mind, wandering again – *What kind of gang would force their members to tag a port-a-potty? How stupid is that? And who would join such a gang? Seems barely human, this kind of behavior. Then again, we are only animals. Is this like a dog marking its territory or what?* Carl's little riff on behavioral psychology is interrupted when he notices he's still wearing his CDC windbreaker. Realizing the jacket might be on the All Points Bulletin no doubt put out for him, Carl yanks off the jacket, almost tosses it down the toilet but, thinking he might need it again, instead stuffs it into his satchel beside his... *Shit! – where's my laptop?* Suddenly flooded with self-loathing, he stares at his sorry reflection again; his better half now seething back with disgust; *You fucking moron; you left it on the seat next to you on the plane, didn't you? How could you be so stupid? If they haven't already figured out which passenger managed to slip through the quarantine, now they certainly will. Fucking idiot!*

After a heavy sigh, Carl composes himself again, finger-combs his hair back to some degree of civilized respectability, slings his satchel over a shoulder, grabs the Fed Ex envelope, then exits.

Stepping from the port-a-potty, Fed Ex envelope in hand, Carl casts a furtive glance in ether direction to make sure he hasn't been detected. A breeze wraps around him, eliciting both surprise and relief that it's not cold; even though he's wearing only jeans, a t-shirt and long-sleeve pullover, and even though the sun is only now just shooting its first few rays of direct light onto the surrounding rooftops, it's not cold at all. Carl crosses the empty street to the Fed Ex box, opens it, glances again at the envelope's tracking barcode, deliberates, but – after coming up with no other viable options – drops it in anyway. Then, as if to assure himself he made the right decision, he mutters some old slogan of Stuart's: *Paranoia will destroy ya.*

Raising his head and looking about, he notices, up the way a bit, a pay phone attached to the wall of a mechanics' hanger. *A pay phone; must be the last one on the planet,* he's thinking as he makes his way towards it. At the phone now he picks up the receiver and listens… surprised to hear that there is indeed a dial tone. There's a sticker on the phone advertising a toll-free number to charge a call to one's home number. Sounds easy. Carl hesitates then begins dialing what seems like a score or more numbers, pauses as if to rest, then continues punching in the remaining numbers. Through some magical passage of electrons through copper and photons through fiber optics and microwave pulses, he hears as the connection is made and the phone on the other end begins to ring. He takes a big, nerve-calming breath as he waits for his call to be answered. As it continues to ring, he hears sirens racing his way. Looking up the street towards the small airstrip servicing all the non-commercial aviators, Carl can see the vehicles responsible for the blaring sirens: two Anchorage Police SUVs escorting a CDC van. But they scream past, not even coming within fifty meters of Carl. Relieved, he returns his attention to his phone call, as now an answering machine on the other end finally picks up: "You've reached the voice-mail for Angela Varella of Aegis Pharmaceuticals. Please leave a message and I'll return your call as soon as possible. Thank you. *Beep.*"

Just hearing Angela's voice pulls tears from Carl's eyes, surprising, even embarrassing him. Finding himself with nothing to say – or perhaps *too much*

the momentum of folly

to say — Carl smashes the receiver against the phone, first just once, then several times before his frustration finally abates. Then, just out of curiosity, he brings the receiver to his ear again — *there's certainly no dial tone now!* — then hangs it back up on its hook.

Moving on foot now, not really sure about where to go or what to do next — thinking maybe it's time to check himself in at the quarantine area — Carl finds himself walking past the shop fronts of dozens of bush pilot offices; one-man, two-man, husband-wife, father-son, widow-daughter operations mostly. Insofar as the office portion of the business is purely functional — most of the money being poured into the planes and Yellow Pages ads and websites — these offices aren't much to look at; just a place to park an answering machine or work on taxes or just stay out of the spouse's hair when not flying. Most of these shops don't even bother to hang business "shingles" out over the door, since rarely do clients even gather here. They're just a door, a window, a desk, a computer, a coat rack, a TV broadcasting the Weather Channel or Sports Center, a hundred or two square feet of cheap carpeting, and, more than likely, a cot in the closet; that's the conclusion Carl is coming to anyway, as he walks past his tenth or so such shop front.

And then, gazing listlessly into yet another passing shop window, Carl sees something through the open Venetian blinds that catches his attention and stops him in his tracks. Indeed, it takes him several beats to even know why it has grabbed hold of him, for all it is is a blown-up aerial photograph — oddly familiar — of some vast snowfield, thumb-tacked now to the corkboard mounted on the wall behind the empty desk. Carl brings his face right to the window so he can better see through the Venetian blinds, so he can better make out the two whalebone crucifixes casting long, crisp shadows across the snow. And then his familiarity begins to make sense; this blown-up photo mounted on the corkboard — though taken from a low-flying plane rather than a satellite — seems to be of the same Eskimo cemetery as those Carl found on the flight to China in Dr. Jenna Williams's manila envelope stamped *Classified*. Carl feels a visceral reaction to his recognizing the photograph — a sinking in his stomach and racing pulse — and he can even feel that reaction becoming heightened when he notices a second photograph mounted beneath the other; this one showing the same whalebone crosses but this time with a rectangular excavation site between them.

And then something else leaps from the deep recesses of Carl's memory; something Stuart muttered about Dr. Jenna's theory that, "...it may not have been the Spanish Flu at all that slammed into those Eskimo villages, but rather some other, much more lethal subtype that was circulating, though not nearly as widely, at the same time...."

"Can I help you?" a male voice, with a distinctively Norwegian accent, calls out from just behind Carl.

Carl manages to suppress his panic well enough to turn towards the source of the voice, a fifty-ish blond man, in jeans and the requisite sheepskin aviator's coat, and a large rucksack slung over one shoulder.

"You scared me. Didn't think anyone was around," Carl replies, with an embarrassed smile.

"You were *hoping* no one was around?" the man suggests suspiciously as he pulls keys from his jacket pocket, one of which he sticks in the dead bolt lock on the shop door, then turns.

"Just the opposite," Carl replies. "I was hoping I'd find you. Are you open for business?"

The man pushes open the now unlocked shop door, replying, "Am now. What'cha need?"

Playing for thinking time, Carl extends his hand for a shake, introducing himself as, "Stuart."

The man reluctantly shakes Carl's hand and introduces himself as, "Olaf, Olaf Kessey."

"Yes, I know," Carl lies with a laugh.

"You *know*? How's that?"

"You flew a group of us, last winter..." Carl now turns and points to the aerial photograph of the excavated Eskimo mass gravesite, adding, "... to there."

Entering his office and tossing his keys on his desk, Olaf says nothing in response to Carl's entreaty. In fact, quite to the contrary, he seems now, suddenly, visibly guarded at the mere mention of the gravesite.

Nevertheless Carl decides to push his luck, "You're Norwegian, right? Remember we spoke about the Sons of Norway camp my family used to go to in the Sierra? You were the one who flew us up to that Eskimo gravesite, weren't you?"

"I don't remember."

"You don't remember flying us up there?" Carl asks incredulously.

"I don't remember the Sons of Norway chat."

Carl smiles and shrugs it off, "Oh. Well, wasn't much of a chat really, it just, I don't know, stuck with me."

"I must've been drunk."

Carl laughs at the joke, or at least only until he realizes Olaf — because of his straight face — maybe isn't joking.

"So — Stuart was it? — what do you want?" Olaf says bluntly.

Carl swallows, deciding to take his biggest risk yet. "I need to go back."

"*Go back up there?* What for?"

"Just some follow-up."

Olaf glares at Carl for an uncomfortably long time, long enough that Carl feels obliged to speak. "You didn't get my email?" he extemporizes.

Olaf shakes his head suspiciously.

"Oh, well, if there's a scheduling problem, I can always hire another —" he begins before Olaf cuts him short.

"You know, we caught a lot of shit for what you guys did up there. Did you know that?" he says, his face already red with anger.

"No, I didn't."

"Well, we did. Hell, I've got Eskimo *rights* groups trying to revoke my license, all 'cause of you jerk-offs!"

"I'm sorry. I don't really know what to tell you."

Olaf continues to stare at Carl. "Same pay?" he asks, his anger apparently beginning to cede to avarice.

Carl nods, "Of course."

The '53 DeHavilland Canada DHC-3 Otter's screaming Pratt & Whitney Wasp radial engine cause the prop to tear hungrily at the air with such torque that in less than one hundred feet of runway the hardy bush plane is off the ground and climbing steeply. Carl sits beside Olaf, both sporting miked headsets.

"Pretty short take-off," Carl remarks, shouting over the engine din.

"That's nothing," Olaf shouts back, "there's a video clip on the Internet of a Super Cub taking off on just eighteen feet of runway."

"*Eighteen feet?*"

"Yah. Check it out."

"I will."

"No, I mean *check it out down there*," Olaf says, pointing out the pilot's window of the already steeply banking bush plane and down to the commercial corner of the airport where the China Air 747 is parked, still surrounded by temporary fencing, National Guard vehicles and guards.

"What's going on?" Carl asks, playing naïve while trying to plumb how much Olaf and, through him, the outside world might know about the situation.

"Some kind of quarantine or something. They're not letting anybody out."

"Quarantine for what?"

Olaf shrugs, "Don't know. Don't care."

It's a beautiful day for flying; sunny, even warm, not a cloud in the sky. The bush plane is headed on a northwest bearing at a cruising speed of 180 miles per hour and an altitude of 3,500 feet. Carl is gazing out towards some smoke from a wildfire in the east. Nodding towards it, he calls out to Olaf, "Fire?"

"Yah. Two hundred forty thousand acres as of yesterday."

"Sounds big."

Olaf shrugs, "Maybe twenty years ago, but not so much now."

"Why's that? – cutbacks in firefighting crews?"

"Naw, naw; climate change. Maybe you've heard of it?" Olaf asks facetiously. "We never use to have fires up here – even when I first came here – the mountains were just too wet. Now with the hotter, drier summers they've become the norm."

Carl looks down to the mountains passing beneath them, surprised by how denuded most of them are.

"Is that why there're no trees down here? – fires."

"Naw, this all is from logging." Olaf glances over at Carl," You're shocked, aren't you? It's not what your Alaskan Getaway brochure sold to you."

Carl nods.

"If it's any consolation, everyone I fly up here is shocked as hell to find out how much of Alaska is logged. The Yukon, hell, all of Canada's the same.

the momentum of folly

Only four percent of North America's native forests are still standing. Between construction and Ikea bunk beds and chopsticks there's just no stopping it. Why, do you know how many acres of virgin forest it takes to put out a single Sunday's edition of the New York Times?"

Carl shakes his head, "How many?"

"A shit-load! Over a hundred acres; something like one hundred twenty, even with fifty-percent, whatever it is, recycled paper tossed in. And that's just Sunday. And that's just the New York Times. Imagine the bite all the papers together take, week after fuckin' week. Check it out...."

Without warning, Olaf puts the plane in a sharp, 360° turn to give Carl a full, panoramic view of what was once horizon-to-horizon uninterrupted forest, but is now a crudely-shaven skullcap, slashed with dirt logging roads and pimpled with smoldering slag piles.

As the Otter's engine whines through the turn, and the wings and frame creak and groan under the stress, and Olaf continues his lament, Carl happens to notice an old thermos, with a red plaid design, rolling on the floor between his feet. He notices it, but says nothing:

"See? It's almost all gone and no one's doing a goddamned thing about it! Tell you what: if they could see what you're seeing, they'd do something about it. First they'd shit their pants, then they'd do something!" Gazing out over the denuded landscape, Olaf shakes his head then adds with a sarcastic smirk, "Oh, well, when it is all gone, least there won't be any more wildfires, right?"

Teller Mission, Alaska. Summer Solstice.

Despite the twenty-plus hours of summer solstice daylight and global warming and sea-level altitude, there's still enough permafrost way up north here — just inland of the Bering Strait — to permit a ski landing if necessary. But, as Olaf explained it, he'd rather not risk it, for fear of getting stuck in the too-soft snow and tundra muck. "Been that. Done there," as he put it. Instead he opts to put the Otter's over-sized tires to good use and land on the pebble-strewn beachhead. It's a bumpy landing by commercial standards, but the Otter nevertheless comes to a safe stop within a stone's throw of Grantley Harbor. And when Olaf turns off the engine, nothing greets the ear but a brain-slapping silence, and nothing strikes the eye but gray-blue seawater gently lapping at the pebbly beach to the north, and a seemingly endless expanse of flat, boggy, thawing snow — starting just a couple of steps from the wheels of the plane — to the south.

"Ah, here we are. Plant a couple of coconut palms and you'd have Paradise!" Olaf quips, as he climbs from the plane.

Carl follows him out onto the snow, slings his satchel over one shoulder, then squints about, understandably disoriented.

"What's your problem? Get going!" Olaf says, half-jokingly.

"I'm not sure where — which way to head; it all looks so different than it did in the winter," Carl says, lying his way through this.

Olaf nods, then turns and points along the beach extending to the Northwest, warning, "Well, you don't want to go that-a-way. That's where the actual town of Teller is — five miles or so — where all the aforementioned pissed-off Eskimos are. So..." Olaf now turns halfway around and points in the opposite direction, "... I recommend you head that way instead."

Carl still looks hesitant.

Noticing Carl's apprehension, Olaf tells him to, "Hold on a minute," then climbs back into the plane's cockpit, rummages around in there for a bit, before

the momentum of folly

emerging holding a handheld GPS device. "Here, take this. D'ya know how to use one of these?"

Carl nods.

"Good," Olaf says as he punches in some preset numbers, then points to the GPS display, shielding it from the direct sun. "Here's where we are and… " Olaf punches in another preset, "… here's where you want to be; exactly, plus or minus three meters. About four clicks that-a-way." he adds, before pointing again towards the southeast and ordering Carl to: "Mush!"

With a thin smile Carl nods then turns away from the plane. But his very first step onto the permafrost sinks his low-top hiking boot a good foot or so into the thawing snow and muck.

Olaf shakes his head at Carl's obvious un-preparedness. "Hey, Mr. Scientist!" he shouts, barb intended.

Carl turns back towards Olaf, who is now rummaging in the open cargo door in the fuselage of the plane. From deep therein, Olaf pulls a pair of old snowshoes from the cargo space then turns back towards Carl.

"Here ya go; Norway's greatest contribution to mankind next to the pup seal club," he jokes, then tosses the snowshoes to Carl.

Carl catches the snowshoes and calls back: "Thanks."

Olaf nods, then can't resist a last joke: "They go on your feet."

If there were difficulties with time continuity in the jungle, they are magnified up here on the edge of the Arctic Circle where the sun just doesn't set — or at least doesn't quite appear to — this time of year. *What time is it, Carl?* Don't ask him; between his irregular sleep cycle since leaving Atlanta — how long has it been now anyway; a week, ten days? — his omni-directional jet lag and, last but not least, the on-going feverish delirium he's battling due to whatever bacterium or virus or both are currently laying siege to his immune system, well, suffice it to say, he'd be the last one to know what time it is, let alone if it's even morning or afternoon. There's the sun, so it's daytime; of that much he's reasonably certain.

Carl pauses his forward plodding trudge through the muck to raise his sunglasses and check his progress against the GPS device. If its frail digital display and unseen satellite gods in the heavens are to be believed, he's about halfway to the mass grave. He turns to check his progress by a more tangible measure:

squinting back from whence he came he sees behind him – no plane, no pebbly beach, nor even a hint of the vast bay sure to be out there – just a seemingly endless expanse of snow bisected by his reasonably straight snowshoe tracks. Turning forward again, he sees more of the same; snow, and nothing but, though this batch unscarred by human tracks. And that's when the thought hits him:

What the fuck am I doing?

It's a pestering thought; one that has crossed his mind more than few these past couple of days:

What the fuck am I doing?
What the fuck am I doing?
What the fuck am I doing?

For whatever reason – call it dog-headed persistence – he nonetheless lowers his sunglasses again, takes a resigned *keep-on-keepin'-on* breath, coughs, and resumes his plodding trudge.

How did it all go down anyway? A tiny whaling village of a hundred-plus native Eskimos and a handful of missionaries dispatched hither to save them, all stuck together out on this frozen isthmus between the Bering Sea and Grantley Bay, when in sweeps the virus, carried on the innocuous runny nose and cough of some one of them who had ventured outside of their otherwise protected enclave and made contact with an infected outsider. What was the religious explanation for this? Were they being punished by their fire and brimstone God? If so, then for what? Must have been something heinous to make their loving creator so pissed-off he decided he should kill off seventy percent of them, including the children. They must have been *bad*. Maybe they hadn't prayed enough. Maybe they missed a Sabbath somewhere during that last, months-long night. Maybe there was some extramarital fornication while stuck out in a hunting igloo. Or maybe, *maybe* some one of them, a sinner by definition, dared to admit, even inwardly, some skepticism as to the existence of their Almighty Lord. Who knows, maybe there was a crucifixion; an obligatory sacrifice of the town agnostic, who felt compelled to shout down from the cross as he was dying something to the effect of:

So, why again am I being punished? Just for being agnostic? Just for admitting, Hey, I don't know if there's a God up there or not? Just for being honest? Wouldn't God appreciate a little honesty, reward it even? The theists and atheists amongst us; now surely they deserve punishment

the momentum of folly

for their equally presumptuous positions; for professing to know that which is wholly unknowable — that thing they call the Truth. That's arrogance at best, dis-honesty at worst, is it not? My God or lack thereof, why hast Thou forsaken me?...

It's plausible such a scenario might have happened, Carl flatters himself as he wanders into what remains of Teller Mission; he has witnessed a town in the process of becoming a ghost town before and, hence, knows from experience just how real the Apocalypse can be. Coughing somewhat regularly now, he continues his slog up what might have been called *Main Street* or even *Only Street*, defined today only by the skeletal wood and concrete and steel remains of a scant few buildings and shops and homes. Not much has survived the nine decades of harsh winters, salty summers and inattentive vacancy. And, who knows? – perhaps the ruthless seasons were not the only cause for the destruction. Perhaps the villagers are to blame, perhaps having torched the town as they fled in terror in order to exorcize the demon scourge. That made sense; can't be leaving a perfectly good town to demons.

As Carl slogs past something that looks like it might have been the church – *Of course they wouldn't burn that!* – he can almost hear the fervent praying that must have echoed in there those long November nights; one healthy person praying as three others coughed or gasped or bled in the same hard, cold pew. And there's a hollowed-out shell of a building that looks like it could have been the town infirmary, intended to treat only the random harpoon mishap or pregnancy or emergency appendectomy, but this fortnight overflowing with the dead and dying. And there's a mother, probably herself just a girl and barely one generation out of her native Eskimo skins and igloos, now dressed like a proper Christian and weeping and waling while crawling on despondent hands and knees through the snow as the townsmen drag her daughter's still-warm corpse away – her daughter who only twenty-four hours before exhibited no symptoms of the illness whatsoever, her daughter who had only just days before joyously received that beautiful fuchsia dress for her birthday. And now here she is, dead but thankfully beyond suffering, being dragged the short distance out of town – out of this *waling village* of fire and ice and darkness – and towards the cemetery and the hastily dug mass grave therein.

It is only the otherworldly beeping of the GPS device tucked away in Carl's daypack that yanks him out of the horrific tragedy, that hell on earth which had brought this town to a life-less end back in November of 1918. The beeping causes the cold and burning night conjured by his imagination to instantly vanish and be instantly replaced with the bright and preternaturally warm reality of the here and now. Pulling the GPS device from his pack, Carl pushes a button to turn off the beeping. That done he checks the digital display and sees that it matches the preset destination coordinates. Looking up he finds himself standing in a subtle, rectangular-shaped depression in the snow which Carl guesstimates measures some five meters in width and fifteen meters in length.

And then he sees something that confirms he has found what he is looking for, that he has indeed arrived. It's the two aforementioned whalebone crosses, of course; one posted at the eastern end of the rectangular depression, the other at the western end — the native crucifixes first shown to him in Jenna's satellite photographs, then again in the *before and after* photos thumb-tacked to the corkboard in Olaf's bush pilot office at the airport. *There they are; the crosses!* If there is such a thing as being able to feel death that is exactly what Carl is feeling, straight up through the soles of his boots. If there is such a thing as a paranormal vortex down through which all life on Earth must twist and funnel until it is no more, he is standing in the very midst of it.

Looking about, Carl spots a rusted shovelhead sticking out of the snow, its handle long ago rotted away. He picks it up with his bare hands — it feels cool but not cold — rolls up his sleeves, takes yet another courage-mustering breath, and begins digging.

The sun is still not at its apex in the sky. Nor will it appear to ever quite set today. Some hundred miles north of here — at a latitude of sixty-six degrees, thirty-three minutes and thirty-nine seconds north of the equator — it truly won't set at all. Hence the moniker, *Land of the Midnight Sun*. Hence the distinction, *Arctic Circle* — named after the Greek constellation *Megale Arktos* — the Great Bear — or the Latin *Ursa Major*. Up there, rather than setting, the sun will only drag its fat belly across the north-north-north-north-north-northwestern horizon for a couple hours or so, then slowly take to lumbering wing again in the north-north-north-north-north-northeast once the planet has pivoted sufficiently beneath it, with its northern axis tipped as directly towards the sun as it will get over the course of the year. But that matters only to the seven hundred thousand or so folks — scattered between Russia, Canada, Alaska, Sweden, Norway, Finland, Greenland, and Iceland — who live on or above the Arctic

the momentum of folly

Circle. But down here, just below the Arctic Circle, the sun will indeed briefly dip beneath the horizon even though, due to the phenomenon of atmospheric refraction, it may not quite appear to. When that's the case viewers may *believe* they still see the sun, when in fact they are only looking at a bent-over-the-horizon reflection of it. But isn't that true of reality in general? What can anyone *really* hope to see? What appears as it *really* is rather than merely as it is reflected within the mind after being bent-over-the-horizon of perception? Is that not what Plato was trying to convey in his *Allegory of the Cave* in Book Seven of The Republic? – "The world of our sight is like habitation within a cave, the firelight there to the sunlight here, the ascent and the view of the upper world is the rising of the soul into the world of the mind. Put it so and you will not be far from my own surmise…"

Who knows? Olaf doesn't, though that doesn't stop him from pondering it like some stream-of-consciousness hallucination as he sunbathes in the nude on an Insulite pad, a can of Ahlafors Ljusa –*Yah, sure, a Swedish beer, but it will do in a pinch!* – stuck in the snow beside him to help him wait out Carl's return. As if further proof of how experienced he is in the art of killing time – hell, he'd smoke a joint if he had one – Olaf also has set a pair of speakers out on the wings of his plane, through which blares the "Classic Rock" station broadcasting out of Nome, Alaska which has just seen fit to usher in the summer by playing the Kinks' *Sunny Afternoon*. Before the song has quite finished the husky-sexy-voiced female deejay breaks in to spew a little news flash before continuing with her "Free Ride" music set.

"Hey, hunter-fisher-dudes out there, there's been an interesting development with that China Air 747 parked under lockdown down there in Anchorage; seems authorities believe that one passenger – a virologist with the CDC no less – managed to slip through quarantine and is presently unaccounted for. So, as if our lives weren't hard enough, they're asking for our help – yes, *our* help – to do *their* jobs. *Dr. Carl Sims is a white male in his late twenties, possibly wearing a navy-blue CDC windbreaker.* Well, that should make it easier. *Though unarmed and nonviolent, he should be approached with extreme caution insofar as he may be infected with a possibly harmful virus. Anyone out there with any information on Dr. Sims' whereabouts should call 9-1-1 immediately.* But enough of that grunt and toil; we've got us a Rock Block Weekend to spin. So, put another worm on the hook and let's kick it off with L-O-L-A *Lola!*…"

Suspicions piqued, Olaf sits upright and turns to stare off in the direction of Carl's snowshoe tracks. Taking another brain-lubricating slug of beer to help him sort through the clues — *Said he'd been here last winter but didn't know which way to walk, said we spoke about the Sons of Norway which I didn't recall, said his name was Stuart but he could have lied...* — Olaf shakes his head, sticks his beer back in the snow, then he reaches for his plane's two-way radio.

Carl is stripped down to his waist and sweating, his jeans soaked from the knees down as he digs away at the snow and slush and tundra muck with the rusty shovelhead he has already grown so intimate with he has given it a nickname — *Rusty*. The exertion has exacerbated his cough to the point where another accompanies each aching, lung-straining breath. Having been digging for better than an hour, his progress is such that he could probably bury a VW Bug in his pit by now, antennae and all. But there's no sense in stopping; not, at least, until he finds what he's come all this way in search of. Taking another over-the-head chop at the hole he, this time, strikes solid ice, the pain of the sudden impact eliciting a fitting expletive — *"Motherfucker!"* Checking his hands he sees one of the half dozen blisters already formed there has torn. He looks about for something that might help protect his hands, spotting his shirts hanging where he left them, slung over the crossbar of the easternmost whalebone crucifix. Clawing his way from out of his excavation site, he trudges over to the crucifix, yanks down his pullover, then skins his t-shirt from within it. After trying and failing to rip the T-shirt with his hands, he gives the task to his incisors, successfully tearing a couple of rags from it. Tossing the sacrificed t-shirt aside he wraps the strips of rag around both hands in a *better-late-than-never* effort to protect his blisters from further tearing. That done, he picks up the shovelhead again, slides on his butt back into the pit, and resumes the excavation.

It happened, coincidentally, after the very next overhead chop of the shovel: he saw something, some unnatural flash of color through the icy detritus below. Tossing "Rusty" aside Carl drops to his hands and knees and begins brushing the snow and ice chips aside with his ragged hands. Sure enough there's something bright down there, just a few inches deeper in the ice; something made all the more remarkable by the fact its color is one of those you wouldn't expect to find at these latitudes — *fuchsia*. Carl continues with renewed vigor to clear away the snow, polishing the ice to transparency with his hands until he can make out a white, laced collar of what is now obviously a fuchsia-colored dress. He pauses, somewhat taken aback that he has actually found a body. Even his sense of surprise surprises him: *Why should I be surprised? — a mass grave is bound to have a corpse or two, I mean, it only stands to reason. Duh!* Then yet another hesitancy— one that can only be described as reverence — stymies his progress and befuddles him: *What am I worried about? It's only a body; "merely a carbon-based life form," as Spock would say. And I am a medical professional; these things don't bother me....* Carl's little chat with himself seems to work, providing him with the requisite objectivity to continue the task. And so he does, clearing away the ice chips and snow and muck until the peaceful, eyes-closed, perfectly preserved face of the Eskimo girl becomes plainly visible. Something about her face strikes Carl as surreal. Perhaps it's that prick of fear the living feel when they look upon the dead; that reminder that they too are not long for this world. Perhaps it's simply the optical distortion the remaining inch or so of ice causes — her visage wavy in spots, crystal clear in others — that makes gazing upon her feel so unnatural. Or perhaps it's the fact she is, at the same time, both younger *and* older than he; *much* older, in fact – old enough to be his great grandmother. And more than the surreal aspect of it all, Carl also feels an inexplicable sense of guilt; guilt he hadn't done enough to save her, to restore her full and deserved life. He was, after all, a virologist; and this, the agent that deprived her of her modest stay on this planet, was just a little flu bug.

    Carl resumes brushing aside the obscuring snow and ice to eventually reveal the girl's entire torso and, therein, the nearly cubical block surgically cut from her chest. He knew what they were after; her *lungs*, the tissue from which would be their best hope for finding any intact strands of the otherwise fragile virus. And he knew how they went about it; he could tell by the over-cuts at the corners that they had used a circular saw — and probably not some low-powered cordless, but rather some hardy worm-drive plugged in to a generator, the saw rigged with a small-toothed crosscut or plywood blade. Carl knew this because he himself had used this technique on cadavers in medical school, as well as on more than a few autopsies since then. In fact, he was so familiar with the process he could smell that unmistakable burning stench created by the friction of the whirling blade against the resistant rib bones. Was he only *imagining* he smelled that burning stench, or was he actually doing so? Considering the original sawing and biopsy was performed only some six months ago and had since been sealed in solid ice, either scenario was possible. Not that it mattered.

"What I wouldn't give for a biosafety suit right now," Carl mutters to himself, as he considers the thin inch of protective ice between he and the Eskimo girl. Sure, he was among the first vaccinated against the "Swine flu" that circulated in 2009, but this might be a different enough strain of H1N1 that his antibodies might not recognize it. Or, it's even plausible that Dr. Jenna's theory may be right; just maybe this mass grave hides an hitherto altogether undiscovered, much more lethal subtype of influenza which circulated around the same time. Or perhaps it wasn't so lethal in and of itself but was only made so because of its *co*-morbidity with the Spanish flu. Who knew? – certainly not Carl. The best he could hope to accomplish was to get a sample back to the CDC for testing, and to protect himself from the unknown in the process. Hence, in lieu of a biohazard suit, Carl tears another strip of rag from his sacrificial T-shirt, tying this one around his face – bandana style. Sure, it's hokey and most likely ineffectual, but it might just be the difference between catching the bug or not. Next Carl grabs his backpack and pulls from it the red-plaid thermos he obviously pinched from the floor of Olaf's plane. He opens it, gives it the sniff test – clean enough – then sets it upright in the snow beside him. From another pocket of his pack he pulls his Swiss Army knife. After opening its sawtooth blade he positions the knife also, just so, on the ice beside of him. In a final attempt to protect himself from accidental infection, he re-dons his CDC windbreaker, positions the bandana snuggly over his nose and mouth, then lowers his sunglasses. Ready as he'll ever be, as protected as he'll ever be, he lifts Rusty high overhead, pauses momentarily, then forcefully drives its blade down towards the Eskimo girl's torso, then again, then again, then again....

Carl's crude operation and all its gory details are visible in the reflection in his sunglasses, even to the point where – despite their tinted lenses – the flying chips of ice take on a red-ish hue once the shovel head began chipping into the Eskimo girl's chest cavity. The same reflection bears witness to the point when Carl switches tools, setting the rusty shovelhead aside and trading it for his trusty pocketknife. Now begins the most graphic part of the process; when Carl begins sawing bite-size chunks from the various recesses of the girl's lungs then – closing the knife's saw blade and putting to use its tiny tweezers – begins removing the bluish-gray chunks of thawing tissue one at a time and conveying them to the open thermos, carefully depositing each therein before screwing the lid tightly closed again.

From inside the cockpit of a sleek, Bell 429 twin turbine helicopter the tiptops of a pine forest seem to race just under foot as, over the radio, some general weather and aviation gibberish can be heard in both Russian – from across the Bering Strait – and English. After a subtle ascent up a gentle mountain slope, the helicopter's floor seems to fall out as it passes over a granite ridgeline. Seemingly bent on hugging the ground, the helicopter descends with the topography and into a glacial valley, banking sharply to the right to then follow a meandering, bluish-gray river northward.

The sun, even for way up north here, is finally settling low in the sky. A bonfire – fueled by scrap wood from the cemetery's fallen-down tool hut – blazes, the picked-up wind whipping the flames around the half dozen 55-gallon steel barrels stood upright and ringed tightly around it, each barrel premeditatedly positioned near the edge of Carl's re-excavated part of the mass grave. Carl scoops a last shovelful of snow into one of the barrels, the splashy overflow from which falls into the bonfire causing a small cloud of steam to join with the wind-diffused smoke rising into the sky. With all of the barrels now full of mostly-melted snow water Carl tosses Rusty aside again, this time for good. Then, after a brief double-checking of his rationale, Carl tips one barrel after another towards the hole, thus submerging the Eskimo girl's corpse beneath the hundreds of gallons of ice water; water that *hopefully* will soon – evening temperatures willing – freeze back to ice and thus re-entomb the virus along with its young victim. And the tipped barrels of water fill the VW Bug-sized hole as planned, but cause also an unanticipated consequence; for not only does it bring the corpse of the Eskimo girl plainly into view, but also the corpses of many of her fellow crypt-mates – seven, eight, nine at least – buried alongside and beneath her. It makes perfect sense, of course; the water thawing the snow just enough to allow the trapped air molecules, which makes snow white, to bubble up and away, thus turning what had just been opaque transparent again. And, of course, it stands to reason the bodies would still be here; after all, it's not like this is some regular graveyard like those down in the lower forty-eight where the bodies actually decompose. Quite to the contrary, up here corpses just freeze and stay that way, pretty much forever; the earth functioning more as a sub-zero meat locker than a compost heap. However logical the presence of these entangled corpses may be, the visceral impact of actually seeing them, even on the objective perspective of a scientist, is chilling; layer upon layer of twisted, cyanotic, stacked, tossed, entwined bodies descending deeper and deeper into an unfathomable icy darkness, as if all the way down to Hell.

An icy wasteland now slips just beneath the helicopter, with only the occasional clump of brush sticking up through the snow, or the biting in of a protected inlet's coastline interrupting the otherwise flat pate of arctic whiteness. The guy riding shotgun points up ahead through the windshield towards Olaf's DHC-3 Otter, still parked out on the pebbled spit where the tundra meets Grantley Harbor. The pilot nods then adjusts the helicopter's flight path so to pass them directly over the seaplane. And as they do, they also pass directly over Olaf, now dressed again and standing on top of his plane's wing. After waving his arms to make sure he's caught the helicopter's attention, Olaf then turns 180° and directs them out along the trail of Carl's snowshoe prints, towards the faint blur of smoke rising in the not too distant east.

Carl is on snowshoes again, coughing with more frequency and ferocity than even just a few hours before as he trudges back along his own tracks, making his way from the cemetery back the kilometer or so towards the ghost town. Between the late afternoon sun and the moving-in of a high ceiling of barely visible cirrostratus clouds, the temperature has dipped considerably. Though the prospect of being inadequately clothed against the chill of evening makes him understandably anxious, it also brings the bonus perk of making the trek considerably easier by giving the previously too-soft, too-deep slush a supportive icy crust atop which to walk. The cool air also brings welcomed relief to his increasingly feverish brow, as does the occasional gust of wind that helps evaporate the sweat from his scalp and clammy armpits. Still, every third or fourth or sixth step or so, his snowshoes break through the crust causing him to sink through and even stumble. But this unpredictable inconsistency is a small price to pay, he figures, when compared to the *predictably* deep trudging effort required on the trip out. And perhaps by the time he passes through the ghost town and is headed back the remaining three kilometers towards Olaf's seaplane, the crust will be firm enough that he won't break through at all. Maybe it will become firm enough to allow him to take off the snowshoes altogether and just stroll back along the homestretch on his hiking shoes. Wouldn't that be nice? After all, it's an outright pleasant day, it truly is. And if only he wasn't so sick, and if only he was able to push to the back burner the rather troublesome fact that several branches of the Federal Government were after him, and if only he could suppress that nagging suspicion that someone, or *some-ones*, have gone to great efforts to collect then test then possibly release one of the most lethal and contagious pathogens known to humankind, well, then the trek, this little stroll in a big, big park, might even be *enjoyable*. If only.

"Late afternoon – *phffsst*, it might be ten p.m. for all I know," Carl ruminates as he stares, without even having to squint, at the pale sun still a good two fists above the gray horizon and ringed by a faint rainbow caused by the cirrostratus's ice crystals. And that's when he first hears the popping *whop-whop-whop* of the approaching helicopter's blades chopping through the air. He doesn't see it yet, but it sounds like it's coming right out of the northwest, right out of the sinking sun. Pausing, he just stares towards the sound. And something about it – well, he *is* a fugitive after all – troubles him. The thermos in his daypack is jabbing uncomfortably in his spine, so he shimmies a little to jostle it into a better spot, and that's when he sees it; the sleek, black 429 Bell helicopter, rising above the snowy hillock just ahead of him and much closer than he assumed.

Trapped out in the open, there's not much Carl can do but hope the helicopter has come to aid rather than to arrest him. But as it slows to a sudden hover just some thirty meters away, then turns profile to him and slides open its side door to reveal another two men – somehow militaristic-looking despite their plain-clothes dress – each poised on one knee, one with a futuristic-looking XM8 compact assault rifle and the other with what looks like some big, ol' elephant gun, Carl's naïve hope that they have come to aid quickly wanes. Instinctually he throws up his hands in a gesture of surrender. But the helicopter, hovering just a few meters off the snow by now, begins to sidle slowly towards him, the bright red dot of the XM8's laser scope occasionally stinging Carl's eyes as it dances about his forehead.

"I'm unarmed!" he shouts at the crew, stoical behind their mirrored sunglasses.

But on towards him the helicopter sidles.

"Hey, it's cool! I'm unarmed. I'm, like, being totally compliant here!" he shouts again, though doubtful if they can even hear him.

It's the big, ol' elephant gun that fires; but not with the reverberating *boom* one might expect, but rather with only a light *pop* and a subtle cloud of smoke at the muzzle. But this is followed immediately by a painful impact to Carl's left thigh, striking him like a juiced swing of a baseball bat. Screaming in pain and grabbing his thigh with both hands, Carl looks down, fully expecting to see a blown-off stump of a leg or, at very least, a lot of blood. But instead he sees something that doesn't quite register at first, but then he gets it; it's the frilly end of a tranquilizer dart.

"What the fuck?" he shouts to the helicopter's robotic crew.

Still clutching his throbbing thigh, he narrows his puzzled gaze on them, trying to plumb their motivation, their *raison d'etre*, as he already begins to feel the tranquilizing narcosis numbing his brain from the outside in.

"Who are you?" he shouts. "What do you want?"

Rather than replying, the helicopter only continues to sidle toward him, rifles' aim still fixed, that pesky red dot still stinging his eyes.

"Fuckin' jerkasses, I'm *unarmed!* See?!"

As his pleas seem to do nothing towards dissuading the helicopter's menacing advance, Carl does what any animal might when so threatened – he panics. Which direction does one run in these types of situations? – *away*, always and directly *away*. But if trying to flee from a helicopter wasn't already a nigh-futile proposition, his attempt to do so here and now is exasperated as much by the lack of cover proffered by the wide-open tundra as by the fact that his snow shoes now break through the icy crust with every desperate, stomping heavy-footed step.

Enjoying the clear advantage, the helicopter begins wrapping tight circles around Carl, continually cutting him off while always managing to keep the riflemen's door facing him. Even to Carl it's beginning to feel like a game of sadistic cat and wounded mouse, which is never much fun for the latter. He trips, he stumbles, he falls, he clambers back to his feet again and changes direction for the umpteenth time, but still the copter manages to tighten its circle around him. With their rifles still trained on him but not firing, the two goons in back seem to be just biding their time until the tranquilizer takes full effect. Carl trips again, this time caused by the crippling effect the drug is beginning to incur on his motor abilities. Coughing violently from the gasping strain on his lungs, Carl spits up a frothy, bright-red hack of blood. And there's more where that came from, but he knows he hasn't the time to worry about it right now. Clambering again to his feet, he tries throwing one numbed leg out in front of the other in a futile attempt at a run, only to fall again. On his back now – arms raised in submission, feeble legs plowing him backwards through the snow – he shouts pleas out to the deaf crew: "Alright, I give up! I surrender! You win! Peace!" he adds, flashing desperate peace symbols to see if that might work, though it doesn't seem to.

Carl then notices the guy riding shotgun speaking into his headset, and soon thereafter the others, seemingly heeding his order, promptly don gasmasks. Carl shakes his head as he realizes what they must be thinking, then shouts out: "No, I'm not infected! *I am not in-fect-ed!*" But if they hear him, or even comprehend his wild gesticulations of surrender, they really don't seem to care, as the helicopter continues to creep towards him with its crew's rifles still trained on his forehead and torso.

In frustration, Carl tries snowballs. It's good snow for snowballs, and he manages to hit the chopper's windows with two, even slipping one through the open door, before the drug renders his arms useless as well.

Perhaps waiting for this stage of narcosis, the helicopter's skids finally settle onto the snow, the pilot careful to keep the rotors spinning with enough torque to keep the craft's weight from breaking through the fragile crust. The two militaristic goons hop from the door and assume one-kneed shooters' positions, providing "cover" as the guy in the co-pilot's seat – seemingly the operation's boss-man – opens his door and steps out. After first walking with his head lowered so not to be decapitated by the whirling blades, the boss-man straightens up, pauses, then proceeds calmly on towards Carl.

Oddly, this guy – handsome with graying-short-cropped hair and four or five-day growth of salt-n-peppered stubble – wears no bio-mask or any such protection; a fact not lost on Carl even as the drug begins to cloud his mind. And despite the fact the man is obviously unarmed, Carl – now half-paralyzed – nonetheless tries to push a feeble retreat from him, plowing himself caterpillar-like though the snow on his side with his one good leg. As the man comes up to Carl and settles down on one knee just beside him, Carl can feel his own pulse racing. And perhaps in his mind he is still mustering a fair retreat though, in reality, his one good leg is only barely scratching at the snow by now. Fortunately, like some powerful codeine and alcohol-laced cough medicine, the tranquilizer has suppressed his agonizing coughing. If only for that, Carl is thankful. Staring up at the man – having to squint now due to the tranquilizer's dilating effect – about all Carl can see of this world any longer is the man's face and the inscrutable smirk there upon, the narcotic having pretty much fuzzed-out everything else. And the face seems vaguely familiar to Carl, *or is that merely an effect of the drug?* – that's what Carl is asking himself when he notices the man has begun to speak, the man's words seeming to come tumbling out even before he opens his grin, as the drug's hallucinatory side effects begin to pry out-of-synch Carl's auditory and visual senses.

Despite everything, Carl can make out what the man is trying to tell him, even as each muffled, thickly Parisian-accented word swims and echoes within his emptying brain: "Dr. Sims, I presume?"

Carl pants like a dying hound, the narcotic allowing him to stare out to this foggy universe through just one eye now.

"I am Dr. LaFond; *Henri* to my friends, and hopefully someday to you as well," the man says, as he pulls a hypodermic needle from his shirt.

Even in his delirium Carl now manages to place the man: he's the biologist who was monitoring the dying frog in that live NPR videocast from Costa Rica. What, where, when, how Carl recalls all this is beyond ratiocination at the moment, but he remembers.

"And don't worry about the tranquilizer dart: diazepam, harmless. As is this," Henri adds, lifting the needle into Carl's narrow field of focus. "Xylazine/ketamine – standard large critter veterinarian anesthesia. You'll be out for some time," he adds with a reassuring smile before clutching the needle between his teeth to free his hands in order to roll up Carl's sleeve. With that done, he takes the needle from his teeth again and presumably injects Carl's forearm, though Carl can neither see nor feel it by this point of sedation.

Henri smiles again, his face now just a foggy glare, his voice a disjointed otherworldly mumble as he assures Carl, "There, *finé!*" Then, just as all light begins to fade from Carl's world, Henri – seemingly unable to leave well enough alone – twists his smile into a smirking grin and adds, "And, believe it or not, this has nothing to do with you fucking my wife."

WHO Infectious Disease Facility, Sao Paulo, Brazil.

On one wall she has thumb-tacked pictures of suffering; enslaved workers, political prisoners, tortured soldiers, displaced families, starving children... starving children mostly. Some of the pictures are cut from glossy magazines, others from newspapers, some she took herself. All the pictures site current atrocities – a little conflict spun out of a land-grab on the Columbian-Ecuadorian border here, a massive famine relief camp in Darfur there – nothing historic. That was the promise she made to herself: to keep this little memorial of hers current in order to remind her that many of these people staring down from the walls at her might still be alive. And that's what keeps her going; the fact that these people are suffering right *now*. She has similarly covered the adjoining wall with photographs and articles of animals. These she has divided into three categories – *threatened, endangered, extinct* – with all the usual suspects posted beneath each. Why there's even a photograph of that very last spotted tree frog – *Litoria castanea* – recently moved from the *endangered* to the *extinct* column. But there's no sorrow to be found in the eyes of these animals and their pups; only innocence and the inability to understand whom exactly to blame for their demise. And on the third wall raw scientific data are the featured theme; cryptic graphs and charts of increasing concentrations of toxins and gases, percentage square kilometer decreases of natural habitat and ice caps, rising sea levels, dropping aquifers; doom and gloom – those sorts of things. But on the fourth wall, the one with the only door leading in and out of this small office space, she has just one huge, decade's old photograph; that of a verdant natural valley replete with a pristine waterfall, forested mountain, and glacier-capped peaks back-dropped by a clear, cobalt-blue sky. Yes, the poster came off the wall of some refurbished bar somewhere; the back-drop of a beer advertisement lending testimony to its beverage's purity; *"From the land of sky-blue waters."* If you were to ask her where this picture is from she couldn't tell you, not even to the continent; she's never been there. For all she knows, it may no longer exist, it may now be just another paved-over and trampled-under paradise, but it just makes her feel good looking at it. And whether it still exists or not doesn't really matter. For to her, rather than it serving as a tombstone for what *was*, it instead serves as inspiration for what *can be* once again; a restored wilderness, a sustainable ecosystem, a healed planet. That's her goal. That's her reason for being.

Dr. Jenna Williams' voice can be heard before she enters through that aforementioned only door, beneath that aforementioned poster of that pristine wilderness scene. She's just outside of the small office; out in the hall and speaking on a cellphone, her voice and bits of the conversation growing ever more audible as she draws near. "Do you have him?... Right.... No, keep him sedated.... I understand, but please don't...."

Dr. Williams enters the office, dropping a large duffle bag onto the floor then slinging her daypack onto a coat rack. All this was done with a rote carelessness that might have gone unnoticed if not for the discernable care she takes for her next action; that being her cautious setting down of the titanium briefcase – the one plastered with biohazard warnings and decals – onto her cleared-off desk. Her stress and weariness is evident both on her face as well as in her voice as she settles into the swivel chair, boots up her computer, and continues the conversation, beginning with a burdened sigh.

"I know. I know. But just don't. Please.... Well, is there anyway you can bring him *here?*"

This last question begets a long pause from the other end of the phone call.

As Jenna pivots in her chair, Dr. Henri LaFond's French accent can now just barely be heard seeping from out of her cell phone.

"Seems to me an unnecessary risk," Henri says.

"I realize that."

"Can you be sure this isn't just wishful thinking on your part?"

Jenna ponders the question thoroughly, her goal being absolute objectivity, especially towards herself.

"Wishful thinking? No, I don't believe so," she replies.

"Believing is great, but how can you be *sure?*"

"I knew his father."

"So you're hoping the apple hasn't fallen far from the tree, is that it?"

"I think he can be reasoned with, yes. In fact, I think we can use him."

Now it's Henri who hesitates before speaking: "Well, for the record, I think it's a mistake."

Jenna takes a breath as she weighs Henri's objection, then overrides it: "Just bring him with you. We'll deal with it here."

Hartsfield-Jackson International Airport, Atlanta.

It's some inconvenient hour of the night when the windowless L-1011 DHL cargo jet touches down. And within minutes the plane is parked and being hastily disemboweled of its contents by trucks, conveyors, and bleary-eyed employees. Everything rush-rush. Over Night. Urgent. Special Delivery. Priority. First Class. Next Business Morning. When it absolutely positively needs to get there on time. *Blah-blah-blah.* Just fussy humans making their fussy demands.

But of all the hundreds of thousands of parcels coming off this particular plane, and even of all the millions more coming off the hundreds of thousands of cargo planes just like it the world 'round, none is as important as the one presently being unlatched and hand-carried by a special courier here and now; the one locked within the *other* crash-resistant titanium case and plastered with biohazard stickers. Verily, even if it were possible to ship or mail or Fed Ex, say, a nuclear warhead, this little titanium case would deservedly, or at least *should*, warrant higher priority by virtue of its potential devastation. This little flu bug....

Dr. Bronwyn Galloway may be head of the National Center for Immunization and Respiratory Diseases and all that, but she's also a mom. And insofar as her two daughters are eight and ten, there's plenty of petty quibbling of the *finish your homework, brush your teeth, leave your sister alone, lights out, don't make me come in there!* variety that goes on most every night at bedtime, and tonight is no exception. And, of course, the stress of it all makes her want to choke her husband; not because any of it is his fault, but just because he's there and thereby blamable and thereby strangle-able. It's the misplaced anger thing, and she's got it big time right now, to the point where she and her husband are shouting at one another, not caring that their beautiful little daughters are listening from their terrified little beds. Two educated, should-know-betters yelling at each other at the top of their lungs. Neither of them can take it any longer. One of them is going to sleep on the couch and move out in the morning. That much they can agree upon. But then the phone rings and everything that's happening in this tiny household becomes instantly unimportant, all that blistering rage becomes what it really is — petty.

Normally Bronwyn would not answer the phone at this hour; ten at night — on a school night, no less — who would? No doubt it's just another telemarketer blatantly violating the Do Not Call laws. It was only because the phone's caller I.D. showed the call to be from "Bruckner, Hans" — *aka* Hank Bruckner, her Head of Terrorism Preparedness and Emergency Response — that she did answer. And why would that make a difference? Because Bronwyn knows Hank has two quibbling grade school kids of her own he's no doubt trying to get to bed. As well as a spouse, and all that goes with that. So, obviously, he wouldn't be calling — and from his cellphone no less — unless there was something of the *utmost importance* magnitude going down somewhere in the world, something only she and maybe a handful of others could do anything about.

"What is it?" she says, answering the phone as expediently as possible.

And Hank's reply is similarly to-the-point: no *Good Evening*, no *How ya doin'?*, no *Whad'up, dawg?* and especially no *How're the hubby and kids?* Thankfully Hank's professional demeanor allows him to skip over such trivialities. In fact, his job demands it. He simply would not have made it this far up the CDC ladder if he couldn't keep a conversation succinct.

"We're not sure yet. All we know is Carl Sims just sent it back from Laos."

"*Laos?* Thought he was in Guangdong."

"Yeah, well, there's that too. How soon can you meet me in the BSL?" Hank asks.

Bronwyn glances at the clock, and then across to her husband, just emerging into the garish light of the kitchen but already rolling his eyes as he bounces and gently carries their crying eight year-old back to bed.

"Ten minutes."

The pounding on the safety glass of the automatic, identification-card-activated, double-sliding entry door is followed by an angry: "Let me in!"

Just inside the doors the night shift receptionist glances to the night shift security guard. Both know the clearly stated rule — no entry without a CDC ID Security Pass — but both also know *who* this is doing the pounding; Dr. Bronwyn Galloway, the head of the NCIRD, the one who just Monday morning gave them the stern *no-one-but-no-one-comes-through-these-doors-without-a-security-pass* lecture. Could this be some sort of security test? Then again both also know the guards at the gate also must have let her in, so the infraction wouldn't be all theirs; if heads are going to roll at least theirs won't be the first into the basket.

"God damn it, let me in!" Bronwyn shouts again, this time kicking at the glass as well as pounding.

The security guard shrugs to the receptionist, who takes a deep breath then nods back then, finally, presses the button that opens the doors.

"Good evening, Dr. Galloway," the receptionist tries, adding a sheepish smile in an attempt to patch over their blatant infraction of the security rules. But Bronwyn simply blows past them, sans any greeting other than a seething glare.

Bronwyn pushes through some double-hinged interior doors and enters the main corridor leading into the heart of the compound. It's all antiseptic linoleum and institutional green drywall and antiquated, occasionally flickering, T-11 florescent lighting complete with humming PCP ballasts, but in its unpretentious, no frills, nauseating kind of way, it's somehow welcoming to her, downright homey even. She rounds a corner, pushes through another pair of double-hinged doors, and proceeds down another corridor. Her route carries her past Hank's open door, with him visible within, standing as he reads from a clipboard.

"Hank?" Bronwyn barks from the hall, without even slowing her pace, her monosyllabic beckoning merely a politely efficient way of inviting him to join her, which he immediately does, matching her gait stride for stride down the next corridor.

"Ain't this a bitch, " Hank comments, as he hands Bronwyn the clipboard.

"Is this from the WHO?" Bronwyn asks, as she begins to scan the data.

"Yeah, just their preliminary analysis."

"Did they get a sample before we did?"

"I don't think so," Hank says, already on his heels.

"And yet they've already done tests."

"Yeah, well, maybe if our courier didn't have to deliver pizzas to make ends meet."

Bronwyn cuts Hank a glare.

"Uh, that was a joke, Dr. Galloway.... Sort of."

They come to an airtight door stenciled with the bold, bright red words, "Bio-Safety Level 3 Lab." Deferring to both rank and male-female etiquette Hank steps back to allow Bronwyn to swipe her I.D. through the security lock before him.

But Bronwyn doesn't step forward.

Hank studies her, concluding, "You forgot your I.D."

Embarrassed, but certainly not one to show it, Bronwyn says nothing.

"You appoint me Head of Terrorism Something Evildoers Preparedness Something-or-other, and you want to slip through on my I.D.?" Hank asks incredulously.

This time Bronwyn barely musters a sheepish nod.

Shaking his head, Hank swipes his I.D. badge through the security lock then opens the door for Bronwyn, the two exchanging a glance in appreciation of the irony of it all as she steps past him and through the door.

Upon entering the antechamber of the main laboratory Bronwyn and Hank immediately commence the BSL-3 routine: peeling from out of their lab coats, scrubbing their hands up to their elbows, drying off with hot air driers, then donning surgical gowns, face masks, gloves, hair caps, and booties. With more than forty years at the CDC between them, this is something they do as routinely as brushing their teeth, and yet with practiced care so no mistakes are made. As they finalize their "BSL" – or, as many herein the Coordinating Centers for Infectious Diseases facetiously refer to it, *"BS"* – preparations, they resume with Bronwyn's updating.

"Any suspects yet; SARS? Coronavirus?" she asks.

Hank shakes his head. "It's definitely an influenza."

"Avian?" Bronwyn asks, more than a hint of worry in her voice.

"And not just any avian," Hank avers, reticently.

"The Bird flu?"

Hank nods. "The crown jewel; H5N1," he responds, handing her the clipboard holding the WHO's preliminary analysis.

Bronwyn sighs deeply as she takes the clipboard and begins to skim through the WHO data. "And it's spreading human to human?"

"Very much so."

"Do they have any idea why?"

Hank shakes his head. "No, other than it's finally mutated to the point where it can readily make the leap from birds to humans."

"Any hope for cross-protection from our current vaccine?"

"There's always hope, I guess. But insofar as H5N1 isn't a component of our trivalent, said hope is probably slim."

"So, we're talking about tossing our current vaccine and starting a new one from scratch — *again*."

"Either that or risk yet another low-efficacy year."

"It'll set us back months."

Hank nods, adding: "I'm hoping the *better late than never* maxim might apply here."

"It's times like these I find myself wishing 2009's Swine flu had lived up to it potential."

"You're worried the public won't take us seriously and line up for their flu shots?"

"They're inured, desensitized. Would *you*?"

"We can't worry about that right now," Hank says, trying to keep his colleague focused.

Knowing he's right, Bronwyn nods, but still can't suppress a defeated sigh endorsed with a succinct: "Fuck."

With that, Bronwyn and Hank take a last breath of unfiltered air, pull their surgical masks over their noses and mouths, don clear plastic safety glasses, then enter the Bio-Safety Level 3 Lab, a slight man-made breeze sucking past them as they move through the airtight doors and into the negatively-pressurized room.

Once inside the lab, Bronwyn and Hank are joined by Ross Corman; similarly suited-up and entering from the adjoining vault. He carries the titanium case shipped by Carl the day before from China. Greeting Bronwyn and Hank with barely more than an acknowledging glance, he sets the titanium case on the lab counter between them, pulls out a utility knife, opens its blade, then awaits Bronwyn's approval to proceed. Sans hesitation, she gives the go-ahead nod, after which time Ross cuts the case's security seals with the knife, opens the case, and removes the milled aluminum case within. Ross then pauses to toss Bronwyn another glance over their facemasks, and once again she nods the tacit go-ahead granting approval to proceed through the next layer of protection. Heeding, Ross opens the milled aluminum case, lifting from it the rack containing the three vials of the pale, reddish-yellow blood serum, which he then carefully sets on the lab counter top.

Bronwyn squats a bit to bring her eyes to the level of the vials to visually inspect the otherwise perfectly normal looking serum. "So, what else do we know about it?"

"You read the WHO's preliminary analysis?" Ross asks.

Bronwyn nods, "Some variant of H5N1, right?"

"Uh, right; except not according to the notes e-mailed by Carl."

"Why, what's he say?"

"Just that it didn't match anything in the field database for H5N1."

The contradiction gives Bronwyn pause.

"Do you trust his field work?" Hank asks her.

"He's a good scientist."

"But none too happy about working in influenza, as I recall."

Bronwyn looks from Hank, then back to Ross. "So, what else did Carl report?"

Ross spins his nearby laptop towards him and reads Carl's email notes to Bronwyn and Hank. "Unidentified influenza, isolated in Laos. Sixty-six percent mortality rate," he conveys, trying not to over-dramatize the raw data.

"*Sixty-six* — that can't be right!" Bronwyn says, reeling.

"Maybe he meant *point* sixty-six percent; putting it more in last season's Swine flu ballpark," Hank suggests.

"You would think; if he hadn't posted it numerically, written it out, *and* expressed it as a fraction maybe," Ross replies, turning the computer screen towards Hank. "See for yourself."

Hank leans towards the screen, "Hmm, you're right."

"Yeah, seems he anticipated our incredulity."

"Still, two-thirds..."

"Sounds conspicuously rounded off," Bronwyn asks.

"That's what I'm thinking."

"Insufficient sampling?" Ross asks.

"That'd be my guess."

"How big did Carl say this village was?" Hank asks.

"A hundred or so."

"So, they may well have all been related, for all we know."

"Suggesting a genetic predisposition?" Bronwyn asks.

"Depending on its isolation, it's certainly possible. Then again, we could be talkin' co-morbidity."

"With an antibiotic-resistant pneumococcus?"

"Or a viral pneumonia, or an RSV, or another influenza; any number of possibilities – *too* many."

"So, who do we believe; Carl's *unidentified* influenza or the WHO's H5N1?" Hank asks.

"The mortality rate certainly supports the WHO's assessment," Bronwyn deduces.

"Whereas the morbidity rate –" Hank looks to Ross for the number.

"Nearly one hundred percent, according to Carl's report," Ross adds.

"The morbidity rate supports his," Hank concludes.

"Where's Carl now?" she asks.

"Missing," Ross answers.

"*Missing?*"

"Missing where?" Hank chimes in.

"Well, if we knew *that* he wouldn't be missing, now would he?"

Bronwyn levels a scowl at Ross.

"Sorry, thought we could use a little levity. Guess not."

"*About* where?" Bronwyn asks, refining the query.

"Somewhere in Alaska we think," Ross answers.

"*Alaska?* What, did he feel like he earned himself a little vacation after all his hard work in Asia?" Bronwyn asks, sarcastically.

"Yeah, well, that part's a bit of a mystery; all we know is he jumped quarantine in Anchorage – *inexplicably*," Ross adds, cautiously.

"So, he's on the loose?"

"Seems so."

"Do we have any reason to believe he may be infected?" Hank asks.

"His roommate seems to think so."

"That crippled kid?" Hank asks, with obvious repugnance.

"Uh, yeah; Stuart, Stuart Chew," Ross adds, to make sure Bronwyn knows who they are speaking about.

"I know who Stuart is," she replies, with a weary edge in her voice.

"Right. Anyway he thought it was a high enough possibility to warrant a quarantine of Carl's return flight to the States," Ross explains.

"So, it was *Stuart* who called it in?" Hank asks, incredulous.

"Uh, yeah. And since there seemed better than the benchmark one-percent chance that Carl might be a carrier, I ordered the concealment."

"Have any of the passengers tested positive?" Bronwyn asks.

"Not yet. Then again, we've only just begun to collect blood samples."

Bronwyn again lowers her eyes level with the vials containing the serum then mutters, "Everyone catches it, two out of three die." She then glances worriedly up to the groaning, rattling exhaust/decontamination hoods mounted in the ceiling above them, shaking her head at the obviously inadequate Biosafety Level Three protection.

Hank reads her mind, "You thinkin' we should move this up to BSL-4?"

Bronwyn nods. "Immediately, if not sooner."

Ross winces in anticipation of the eminent logistical headache, "Level *Four*? – it's just influenza."

"That's right, and we're going to treat it like it's airborne ebola or small pox, or weaponized anthrax because, in reality, this could be every bit as lethal and even more contagious."

"I'll post a bulletin that no one's to work with it in anything less than full biosafety-suits," Hank adds.

"Good. And Ross –"

"Start ordering eggs?" Ross interjects, anticipating the directive.

Bronwyn nods. "All you can get a hold of."

"I'm on it," he says, already turning for the exit.

"Hank –"

"Let me guess: alert all the pharmaceutical companies under vaccine contract for us to be prepared to drop everything they're doing."

"Exactly."

"What about the Pan American and European Health Organizations?"

"They'll need to gear-up for full emergency vaccine production as well. Notify them that we'll be sending the virus within seventy-two hours."

"And the wife and kids?"

"Tell them you love 'em –"

"Get all their preemptive spanks and kisses out of the way."

Bronwyn nods at Hank's interjection, "... but not to expect to see much of you for the indeterminable future, 'cause daddy's got to save the world."

"I'll go put on my cape," Hank quips, as he too exits.

Alone now, Bronwyn lifts one of the vials of serum, stares at it reverently and mutters quietly to herself, "God help us."

WHO Infectious Disease Facility, Sao Paulo, Brazil.

In the beginning? What was there? Hot gases? Dark energy? The Word? From out of what vague randomness did this all come to be? Did the universe emerge from out of a Big Bang 13.7 billion years ago? And, if so, what lies out there beyond its outermost fringes? What existed of the universe before the Bang? And what, after it implodes upon itself again, will there be after it? Or was that merely the most recent of a series of big bangs – of violent expansions and contractions – extending infinitely in both directions, past and future like an endless string of pearls? Or is it even relevant to think in terms of time and space? If indeed this all began with the "Word" – or, probably more accurately, a *thought* – aren't these concepts of *time* and *space* just *bricks* and *mortar* of that thought? And if this is all a dream or illusion or subjective construct as many religions and philosophies posit, are not the concepts of time and space and even God, merely components of the illusion? What other theory could support why the universe is purported to extend infinitely both outwardly and inwardly; having no periphery to its vastness nor subatomic limits? How else can we explain the *a-world-without-beginning, a-world-without-end* nature of time unless this is all, as they say, *just a dream?* It would seem, *rationally*, one must either subscribe to the possibility of a subjective reality or else buy the immeasurably slim odds that he or she just happens to be alive here today; the odds of which, under the best of circumstances, are one in some two hundred million, assuming a seventy-year or so average lifespan up against a minimum 13.7 billion years-old universe. But if time is indeed infinite then the odds of being alive – and not already dead, or yet to be born, or never to be born – here and now drops precipitously towards absolute zero. But, of course, the *Merrily, merrily, merrily, merrily, life is but a dream* theory then begs the question: *Whose* dream? And if one is to ever finish unraveling that Gordian Knot – that *mindfük* – they may then want to ponder what might exist beyond said Dreamer and its Dream. Is there a God? And, if so, is

the momentum of folly

God the Dreamer of this dream? Some might interpret the infinitesimally slim odds of there being life or consciousness as proof that there indeed must be a God. But if we were to step back from the question a bit – perhaps a dimension or two or eleven – we would deduce that it doesn't solve anything to believe in God; it only temporarily obscures the fact that the existence of God – particularly a god of order, a god of consciousness, an anthropomorphic god – is equally as infinitesimally *im*probable as our own odds of being here. Hence, it could be argued that both our God and we owe our existence to yet a higher deity, one who could go by the moniker *Slim Odds*.

So then, what is reality? A *nothingness* that just *is?* Or a *somethingness* that just *isn't?* If there is indeed a model for how the universe began – a micro for this macro – it may well be in the process of being re-imagined within Carl's brain at this very moment, as *his* universe is being reconstructed therein, brick by brick, dimension by dimension, theory by dogma, desire by fear. The first of Carl's senses to return was that of sight. It came in the form of a faint light, shifting and flickering, diffuse and gray, penetrating right through his closed eyelids. The next sense to return was auditory, as sounds began to seep in. These came in the form of voices – quiet, distant, detached – their words beginning to emerge from an otherwise cacophonous mishmash. But these – both the visible and auditory senses – were quickly usurped by the sensation of pain. Bone-crushing pain. Everywhere.

Carl's eyes flutter a bit before fully opening. When they finally do, and once they eventually focus, he finds he is staring towards an old but functioning television mounted on a cart. As his wits return he is struck by the realization that someone must have went to considerable effort to try to make him comfortable, to prop him upright in bed to keep fluids from pooling in his lungs, to stick an I.V. in his arm, and even to wheel the television into this dimly-lighted room and position it just so for his... for his what? – *entertainment?*

He was aware enough to realize he was bleeding; epistaxis, petechial and subconjunctival hemorrhage – bleeding from the nose, ears, and lining of the eyes – and probably, though he didn't care to check, from his rectum as well. He wasn't bleeding a lot, but enough to let him know he was either suffering from a co-morbidity of pneumonic plague and Ebola, or mustard gas poisoning, or, most likely, a particularly nasty flu bug. And though his lungs and ribs ached – no doubt from endless coughing – he seemed now to be under some industrial-strength suppressant, for each breath, albeit shallow and painful, came without interruption.

The television demanded his attention if only because it was the predominant source of light – baring the negligible luminosity from the scores of tiny green, red, amber, and blue diodes of the sundry machinery and monitors stacked and scattered about – in this apparently vast but otherwise dark room. Whatever and wherever this place was it had the sterile ambiance of a hospital room, but thankfully without the tight walls and stingy square footage. To Carl it seemed to be a lab of some sort, dedicated to medical science. It also appeared – by its seeming enormity and all the gleaming gadgetry – to be fairly well-funded, though the proof of that still lay out there in its dark periphery. For now the only thing that mattered about this place to him, aside from the fact that it seemed to be keeping him alive, was the television monitor. And his interest in it was understandable, for it was showing something that had only appeared to him once before in his already distant youth and ever since then only in his nightmares. It was showing the grainy, hand-held video of his father and two aides addressing a crowd from a crude stage at that afore-glimpsed outdoor rally in that anonymous third-world village. Back dropped by the *Just Two!* banner with its logo of a two-child family superimposed over a photo of the world, Carl's father stands center stage holding a cigarette-pack sized electric metronome to a stand-up microphone. At first it's only the metronome's steady 2.37-beeps-per-second beeping that can be heard, the beeping carried out across an audience of several hundred through a cheap, crackling loudspeaker P.A. system. It amazes Carl that a crowd would be listening so raptly, so seemingly mesmerized, to a lone man holding a metronome. And the steady beeping went on and on for several minutes before his father interrupted it to explain the reason for it.

"This beeping sound," he asks the gathered, "...anyone know what it represents?" After he speaks, one of his aides leans in to share the microphone and translates his words for those in attendance – the majority likely – who don't understand English.

From the audience comes no response, other than a few shrugged shoulders and shaking heads.

And so Carl's father explains, making certain to speak slowly enough to allow the interpreter time to repeat each statistical example in individual parcels:

the momentum of folly

"Each beep represents another person being added to our human family here on Earth… 4.17 births less 1.8 deaths for a grand total of 2.37 new humans each and every second… another full classroom every average breath… 10,440 per hour…. 250,000 – a good-sized city – every day." He pauses to let the figures sink in for a bit, the metronome continuing to spill out of the speakers and washing over them though with much more of a ominous meaning now.

"Which poses the question: How many is too many?" He then switches off the metronome in order to conjure another image in their minds: "If rats come to a small island they will eat all the food available to them and quickly multiply and cause many of the other animals that relied upon that food to die off. Then the rats themselves – though thousands of times their original numbers – will also starve, leaving behind only a decimated island that can support almost no life whatsoever."

He pauses again to allow his interpreter to catch up with him, but for not so long this time, as this *multiplying-rats-gobbling-everything* is an easy image for these villagers to comprehend, as for any people living so close to the Earth.

"That's what we humans are doing to our planet Earth. We are eating everything. We are multiplying. We are consuming all that we can, as fast as we can, and the other creatures – the plants, fish and animals upon which we depend – are vanishing. Today there are over *twice* as many people on the planet than when I was born – and I'm not *that* old. That's an amount equal to all of Africa, *plus* India, *plus* China – some three billion in all – added just since I've been around. Problem is: we estimate the world can only sustainably support *two* billion of us. What's that mean? That means everything that still makes this planet beautiful to us will be gobbled up if we don't stop growing. Is that what we want? – a dying world for our children, and a dead world for their children."

The video camera operator pans away from Carl's father to catch some reaction shots of the crowd as the aide translates. Some in the audience seem to greet his dire assessment of the state of the planet with disbelief, others appear to take the concern to heart. Some try to dismiss the strange man's mutterings to their worried children – all seven, eight, nine of them – wrapping them in the solacing knowledge that, whatever the challenge, this is all part of God's plan, and, hence, there's no reason to worry.

As Carl's father begins to speak again, the camera pans back to him. And as it zooms in more tightly, the genetic relationship between Carl and his father becomes apparent; both standing slightly over six feet despite their tendency of to carry themselves slightly hunched over, both lean and handsome in that unkempt scholarly fashion. Even their voices sound similar. And more eerie still, most every mannerism rings familiar, all combining to confirm, beyond a shadow of a doubt, Carl was spawn from these loins. Even Carl can see it, and is shaken by it. Sure, he has seen scores of pictures of his father, and recalls vague memories of time spent with him, but seeing him here in motion, hearing his voice, it makes him so much more… *real.* His father is wearing jeans and a pulled-out light green cotton shirt with the top few buttons undone and the sleeves rolled up. No wristwatch or rings or necklaces or tattoos; nothing pointless or superfluous. Even the beads of sweat across his brow, and wet stains spreading out from his armpits, strike Carl as familiar – *Yep, he's a sweater like me.* And his longish hair – unwashed from perhaps a weeklong campaign of similar speeches – is finger-combed straight back in the unintended "style" Carl often sports.

And now the camera operator, whoever it is, tightens even more on Carl's father's face – uncomfortably tight. There, in his father's similarly green eyes, Carl can see something else, something they *don't* share. For therein Carl can detect the hint of a manic disposition about his father, of which his mother often spoke. Ironically it was the trait that had both attracted Carl's mom to his father *and* had forced them apart, but thankfully one Carl did not inherit. Reading more in his father's eyes than probably would be apparent without the benefit/baggage of family lore, Carl senses his father is tired. Maybe not so much *tired* as *weary*; weary of all this, weary of the hopeless world and all the stupid people on it. This was just the latest of his increasingly more frequent ventures out across the planet, for an increasingly more protracted break from his family and all the creature comfort trappings of the First World. Carl's father and mother hadn't officially separated as yet, but it was beginning to look that way. But with him gone so often now, there hardly seemed to be reason to officially do anything. All he needed was a place to receive the nonprofit charitable donation checks – for $30 or $50 or $100 – that occasionally trickled in to the *Just Two!* home office, recover from whatever bacterium he caught out there in the Third World, wash his clothes, then head back out again to some godforsaken corner that probably can't even get birth control, making his efforts all the more futile. But none of it matters, for he knows he cannot save the world. He knows

the momentum of folly

his mission is merely to plant the seeds for others to take up the cause. And it will happen, maybe not before it's too late, but it will happen. This he knows.

Carl's father again raises the microphone to his lips and continues: "There is, fortunately, a way to avoid this fate. A very simple way, and it can all be accomplished in three generations, or two generations, or even within *this* generation — *your* generation. All we need to do is —"

Suddenly there's another amplified voice that tears through the crowd, more tinny and crackly than the P.A. system carrying Carl's father's voice, but much, much louder — *surreally* loud, in fact, 120 decibels or better — an ear-crushing volume that has become unbelievably routine in the Third World, whether it is promoting a political campaign, religious event, or merely a new type of cigarette. "Brothers, sisters, do not listen to that man," the competing, amplified voice begins, purposely in English, drawing to it both the crowd's attention and the hand-held camera's as well. The grainy video on the television now shows the source of this voice: he's a light dark-skinned, handsome, well-kempt man, meticulously dressed in local tribal ware with just enough Western accents — a wristwatch, expensive sunglasses, pressed pants, polished shoes — to suggest he somehow represents the government, the powers that be. He stands in the back of an open Jeep parked on a slight rise just behind the audience, addressing them through a handheld bullhorn. Accompanying him are two edgy guards in camouflage military shirts and sunglasses — one in long pants and boots, the other in shorts with flip-flop sandals, but both toting the ubiquitous AK-47. In spite of his fearsome entourage, the man speaks in slow, measured sentences. His confident smile, as his attire, suggests to the crowd that he is on their side and, therefore — and quite unlike the stranger standing before them on the dais — has only their best interests at heart. And, as if to underscore this point, he switches languages and begins addressing the crowd in their local dialect, the only exceptions being the few English words for which their language has no suitable translation; *dollars, great Satan, racist*....

Before long the choppy seas of consternation are palpable in the crowd as their allegiance begins to waver between Carl's father and this new but *one-of-them* interloper. Whatever it is he is saying — and Carl's father's translator is trying her best to explain it to him — the man is slowly but surely winning the villagers over. And so, if Carl's father is to hold them, if today's sweat and toil is going to be tallied as a minor victory rather than yet another set-back, he'll have to nip this little insurrection in the bud and quickly. This much he knows, for he's seen it before.

Thus Carl's father raises his microphone and begins speaking again, though this time in a somewhat awkward effort to dispel whatever disinformation the interloper may be feeding the caught-in-the-middle villagers.

"Unfortunately, I can't understand what he is saying, or why exactly he feels threatened by what I'm telling you. But I *have* seen this in other villages and countries on continents the world over. And it's always because there are governments or religions or businesses that have a vested interest in keeping things just the way they are. They want to keep their people – in this case *you* – poor and uninformed and barefoot and pregnant and, most of all, out of the governing process and away from their money and power. Just the fact that they have guns – that they *need* guns – should tell you something. It should tell you that they *fear* what I am saying!"

But suddenly Carl's father's voice goes silent as someone – a confederate of the interloper likely – cuts the power to the P.A. system. From the perspective of the video camera it all looks very confusing; Carl's father's muted attempts to continue speaking, followed by his futile efforts to stay on message by shouting it out to the crowd, despite said efforts being too easily drowned-out by the interloper's bullhorn. Accepting the reality of the hopeless situation, Carl's father simply throws his arms up in frustration. Soon thereafter the camera movements become shaky as the consternation in the crowd manifests into physical pushing and shoving. Here and there chants of descent break out, eliciting the throwing of objects – plastic beverage bottles and such – towards the stage.

While still dutifully videoing the rapidly-spiraling-out-of-control event the voice of the up-until-now-silent camera operator can now be heard muttering, "Oh, no, please no!" Until hearing the voice – a female's – Carl had never given any thought to who had been operating the camera on that day. But now, recognizing the voice, it all becomes clear; it belonged to Dr. Jenna Williams, and no doubt long before she had earned the doctorate title. The revelation that Jenna was present that fateful day, however much it might explain for Carl, does not slow the events playing out on the television screen before him. Quite to the contrary, the pace only seems to quicken, especially as the camera movements become increasingly erratic as what had been an orderly rally turns rapidly towards chaos.

The camera pans quickly back to the Jeep, zooming in time to catch the handsome interloper man calmly pointing directly towards the camera. "Oh, shit. Oh, shit!" Jenna can be heard muttering to herself, as the interloper is seen issuing a discreet order into the ear of one of his AK-47 toting henchmen. The henchman nods in response, prompting an even more troubled, "Fuck." from the still-unseen Jenna.

Now off-camera screams can be heard, which pulls the videographer's attention back towards the dais. There two men and a woman climb from the audience and onto the stage and begin to grapple with Carl's father, ripping at his shirt, striking at him with the microphone stand, then finally shoving him down into the suddenly swarming, frenetic crowd. It all happens with a surreal rapidity; one moment Carl's father is there, the next he simply isn't. Witnessing all this, Jenna — still unseen, never seen — now breaks into a run towards the stage, her camera still turned on but shaking so violently it's difficult to make sense of the jumbled mosaic of images it records. But, however *in*comprehensible the visuals might be, the audio captured by the recording is hauntingly clear and uninterrupted; a steady stream of frantic pleadings — "Stop it! Stop it! Please, no. Get off him! He's only trying to help! Please, stop!.." — as she tries to push and shove her way towards Carl's fallen father.

Then, the sound of a dull thud is captured by the audio. This is followed immediately by the video's visual image tumbling to the ground, then becoming unnervingly static at a ninety-degrees-off-kilter angle. Simultaneously, the video's audio component suddenly becomes muted, apparently broken as a result of the fall. Something tragic has happened, that much is obvious, though it is impossible for Carl to know exactly what. The only clue is up there on the television screen, as the camera's now steady but soundless image continues to record an eerie progression of sandals and worn-out shoes and bare feet, all pressing forward *en masse* like the dumb hooves of cattle in an over-crowded stampede through the red dust. And this dreadful image lasts for a good minute or so before the television screen finally, *thankfully*, is switched off.

Carl swallows painfully, tears streaming helplessly down his face. If there is a hell worse than that which his father suffered, it is his own; stuck here — *wherever* — sick as a dog and having to watch his father's death by mob. Carl turns his head from the television, still not knowing where he is but at least curious enough to look around. Judging by the sparse furnishings – the bed in which he lay, a chair, the aforementioned TV, and an old-fashioned, dial-less telephone intercom – the bedside medical equipment trying to keep his vital signs vital, the banks of Plexiglas windows which completely envelop him in an octagon-shaped-fishbowl-esque enclosure, and the vast laboratory of computers and monitors and counters and centrifuges and refrigerators with clear doors and racks of test tubes and other techy stuff barely visible out there in the dark recesses beyond his personal enclosure… through all these clues he comes to the rational hypothesis he must be in one of the planet's four pathogen confinement centers. And, judging by the ultra-sophisticated, high-tech looks of this particular place, and the single-occupancy-ICU-hospital-room-cum-maximum-security-prison feel of it, but especially by the flashes of purplish light emanating every ten seconds or so from the ring of ultraviolet, virus-killing strobe lights hanging from the ceiling, Carl senses he might very well be in the world's one and only Level Five biological containment facility, intentionally situated far from civilization in the mowed-down jungles of Brazil. Verily, judging by everything he's heard of the place, specifically designed to safely contain and study only the most dangerous of bacteria and viruses, he assumes he must be in the facility fondly referred to as "the Slammer."

Ironically, this is where Carl wanted to work. If given the choice of the top four pathogen confinement centers, this – the *ne plus ultra* of them all – would have been his first choice, since it was the only facility designed for BSL-5 research. And, oh what a thrill and honor that would have been if not for the fact that, instead of being the researcher, he presently seemed to be the *researchee*.

The old-fashion, dial-less intercom telephone beside Carl's hospital bed rings. He stares at it for a beat; not sure if he should answer it, not sure if he physically can. But it keeps ringing and ringing – and by the echoing, antiquated sound of it intertwined with his delirium, it just might be President Dwight Eisenhower calling, or Albert Switzer, or Lois Lane – and so he tries. Fumbling at first, Carl eventually manages to pick the telephone's receiver up and bring it to his ear. But before he can much more than *try* to lick his lips in order to *try* to speak, a voice – an all too familiar voice – greets him:

"Good morning, White Satan."

It takes a moment for Carl's brain to make sense of it; first to place the voice as Dr. Jenna Williams', then to associate it as the same voice belonging to the unseen camera operator in the crude video of his father's death. But once his process of ratiocination connects the dots, Carl pulls himself into a sitting position so he can begin to gaze out into the darkened lab out beyond his enclosure. Still clutching the receiver to his ear, his search eventually finds... Jenna – barely visible in the shadows, a few meters beyond the confinement cell's Plexiglas walls. She sits at a table near a speakerphone intercommed into the cell. For the moment she says nothing, apparently waiting to see if Carl can even speak.

Carl licks his lips then manages an incredulous, "You were there? – when my father was killed?"

Jenna hesitates, but then nods. "A lowly intern. After initially thinking he was a racist – you know, just another whitey trying to keep brown-skinned people from taking over the planet – I eventually came to realize that wasn't the case; he hated everyone equally," she adds, knowing Carl wouldn't be offended by what was obviously intended as a joke.

"A *human* racist," Carl recalls with a weak smile.

Jenna smiles as well. "Yes, that was his comeback; he wanted *everyone* to stop at two." Her smile then slips from her face as she alludes to the television screen. "Suppose it doesn't help any for you to know that that was the worst day of my life."

"Were you hurt?"

Jenna shrugs. "I was struck in the head by something. I was bleeding just enough to enable me to pass for dead. Then, once they were all *preoccupied* with your father, I grabbed the camera and got the hell out of there."

"I was ten," Carl begins to painfully recall. "My mom was watching the video. She didn't know I was behind her."

A tear slips down Jenna's cheek. "I shouldn't have sent her the tape. I just didn't know what to do."

"I don't know; it probably would've been worse *not* knowing, having to try to imagine what happened," Carl replies, trying to envision the scenario differently. "I suppose you had sex with him."

"With you *father?*" Jenna laughs, shocked by even the thought. "No, I'm afraid that wouldn't even have crossed his mind. Naw, he was pretty much your quintessential, single-minded idealist, though it wouldn't be a stretch to admit that he did *impregnate* me with something — *planted the seed* might be a better choice of words."

Carl closes his eyes, resting again. "Overpopulation."

Jenna nods then, after staring at him for a moment, decides to change the subject. "So, any idea where you are?"

Carl answers without even opening his eyes, "The WHO's Infectious Disease lab in Sao Paulo, Brazil; a.k.a., the Slammer?"

Jenna smiles, impressed, "Very good. Although, under full disclosure, I should note that because of funding cutbacks from the U.N. due to the house-of-cards-like collapse of the global economy, the WHO has had to close this facility — *suspend research*, I think was the terminology."

"So, how is it that we are in here?"

"Fortunately no one thought to ask for my set of keys back," Jenna answers with a wry grin.

"Who pays the utility bills?"

Jenna shrugs. "The Brazilian government must figure the U.N. is good for it. But, who knows, if this really is the end of civilization as we know it, this all might become yet another ambitious, Industrial Age relic — like the Super Collider and the International Space Station — for our progeny to strip bare for its metal in order to make their spears and whatnot."

Carl closes his eyes, exhausted, morphined-up. "I feel like I'm in Limbo."

"You *are*, in a way. Any idea *why*?"

"I tested positive to that influenza strain we just *happened upon* in Laos?"

Jenna stares at him, unreadable; clearly not willing to answer his hypothesis either way. Behind her, a light begins to flash above the only door accessing the lab. Jenna glances at it, then turns back towards Carl to ask, "Feeling social?"

"Would it matter if I said no?"

Jenna smiles, "No, probably not." She then pushes a button on her intercom, placing Carl on hold as she speaks with parties unseen in silence. Opening his eyes again, Carl watches as she hangs up the intercom phone, crosses to the entrance, and swipes her I.D. card through the automatic door lock. In response, a red light above the entrance turns green. Jenna returns to her seat as, behind her, the door opens and into the lab walk a woman and three men. Though strangers to Carl, the first three are known to the world of science as Drs. Alyesha Singh, Hiro Nakayama, and Fernando Perez. The last of the four is the only one Carl recognizes; Dr. Henri LaFond. Each carry themselves with the confident demeanor of an expert in their respective field, each taking a studious, even troubled glance at Carl as they take seats around the table with Jenna. Henri is the last to take a seat, choosing instead to approach the Plexiglas wall panel nearest to Carl and stand there with his hands clasped behind his back. He nods and smiles, then raises his voice to shout in to Carl through the barrier.

"Hello again, Dr. Sims. Sorry about, you know, *shooting* you and all."

"Could've been worse, I guess," Carl responds.

"Yes, could've used bullets rather than tranquilizer darts!"

Pleased with his humor, Henri smiles then turns towards his colleagues at the table. He asks them something, which Carl cannot hear. Jenna shrugs then nods in response. Turning back towards Carl, Henri unlocks and opens the hatch door leading into the confinement enclosure. A gentle in-rush of air is heard as the atmospheric pressure within the greater lab room equalizes with that of the slightly negatively pressurized chamber.

The fact that the others seem now willing to place themselves at risk of exposure does not escape Carl. "I take it you've all been immunized," he says, noting the procedural change with subdued surprise.

Jenna shakes her head, "As yet there is no vaccine, or antiviral."

As Carl tries to make sense of why they would be so cavalier as to expose themselves to a potentially lethal virus, Jenna then exasperates his confusion by summoning him to join them at the table.

"Come join us, Carl."

He hesitates. "I thought you said I tested positive," he says.

"Actually I didn't say."

"You suggested as much."

"Suffice it to say; you tested positive for *a* flu but not *the* flu, if you catch my drift." She then beckons him again towards an empty seat at the table, "Please."

Though uncertain if he is even physically capable of accepting the invitation, Carl decides to give it a try. Sitting upright, with a surprising lack of difficulty, he then pulls his legs over the edge of the bed and sets his bare feet on the cool, sterile tile floor.

"You must have me pumped full of pain relievers."

Henri smiles, "Pure morphine. Nothing but the best for our colleagues. Please, join us."

Unable to think of a good reason not to join them — other than the sheer embarrassment of the ties-in-the-back hospital gown they've managed to clothe him in — Carl considers the I.V. catheter attached to his arm.

"Oh, I can help you with that," Henri says, already ducking through the hatchway and entering the chamber. He smiles to Carl as he prepares a bandage from the bedside tray. He then gently slides the catheter from Carl's vein, telling him, "You won't be needing this any longer: feeding yourself from now on. I imagine the opiates have you feeling all warm and cozy."

Carl nods.

"Yes, wonderful stuff," Henri quips, as he tapes a pad of gauze to Carl's arm over the I.V. puncture. Then, after a close inspection of Carl's slightly bloodied face and ears, he calls out back towards the table, "Jenna, dear, could you bring a damp cloth so we can clean him up a bit?"

As Jenna crosses to a lab sink and begins to dampen a sterile cloth, even Carl is aware of the subtle consternation brewing at the table. Perez is muttering something to Nakayama and Singh, who are nodding back in troubled agreement.

Perez then calls out to Henri, "Dr. LaFond, not to be insensitive, but we *are* in a bit of a scheduling pinch here."

"I am well aware of that, Fernando. This will only take a sec. Jenna?" Henri asks, extending his arm backwards for the cloth just as Jenna enters the chamber with it.

"I'll do it," Jenna tells Henri, as she gently pushes past him to get closer to Carl.

"But of course you will," Henri smirks, stepping back to allow her access to their patient.

Ignoring Henri's possibly hurt feelings, Jenna speaks softly to Carl as she wipes the dried blood from his nose and ears. "Looks like you've stopped bleeding. Do you think you can walk?"

Carl does a brief assessment of his faculties and nods.

"Alright, let us help you up," she says, setting the cloth on a tray then taking up one of Carl's arms. "Henri?"

At Jenna's subtle prompting, Henri takes up Carl's other arm and together they help Carl out of bed and onto his feet.

"You okay?" she asks.

Carl nods.

"Okay, easy does it," Jenna says, releasing her hold on him.

As Henri does the same, Carl begins a slow and wobbly shuffle towards the hatch.

"Watch your noggin there," Henri cautions him, placing a gentle hand, cop-like, on Carl's head so he doesn't bump it as he ducks through the doorway.

Stepping from the containment chamber into the greater lab room, Carl soon finds himself facing the other three scientists seated at the table. Pulling a seat out for Carl, Jenna begins the introductions, starting with the only other female of the group.

"Carl, I'd like you to meet Dr. Alyesha Singh, Professor Emeritus Marine Sciences University of Mumbai, and visiting Professor at U.C. Santa Barbara. Alyesha, Dr. Carl Sims."

"Pleased to meet you, Carl," Dr. Singh replies, managing to flash a brief, if perfunctory, smile.

Carl nods back, still not certain what to make of the gathering.

Jenna now turns Carl towards Dr. Nakayama. As evidenced by the beads of sweat sprouting from his forehead, the hands clasped before him, fidgety thumbnails picking at one another, and his downcast, thickly-bespectacled eyes, darting about but unwilling to make contact with Carl's, Nakayama seems the least able of all the scientists to hide his nervousness.

"Dr. Hiro Nakayama, Professor of Climatology, Tokyo University. Hiro, Carl. Carl, Hiro," Jenna says, keeping the introduction succinct.

Though Carl manages a nod, no reaction whatsoever comes out of Dr. Nakayama, making it difficult for Carl to gauge whether the septuagenarian is angry, frightened, socially challenged, or merely shy.

Jenna turns Carl now towards the remaining member of the team. "And last but not least, Dr. Fernando Perez, Political Economics of Natural Resources, Universidad de Lima."

"Carl, it is truly a pleasure to meet you," Dr. Perez says, warmly taking Carl's hand and shaking it, the gesture — actual physical touching — not lost on Carl. "I once hosted a lecture of your father's. And, I dare say, if only the world had heeded his two-child advisory, we might well have avoided having to be here today."

As Carl tries but fails to decipher the exact meaning of Dr. Perez's cryptic greeting, he watches the latter's smile give way to the type of heartfelt resignation one might expect to be shared in the trenches between soldiers about to undertake a nigh hopeless charge. Unlike the scientist before him, Perez's eyes seem unwilling to release Carl's; the lock between them feeling like a portal to convey something of grave, if as yet unspecified, magnitude.

Releasing Perez's hand, Carl replies with a sweeping response directed to them all, "I'm beginning to think you guys aren't with the World Health Organization."

Anxious glances bounce around the table as they all settle into their seats. Henri takes it upon himself to answer Carl's question.

"No, indeed we are not. Nor do we represent the Union of Concerned Scientists, the United Nations Panel on Climate Change, the Sierra Club, the Natural Resources Defense Council, Negative Population Growth, Population Connection, the World Wildlife Foundation, UNICEF, or any of the scores of other such organizations – upon whose boards we probably each sit – futilely trying to save humanity from itself. We just are who we are and who you see here."

"A Union of *Very* Concerned Scientists, if you will," Dr. Singh quips.

"So much so, in fact, that we are willing to actually do something about it," Dr. Perez modifies further.

Carl nods. Even if his head weren't still swimming from the morphine and flu and tranquilizers *et al*, this gathering would, no doubt, seem surreal to him. But it is, and so it does. "To actually do what?" he asks, to no one in particular.

His query is met with silence, of the ilk spun from some solemn vow.

"So, what's the big secret? Why are we here?" he tries again.

"*You're* here by accident," Dr. Nakayama finally snaps.

"Well, my apologies," Carl sarcastically replies. "Just show me the door and I'll be on my way."

"Regrettably we can't do that," Jenna says.

"Why not?"

Carl's innocent question is met with more furtive glances between the scientists.

Henri takes it upon himself to try to explain. "Carl, as you know, we are on the verge of making vaccines through genetic manipulation. This will probably be the rule rather than the exception over the next two or three or four flu seasons. Meaning no more reconnaissance missions to Guangdong in search of emerging strains, no more tedious growing of the virus in millions upon millions of fertile chicken eggs. Instead, the pharmaceutical companies will simply, *preemptively* create them in the laboratory, then genetically match them to any strain that pops up anywhere in the world, suppressing it before it even has a chance to get a chance to get started."

"And if a contagion *does* manage to get started, then there's the rapid advancement of *antivirals* to contend with, and the impact genetic engineering is having there," Jenna adds.

"Basically, we live in an era wherein the eradication of pathogenic viruses is not just a *possibility* but a *likelihood*."

"Which is good, right?" Carl asks, intentionally prodding Henri.

"Well, it would be good; it would be *great* if not for the fact that diseases are about our only hope for keeping human population somewhat in check."

"So, disease is good and *we're* the evildoers; that's what you're saying, right?" Carl asks, allowing his sardonic skepticism to seep through.

Henri sighs, perturbed either by Carl's inability to comprehend the problem, or his unwillingness to do so.

Dr. Perez takes up the slack, "Have you any children, Dr. Sims?"

The question catches Carl off his guard, driving a stake of guilt through him thanks to the none-too-small matter of his and Angela's pregnancy. *Have you any children?* — a good question indeed! After the belying hesitation, he mutters, "No."

"Well, consider yourself lucky. I say this only because many — and certainly all of us here — believe the Earth is in the midst of its sixth mass extinction event. And it's happening despite the fact that this one is entirely manmade and therefore avoidable."

"You sound like my father," Carl says, his remark not meant as a compliment.

"Thank you," Perez responds, taking it as a compliment nonetheless. "Your father was absolutely right about the root cause of the problem, just maybe too trusting of humanity's ability to correct it."

"The future, contrary to what optimists might tell you, is not bright," Dr. Singh takes over. "Humanity has a dismal track record when it comes to addressing any of the big environmental problems confronting it."

"If it costs money, if it impinges at all on the Almighty Economy, it's off the table," Dr. Perez adds, "as evidenced most recently by the utter failure of the Copenhagen Climate Summit to ratify any meaningful legislation regarding greenhouse gas emissions."

"Similarly, if human populations continue to grow anything resembling wilderness will be denuded, all arable land exhausted, aquifers sucked dry, oceans utterly fished-out and polluted, and half of all present life-forms driven into extinction."

Dr. Nakayama jumps into the fray, "There will also be the inevitable famines and wars which break out whenever resources become scarce. But not just in isolated regions this time around, but *everywhere*."

"Basically, unless we do something right now, in *our* generation, we will slip past the tipping point, the *Rubicon*, where the environment simply cannot recover in a way that can support higher life-forms such as humans ever again."

"Or, in more scientific terms..." Jenna interjects, to sum it all up, "... we're fucked."

An awkward silence smothers the table as the scientists' conspiracy is unabashedly laid bare. Carl studies their faces, meeting justified resolve in each. When he comes around to Henri's, Henri explains the rationale behind their endeavor:

"Regrettably this isn't science fiction, Carl. All what you've heard here, all these dire prognostications *will* happen unless we do something about it *now!*"

Carl turns back to Jenna, staring critically at her as he asks: "The Laotian village; you intentionally infected the pig and gave it to those little girls."

Jenna returns his stare unapologetically, "The virus had been dormant for ninety years, it had to be tested."

"H1N1? – the *Spanish* flu?" Carl asked, confused.

Jenna hesitates, then turns towards Henri for permission to fully apprise Carl of their plot.

Henri nods his tactic *go ahead* consent.

Turning back to Carl, Jenna explains: "After the 2009 Swine flu pandemic basically fizzled, I became ever the more convinced the high death rates up in the Arctic back in 1918 meant there had to be something other than H1N1 present."

"And you found it?"

"Yes."

"And was it — *is* it avian?"

Jenna shrugs. "That'd be my guess, but I haven't sequenced the genes. We'll leave that for the experts."

Henri contributes what he knows, "Whatever its ancestry, all we can put together is that it has drifted and shifted to the point where we have not just a new strain, but probably a new *subtype*, and possibly even an altogether new *type* of influenza."

"Which is why it didn't show up on any of our field tests."

Jenna nods. "I still don't know all the *hows* or *whys* or *particulars*; all that matters is that it serves our needs."

"So what now? — release it worldwide to kill off two-thirds of all humans from the planet?"

"That's the plan," Henri confesses.

"But that's genocide."

A silence falls over the room until Dr. Singh takes it upon herself to respond to the charge. "We feel it's genocide to idly sit by and do nothing," Dr. Singh counters.

"Better to cull four billion now than to permit ten to fourteen billion to suffer horribly miserable demises soon hereafter, likely by the end of this century," Dr. Perez chimes in.

"Not to mention the countless species that will go extinct along with them," Dr. Singh adds.

"And that's your justification," Carl says, accusingly.

"However abstract or, I don't know, *cold-blooded* this may sound, this is what the data bears out."

"We're operating under the *God helps those who help themselves* proviso," Henri adds.

"Well, I'm comforted to learn God is on your side!" Carl retorts sarcastically.

"I was being glib, Dr. Sims."

"So was I."

Henri turns towards Jenna, asking with a glower why it was she thought Carl might be of help to them, why it was she wouldn't let him kill Carl when he had the chance.

Jenna acknowledges the miscalculation with a sigh then turns back to Carl. "Carl, none of us here needs to prove his or her life-long commitment to humanity," She now nods towards the scientists seated around the table as she rattles off just some of the awards each has received: "... a Guggenheim, a Medal of Science, various national awards, a couple of Nobels.... Which is all to say, we're good, reasonably intelligent people who didn't come to this decision lightly. We agonized over it. We've thought this out. Not a one of us want to take an innocent life or inflict suffering, but we've each come to the conclusion this is the *only* way of preventing far more death and suffering. Exactly what part of this don't you understand?"

Jenna pauses to check to see if she's getting through to Carl. With no indication either way, Dr. Nakayama takes over the rhetoric.

"Dr. Sims, although it may not seem like it, I *am* an optimist. I believe that – all the petty skirmishes, idiotic consumption and looming environmental catastrophes aside – humanity is actually at a fairly highly-evolved level at the moment, and the possibilities the future holds for us are truly limitless. Look how far humanity has come in the last century; from horseless carriages to interplanetary travel, from abacuses to super computers, from leeches and medical bleeding to cloning and genetic engineering. Imagine where we might be in another hundred years, or a thousand, or a *million*! All we need is a little time and breathing room to work it out."

Dr. Perez now takes up the cause: "At the risk of sounding boastful I think we can agree this grim task we are undertaking here today is likely the single most important endeavor humankind has ever attempted. As to whether our actions are *good* or *evil*, well, we'll just have to leave that debate to the moralists. All that really matters is the fact that it is absolutely necessary, that it is *vital for* humanity's ultimate survival."

Henri sums it all up for Carl: "Basically, I guess you could say, we here regard human evolution as an unfinished process. We're just hoping to give it the opportunity to get there; to *be all it can be* in spite of itself."

Carl makes a concerted effort not to nod in agreement; rationally he knows they are right, but emotionally he knows, or at least thinks he knows, they are wrong. Perhaps in an effort to stall for time he turns back to Jenna. "What about the samples of the virus we sent back to the CDC and WHO? Won't they already be –"

the momentum of folly

Anticipating Carl's question, Jenna cuts him off, "We sent them *a* virus, but not *the* virus, if, again, you catch my drift."

"We sent the wrong strain?"

Jenna nods, "A nasty but previously known one."

"Let me guess; H5N1?"

"Yes, the scariest of the known avian subtypes," Henri adds.

"The plan was to get the CDC and WHO's attention;" Jenna explains, "lead them to believe the dreaded Bird flu finally accomplished the antigenic drift mutation making it capable of the inter-species leap to humans – just as they had always feared."

"And while they all are in full emergency production of the vaccine based upon that certainly lethal but – unbeknownst to them – still-not-so-very-communicable H5N1 strain you and Jenna sent them, we will be releasing its *much* more lethal cousin – the very strain you witnessed ravage the Laotian village."

Carl nods, then turns back to Jenna, "Kind of like tossing two snowballs at 'em."

Jenna returns his stare; saying nothing, not needing to.

Henri crosses back to the hatch entry to the Slammer's chamber, and pauses there to turn back towards Carl. "So, Carl, if you please…"

"You want me back in there?" Carl asks incredulously.

"I'm afraid it's necessary; you might try to stop us."

"When do you plan to let me out?"

There follows an awkward silence.

"I see," Carl deduces.

Jenna tries to allay his fears. "We think the facility's doors will automatically unlock once the power grid goes down and the back-up diesel generators run out of fuel."

"You *think*?"

"That's right. After which time you should be well enough to just walk out of here."

"But by then it will be too late."

Jenna nods, "If all goes smoothly."

"Personally, I wouldn't be in such a hurry to get out of here, if I were you, Carl," Henri adds. "There's plenty of food and water, making it just about the safest place on the planet for the non-infected to hunker-down."

"Why not just kill me?"

"Because we're not murderers," Jenna says.

Carl could challenge that claim, but he knows she is only stating what she believes to be true.

"Now, if you please…" Henri says, beckoning Carl into the chamber.

Carl hesitates. Purposely avoiding their eyes, he rises from the table in apparent compliance, but then suddenly turns and bolts towards the lab's only exit. Still physically hampered by illness and narcotics, his stumbling flight sends him crashing into a cart, knocking empty flasks and Petri dishes smashing to the floor. Knowing they will soon try to thwart his escape, he claws his way on hands and knees for the door.

"What's he doing?" Dr. Singh asks no one in particular.

"Trying to flee, apparently," Dr. Nakayama opines, with a sad calmness.

Upon reaching the lab door, Carl grabs hold of the handle and pulls himself to his feet. But then, tug as he might on the handle, he finds the door magnetically-locked and his efforts to open it — at least by sheer, brute force — hopeless.

Dr. Perez can't help but smirk at Carl's pathetic attempt to escape. "Dr. Sims, please; this cell was designed to contain even rabid *gorillas*, I doubt you'll have much luck."

Resigned to the fact that his efforts to pull the door open are futile, Carl turns back for the table; lumbering now defiantly straight towards them, his head listing forward and sporting a look of crazed determination.

"C'mon, Carl, don't be stupid. Get back in the chamber!" Jenna shouts, but to no avail as Carl continues straight towards her, his focus fixed on the I.D. card hanging from her neck.

"He's after your card!" Dr. Perez shouts, but before any of them can react in time Carl grabs hold of Jenna's I.D. and attempts to yank it from her neck.

"Stop it! *Stop it!*" Jenna shouts, choking painfully as Carl tries first to break the nylon strap then, when that fails, to pull it over her head. Jenna manages to get just enough of her hand on the strap to keep Carl's efforts from breaking her neck, and giving the others time to jump into the fray; Drs. Singh and Nakayama helping the tug-of-war over the strap from Jenna's side, Henri and Dr. Perez grabbing hold of Carl from the other direction and wrestling him to the floor, face down against the cold tile.

"Carl, Carl, Carl…" Henri mutters, shaking his head as he grapples his way on top of Carl; knee on the small of his back, his right arm wrenched up behind him. "Did you think we were going to let you just walk out of here?" As if to force an answer out of Carl, Henri applies more pressure on his arm, torquing it towards its breaking point. "Eh?"

Carl groans in agony.

"That's enough, Henri. Let's lock him in the chamber and get on with it," Jenna says, recovered and climbing back to her feet.

But, rather than letting up on Carl's arm, Henri wantonly applies even more pressure, causing Carl to clench his teeth in pain.

"C'mon, Henri, just get him in here!" Jenna tries again, now standing at the Slammer's open hatch door.

But again Henri ignores her, instead leaning towards Carl's ear and whispering, "Hear that? — she's on your side. Go figure, eh?" With that, Henri buries his knee further into the small of Carl's back as he increases the upward pressure on his arm.

Now even Dr. Perez pleads for mercy, "Henri, please, let's just get him into the cell!"

"Sure thing, Fernando…" Henri answers, seemingly ready to comply, until he abruptly forces Carl's arm further up his spine until his elbow breaks, the nauseating snap heard by all.

Carl screams in agony.

"There; that *was* about you and my wife," Henri hisses into Carl's ear before finally climbing off him.

"Jesus, Henri!" Dr. Perez says.

"You motherfucker!" Jenna adds, glaring at Henri as she joins Dr. Perez in helping Carl to his feet.

"Oh, I see; he fucks my wife yet *I'm* the motherfucker," Henri snorts, after Jenna as she and Dr. Perez help Carl back into the chamber and sit him back onto the bed.

"You *told* him?" Carl asks Jenna, incredulously.

"Of course. Just didn't expect he'd be such a baby about it," she replies, ripping a pillowcase with her teeth, then fashioning a crude sling from it. "This should take some of the weight off your elbow," she says, slipping the sling over Carl's head and gently tucking his arm into it.

As she manipulates his arm into the sling, Carl tries to suppress the pain, but as it proves just too much to bear he finally screams in agony.

Out in the lab, Henri shakes his head scoffing at Jenna's attempts at making Carl comfortable as he crosses the lab towards a refrigerated cabinet labeled with biohazard warnings. "A *sling?* You've signed on to kill billions of people and you're fretting over your boyfriend's little *ow-ee?* Give me a fuckin' break! Maybe you'd like to hang around and take his temperature?" he rants as he unlocks the cabinet and pulls from it a hardened, plastic case. "Well? Would you? It can be arranged, you know."

Slamming the cabinet door, he now carries, with a seemingly reckless carelessness, the hardened plastic case back towards the table, redirecting his diatribe now towards Drs. Singh and Nakayama, "I hope the rest of you have thought this through. I really, really, *really* hope you all have thoroughly wrapped your heads around all that you're about to *bring down* over the course of the next few days, weeks, months, whatever, because – a little F.Y.I. here – little *Carlito's* arm there and all his tears and suffering are just a drop in the proverbial fucking bucket in comparison." Henri then sets the case, not gently, onto the table amidst them all, adding with ominous understatement, "Just a teensy-weensy drop in the big-fuckin' bucket."

Henri then pulls out a seat for himself, sits, folds his hands on the table, cuts Dr. Perez a little glower of disappointment as he returns to the table, then calls out with sarcastic impatience to Jenna still in the chamber attending to Carl, "Jenna dearest, care to join us?"

Jenna fills a hypodermic needle from a small vial of clear liquid. Removing the needle, she taps it to remove any air bubbles, then gently inserts it into a vein in Carl's trusting, compliant forearm, assuring him, "A little more morphine to take the edge off while you lick this little flu bug. Sorry I can't do anything more for the arm." After emptying the full contents of the needle into his arm, she removes it. With that done, she then lifts his face towards hers, smiles sadly, then utters an unconvincing, "See ya."

Not one to lie, nor feeling particularly amiable towards her, Carl says nothing.

Jenna sighs sympathetically, nods, then rises from the bed and exits. After passing through the hatch she closes and locks the door, tests it with a tug, glances in a last time at Carl, then turns away to join the others at the table.

the momentum of folly

From Carl's perspective, he can now only read Henri's lips as he sarcastically welcomes Jenna back to the table with a disingenuous, "How nice of you to join us." He then slides the hardened plastic case across the tabletop to Jenna. After catching it, she swaps a brief glare with Henri, then pulls her eyes away and down to the case. Trying to clear her mind of all the unintentional emotional baggage cluttering the event, she takes a deep, calming breath then slowly releases it. Refocused on the matter at hand she opens the case and pulls from it a single, clear, 50 ml. polystyrene test tube containing the translucent, rusty-tinted, slightly cloudy, rather inconsistent, serum fluid.

Dr. Singh pulls a common, small, white, plastic generic version of a nasal spray inhaler from her pocket; empty and innocent enough looking except for the curious fact she has taken the precaution of double sealing it within two zip-lock baggies. She removes the inhaler from the baggies then passes it to her left to Dr. Nakayama, who unscrews the inhaler's cap then sniffs the container. Satisfied – apparently with its cleanliness and lack of residual chlorine disinfectant – he passes the inhaler along to his left to Jenna.

Without trying to over dramatize the event, Jenna uncorks the vial and carefully decants it into the nasal sprayer. With every drop from the vial fitting nicely inside the container's little 80-ml. tank, Jenna screws the inhaler's sprayer cap back on. After glancing quickly around the table – as if in a last check to make sure everyone is still on board – she brings the inhaler to her nose, tilts back her head, gives it a quick squeeze, and takes the deep shot of misty serum up her right nostril. Snorting that first shot well up into her sinuses, she brings the inhaler to her left nostril and repeats the process. Sniffling the mist deep into her lungs, Jenna raises her brows in a quasi-anticlimactic expression and mutters, "Well, that's that."

That done Jenna passes the sprayer back to Dr. Nakayama. Dr. Nakayama removes his eyeglasses and sets them on the table. Closing his eyes, he pauses; not so much in hesitation as in silent prayer, perhaps to that cultural gene trait that made *hari kari* such an honorable deed. The moment completed, he calmly picks up the sprayer, takes two quick snorts, then passes it on to Dr. Singh. That done, he takes up his glasses again, dons them, and only then finally opens his eyes, perhaps hoping to tuck his participation in the conspiracy into a purposely blind and thereby deniable fold of his memory. Over to Dr. Nakayama's right Dr. Singh dutifully snorts down her double-shot dose, then slides the sprayer across the table to Henri.

"No, thanks. I'm good," Henri says, pretending to politely decline the offered sprayer with a slight shake of his head. But as his perhaps-a-bit-too-wry gallows's humor is met with decidedly un-humored glowers, Henri sighs, then mutters, "You nerds are no fun." He then picks up the inhaler, takes his two shots then, just to underscore his commitment, takes a third, before passing the sprayer on to Dr. Perez.

Dr. Perez pauses as he takes hold of the nasal sprayer, "I feel something should be said. Basically, I guess, I would like to express just how *privileged* I feel to be among such committed scientists – humanists, really – who have risen above all of our respective cultural dogma to be willing to sacrifice our lives for what we all believe to be the greater good. Thank you for your courage. Thank you for your rationality. It is truly a great honor to be part of this. *Gracias.*" And with that and a respectful last bow of his head, Dr. Perez takes his two snorts of the virus-infected mist, sniffles it as deeply into his body as he can, then hands the empty sprayer back to Dr. Singh.

"I'll make sure this isn't found," Dr. Singh says, as she slips the sprayer back into a zippered pocket under her sari.

Henri pulls up Carl's daypack onto the table and pulls from it the red plaid thermos bottle Carl stole from Olaf's airplane. After unscrewing the cap, he slides the Thermos to the center of the table and sets the top beside it. He then pushes the intercom button on the desk phone, thus reestablishing communication with Carl within the chamber. "Dr. Sims, I'd like to personally thank you for being our scapegoat."

"For bringing you the virus?" Carl asks, already groggy from his second dose of morphine but still managing, forcing himself actually, to follow the conversation.

Henri nods, "We already had it, of course, but now it will appear as if you were the sole carrier."

"And your excavation of the mass grave; I suppose that never happened."

"Exactly, which could prove quite helpful should any litigations or prosecutions dog us in the event any of us survive."

Henri then purposely knocks over the thermos, its blood-tinged fluid and chunks of lung tissue spilling out across the table. Regarding the spilled mess with outstretched hands, and a wink meant just for Carl, Henri makes a sweeping proclamation: "*Voilè!* — a plague begins."

Someone at the table pushes the intercom button off again, returning Carl's cell to insulated silence. And though he's fighting to stave off the effects of the morphine and stay awake, Carl is vaguely aware that the scientists have mustered some form of exodus; seemingly scurrying about, hectically attempting to cover any trace of their conspiracy while intentionally leaving behind planted evidence suggesting an accidental viral containment breach.

Within a couple of blinks and drowsy dips of Carl's head all the scientists seem to have exited, with the last one of them apparently having switched the lights off again returning the lab to its barely-lighted dimness into which he had first awakened. But then, Carl becomes aware of Jenna's presence. Forcing his eyes open, he sees her standing just outside the Plexiglas cell wall though, aware of his own sedation, he cannot be wholly sure he isn't just dreaming her up. Nevertheless, there she is. She smiles, only making her image look all the more chimera. Carl struggles to bring words to his fumbling lips in a nigh futile effort to speak.

"What... what would you like me to tell them?" he finally manages to ask.

Jenna smiles thinly and shrugs. Resigned to the likelihood history will never quite understand or forgive her sacrifice, she tells Carl, "I don't know. Maybe just try to explain we did it for them."

"For *them* or for *you*?" Carl asks, skeptically.

"Considering there's a very good chance I'll die from this, and the fact that I'm an atheist and thus don't believe in any heavenly reward or afterlife or any of that, I think we can conclude I am indeed doing it for *them* and not for *me*."

"So, only an atheist can be capable of genuine altruism."

Jenna thinks about it, then nods, "I suppose you're right."

"Gandhi? Martin Luther King, Jr.? Mother Teresa?..." Carl mutters, seemingly sleep-talking.

"Self-serving, heaven-seeking posers," Jenna quips.

Carl manages a grin, still enjoying her wry humor.

After Jenna's smile fades, she places the palm of her hand against the Plexiglas, as if to touch it to Carl's. But Carl is too far gone to return the gesture, let alone stay awake. Instead, his eyes drop closed for a final time and he falls against the glass, just opposite Jenna's hand. And for a moment he just leans there, face squished against the glass, until gravity and flaccid unconsciousness finally drag him to the floor. Sleep, sleep has enveloped him. Sweet sleep has gently whisked him away from this miasma of anguish and suffering, and tucked him back into that fluffy world from which no harm can come. Sweet, forgiving, equitable sleep.

Sao Paulo International Airport.

Ten hours after willingly inhaling those two snorts of the lethal, thriving flu virus, Dr. Fernando Perez steps into line at the Brasilia Air check-in window. He had thought about roaming the vast Sao Paulo open market first, or even paying a scalper whatever sum necessary in order to catch this afternoon's Brazilian National Soccer team's exhibition match against Argentina, but even though he'd be amongst 80,000 screaming, sweating, rubbing-together fans, this wasn't an effective way to spread the contagion. They had already run the computer models, so they knew this. It wasn't a *bad* way to spread it, of course; as long as his cells were erupting with the virus — as they indeed were by now — there was a good chance everyone present in the stadium would take at least one strand of the virus into their lungs during their two hours there. The problem was, it just wasn't likely they would take in *enough*. Although a single, complete virus strand *is* enough to pass along the infection from one human to another, ideally it would require some 30,000 individual strands of the virus to insure transmission. 30,000; that is the approximate dosage one might expect to receive if, say, riding for ten minutes or so in a bus in which an infected passenger has coughed or sneezed. That would insure transmission best. That would be pretty much ideal. Thus it was determined the single most feasibly effective way to infect the greatest number of strangers was through prolonged contact in closed quarters; the kind one experiences in airport shuttle buses, passenger trains, commercial airplanes, or even via — though to lesser degree of efficacy — indoor concerts or lectures or plays or films or sports events. Infect the passengers and audience members, and allow *them* to do the dirty numbers work for you. Let them bring it home — "Hi, daddy. How was your trip? — then they infect their kids, then the kids bring it to the Petri dish-like environment of school where the virus is effectively passed via snotty noses and pencils and drinking fountains and keyboards and, yes, doorknobs. Then let those newly infected kids bring it back into their homes where they pass it on to their siblings and parents, anon anon.

the momentum of folly

Workplaces, school buses, churches, elevators, doctor/dentist waiting rooms, teens making out in cars, etcetera; small batches of prolonged, intimate contact – that's how it's done best.

Dr. Perez sneezes across the check-in counter, deliberately missing his handkerchief. There are plenty of germs on the counter now. He knows this for a fact. He can practically see them. The check-in employee – "Maria" by her name tag – makes a reasonable attempt to smile despite the face-full of sneeze germs she just received. She was, after all, hired because of her bubbly, genial nature. That characteristic together with her good looks will make her an ideal "carrier"; women will want to associate with her, babies will trust her, men will tend to lean in over the counter in order to flirt, and, with any luck at all, she is sexually active. If there are, say, a million other check-in employees like her scattered across the globe – not to mention the requisite waitresses, receptionists, baristas, strippers, real estate agents, teachers, masseuses, strippers, librarians, nurses, dental assistants, baby sitters, bartenders, prostitutes, flirty sales reps, and, say, strippers – then this problem is solved; humanity is saved. But for now "Maria" just smiles politely as she takes his unusually thick stack of tickets and begins looking them over.

"Wow, Mexico City, Bogotá, Buenos Aires, Guatemala City, Quito, Santiago, Lima, Havana, Caracas, Montevideo, La Paz; you must really like to fly!" she comments, with genuine amazement.

Dr. Perez musters a smile and nods, adding a cryptic, "More than you know," before blowing his already runny nose into his handkerchief.

Maria gives him the boarding pass for his first flight, politely smiles again – her job – and tells him, "Gate 77."

"Gracias."

"De nada."

Off in another wing of Sao Paulo's sprawling airport, Dr. Nakayama pushes in through the door of a somewhat antiquated men's restroom. He checks himself in the mirror and notices the first beads of perspiration have begun to break out across his forehead. He feels it with his hand. Yes, it's a bit warm. Feverish. His nose is also runny, evidence of the beginnings of an upper respiratory infection and the body's frail attempt to expel it. He inhales deeply a couple of times checking for lung congestion, but there is no indication of such as yet, nor of a cough, though his throat is beginning to feel a bit scratchy. Together these symptoms make the conspiracy suddenly feel real to him. Very real. Despite all the planning and preparation, somehow it only hits home now. He takes a breath and, still staring at himself in the mirror, mutters a purportedly ancient Japanese saying roughly translated as, *This is it*. Though he learned the saying, not from his father or some wizened elder master, but instead from some cheesy, circa 1970 Samurai martial arts film, it has always worked for him.

Dr. Nakayama takes out his wallet and opens it to the pictures of his two grown children; son and daughter, bespectacled professors both. Accompanying them are photos of their respective offspring; two grade school children each – punked-out with blue, green, pink, and white spiked hair, Ipod ear buds, some facial metal already, but smiling nonetheless. Dr. Nakayama looks at his four grandchildren with stoical detachment. He takes the Samurai's requisite seven breaths, then tosses the photographs in the trash. *This is it*.

Refocusing away from his reflection in the mirror, he sees the twenty porcelain urinals hanging on the opposite wall behind him. Two men are presently putting the urinals to use, courteously spaced with one urinal between them. After pondering the situation briefly, after exploring the ramifications of his newly revised *raison d'etre* – to pass on the infection to as many people as possible – Dr. Nakayama turns from the mirror and walks up to the urinals, deliberately choosing the one wedged just between the two men, violating the unwritten etiquette of urinal "space" and no doubt arousing unspoken chagrin. Without looking at his "neighbors," he exhales forcibly a few times, as if trying to hack up mucous from deep in his lungs. After some uncomfortable and disapproving shuffling of feet, the others finish their "business," flush, and move on to the two dozen or so sinks mounted on the opposite wall, leaving Dr. Nakayama alone now at the urinal, seemingly oblivious of his antisocial behavior. This motif – that of the absent-minded professor, the socially inept scientist, the brilliantly aloof idiot/savant – this will work well for him. It's a stereotype people know and forgive; hence, he probably won't get shouted at or punched when he violates someone's space. This caricature has already been sold to the public as laughable and fuzzy and harmless, thus it will functionally serve the cause. He'll go with it.

Once the other two men have exited the restroom, Dr. Nakayama hacks out a spit, intentionally aimed at the white tile wall directly in front of him. As he

the momentum of folly

similarly finishes his *business* he ponders the mucous spittle clinging to the tile before him. That snotty little spittle: is it vile and disgusting, or a coveted vessel of hope? Clearly beauty is in the eye of the beholder. After zipping up and *not* flushing – splatter being yet another effective means of conveyance – he reaches out with the palm of his right hand and deliberately smears it with the spittle. Then, with that hand, he proceeds down the line of urinals intentionally grasping the handles of each, knowing the virus will wait there – like passengers for their bus – for up to two days, or, short of that, until cleaned off by a minimum wage janitor with a maximum strength disinfectant. Dr. Nakayama now turns towards the row of sinks. Stepping up to the sink furthest to the right, and resisting the instinct to wash his hands, he takes deliberate effort to touch its hot and cold knob handles. He then works his way up the row of identical sinks, fondling the handles of each. That done – and his newfound *business* here in the restroom truly accomplished – he picks up his briefcase and moves towards the exit. There, just before he is about to push through, yet another opportunity presents itself; this one in the form of the rectangular brass plate mounted on the swing-hinged door. This will be a good one. Without even having to think about it this time, Dr. Nakayama spits into his open palm, which he then presses against the brass plate. That done – mission accomplished – he pushes on through door and exits the restroom.

Just outside the restroom now, Dr. Nakayama pauses to shove his thick glasses back up his sweaty nose, then looks both to the right and left along the wide, busy, departure concourse corridor. And though his countenance may appear expressionless, his mind is churning: *So many opportunities, so little time.*

The airport's ubiquitous Public Address speaker then chirps, in Portuguese, some pertinent departures update, which it repeats in Spanish, then in English, "Now boarding Flight 2122 for Tokyo and Seoul, Gate 28."

Dr. Nakayama pulls his boarding pass from his jacket pocket then – setting a course down the exact middle of the corridor and deliberately against the flow of the other pedestrians whenever possible – he begins walking towards his appointed departure gate, muttering in Japanese to himself en route, *This is it, this is it, this is it....*

Dr. Singh happens to notice Dr. Nakayama walking past, appearing like some catatonic automaton mumbling to himself as he walks against traffic up the center of the terminal corridor. And though he may look like a stranger she knows, in reality, he is closer to her in many ways than her siblings, sharing something closer than mere DNA – an idea, a purpose, a hope. After Dr. Nakayama walks past and disappears in the crowd of travelers, probably never to be seen by her again, Dr. Singh resumes what she had been doing; ostensibly reading the <u>Delhi Times</u>, but really just weeping to herself. She sits in a departure gate amidst hundreds of other Indians waiting for the same delayed flight. Alone in the crowd. Like them, she is dressed in a colorful sari. She has the ruby glued to her forehead, the heavy eyeliner, the fine gold jewelry, et al. She can *pass*. Maybe it's the Indian children laughing and chasing one another around the rows of seats that has elicited the remorse she feels churning within her. Maybe it's genuine shame. Or maybe it's her own fear of death, but she doesn't think so. The headline of the newspaper proudly announced India's population has just surpassed China's for the first time. 1.28 billion. This is heralded as a proud moment for India. "We're #1!" – the headline boasts. Quite contrary to feeling any patriotic pride for the momentous occasion, Dr. Singh is thoroughly embarrassed by it. *What's there to be proud of? – that we can live in utter squalor and stupidly reproduce like rats?* Beyond embarrassment, she is infuriated. In her mind any hope for her nation to get a grip on its population explosion died with the suicide bomb attack on its seventh Prime Minister, Rajiv Gandhi, for he was their only leader to ever attempt to do anything about it. During his administration it was unspoken policy that anyone hoping to get a government job had to practice family planning. Vasectomies and birth control were encouraged. When this dirty little secret was revealed he was vilified. *What an intrusion! What an outrage! What a despot!* Fortunately he had died before they could stone him to death and drag his corpse through the streets in the name of human reproductive rights – in the name of God's will. After Rajiv's death, well, there was just no mentioning the burgeoning population problem. It was swept under the rug. The people were free to pursue happiness, and if that meant having six, seven, fifteen children, well then, so be it. If it meant surpassing Japan's greenhouse gas emissions, just as China had surpassed the United States back in 2008, well then, so be it. If that meant the utter destruction of any Indian wilderness, the denuding of the Himalaya, the sucking-dry of any remaining aquifer, and the extinction of the Indian elephant and the Bengal Tiger, well then, so be it. If it meant even greater tensions with Pakistan and the Tamil Tigers, well then, so be it. If that meant another famine and all the suffering that comes with that, well then, so be it. *Fuck it, nobody's gonna tell us what to do. We're #1!*

Dr. Alyesha Singh never had children, never even considered it. Still being under thirty, it was not a matter of her biological window closing. Rather, it was the plain and simple reality of the state of the world into which she would be bringing a child. And who with open eyes and a heart could do that?

There is a mythical image of India she shares with probably everyone in this departure gate; of a land just barely still attached to the temporal world, on the very threshold of transcendence. In that mythical image Dr. Singh is bejeweled and sparkling, her vividly colored sari and long silky hair flowing weightlessly. And she is just emerging from the pristine, crystalline waters of the Ganges River in Varanasi, where life, Hindus believed, began. She is radiant, of course, and beneath her wet homespun cotton there's the swollen belly of a second trimester pregnancy. The Goddess Shiva is rubbing Alyesha's belly and smiling approvingly. Blue Vishnu extends his gleaming sword down to her from Nirvana. And this is a daily activity; she is merely taking her morning bath here in the holy river and will thereafter float back to her cool marbled Taj Mahal-esque home and dine on fruits and curried nuts and nectar and play the sitar. She is in utter bliss, but such is mythical life; the way it was intended, the way the travel brochures portray her homeland.

But the reality of India is a bit different. What with two-thirds of the Himalayan glaciers that feed the Ganges now melted, the mighty river is barely more than an all-but-dry creek these days. Rowboats lie grounded on cracked mud banks. But, oh, are the cremation ghats still busy! Smoke fills the air with the putrid burning stench of bodies; bodies which arrive on trains, rickshaws, and the roofs of taxis, bodies of those who had come here to Varanasi to die in the hope of being whisked promptly from this tedious treadmill of death and rebirth, and up into Nirvana forever more. But, like everything, it's all a matter of perspective. Ask one of the hundreds of stray dogs that live near the Ganges cremation ghats what they think of the filthy place, and they'll tell you that it is indeed Paradise. But this is only because they feed – and feed well – on the incompletely cremated human remains – hips, internal organs, skulls, and whatever might still be found therein – that the fire tenders flick into the holy river with their long, fire-poking poles. *Fetch!* But for humans this place is no Paradise. In reality the Ganges is far from blue, and probably will never be again.

In reality it is little more than a culvert for raw sewage in the dry season, and a relentless, unchecked, erosive, muddy torrent in the monsoon. And the sky? – hardly ever blue anymore either. Brown. Brown like the water. Brown like the dust-dry soil. Brown like her people.

But are they really *her* people? Some still perceive ethnic distinctions – Indian, African, Latino, Caucasian, Asian, Arab, Aboriginal, Native American, etcetera – as if they had always been different from one another, as if sprouted up from the slimy pond in the land where they now reside or else planted there by God. But scientists, or anyone curious enough to look into it, know such racial distinctions only evolved in the last 70,000 years since humanity's initial exodus out of our common African homeland. In reality, every human is of African descent, the only subsequent racial distinctions determined by *when* each ethnic group's ancestors emigrated out of Africa and *where* they settled. And as it happened, a lot of them settled on the southern Asian subcontinent – hugging the Indian Ocean as there were glaciers just to the north of them – and in India in particular. And there they multiplied for some 40,000 years until they finally ran out of room and burst at the seams. Which is why, here today, in this sprawling airport departure gate, their relocated progeny can be found; some now calling themselves *South Americans of Indian descent*, some – particularly the free-floating Gen X and Gen Y'ers – preferring the label *World Citizens* as they jet about the globe on the fumes of prosperity – mixing it up, killing time, searching for purpose.

The call comes in: "Pre-boarding of Air India flight 1221 for Dhaka, Calcutta, New Delhi, and Mumbai," first in Portuguese, then Spanish, then English.

Dr. Singh rises from her seat. As with all her fellow passengers, she feels that naïve compulsion to cut in line and be among the first on the plane, just as they'll all spring to their feet prematurely in the futile desire to be among the first off again some fourteen hours hence. But she resists the pull, the temptation. Instead she just stands and patiently waits, letting the others cut and shoulder past her. It's all right; no one's really going anywhere. She's feeling a bit lightheaded, a bit warm as well. Maybe this is how it feels to be pregnant, she muses. Then again, she *is* pregnant, in a manner of speaking. It's been, let's see, eleven hours since she took in the virus, so right about now the first cells in her lungs are erupting, releasing into her body a thousand subtly different mutations of the strain exhumed from the Eskimo mass grave – giving birth.

the momentum of folly

And then the call: "Final boarding for Air India flight 1221 for Dhaka, Calcutta, New Delhi, and Mumbai," first in Portuguese, then Spanish, then English. This time Dr. Singh notices the person making the announcement; a young check-in gal – sweet, bubbly, Brazilian, looking proud of her smart Air India uniform, her life and the world still ahead of her.

Every other passenger is now through the gangway and on the 747, but Dr. Singh is still lingering in the departure gate – expressionless. The Air India check-in gal is about to close the gateway door when she notices Dr. Singh still standing there in the now emptied room. She smiles, and politely nudges the obviously preoccupied professor back to the here and now: "Señora? Time to return to your beautiful motherland, home of the Ganges."

Dr. Singh stares at the employee – just a girl really – her beatific smile, wise well beyond her years, perhaps even beyond this lifetime. "Could she know?" Alyesha asks herself. "Is she some demi-god somehow participating in this plot towards the common good on another temporal plane? Is there magic in this world after all; work being done by *others*? And, if so, are they my instrument or am I merely theirs?" All this is what Dr. Singh is pondering behind the ruby stuck to her puzzled brow, as the girl holds open the door for her – the *gateway* – and beckons her forth with a polite nod of her beautiful head, and that radiant, calming, otherworldly smile.

Dr. Henri LaFond steps through the end of the gangway tunnel and onto the plane. Like just about all his fellow passengers he doesn't think much about the plane itself – never really even sees it – just walks into it blindly, hands his boarding pass to the sexy Air France flight attendant, tells her what he'd like to do with her all in a flash of a devilish grin, then begins down the aisle towards his personally selected seat. Like the other passengers, the plane is just a means to an end, however different their *ends* may be.

"Window or aisle?" he was asked by a travel agent, some months ago already.

"Neither, please. Call me weird if you must, but is it possible for me to have the seat smack-dab in the middle of the plane?" he responded, in what already seems like another lifetime.

Henri had his first baby teeth at three and a half months, walked well before his first birthday, and had his first wet dream – remembers it well – before his twelfth, so it comes as no surprise to him the virus has already taken over his lungs. That's just how he's always been; naturally impatient. The fact he's already sweating profusely has turned some heads as he bumps and shoulders his way down one aisle and up the other, seemingly lost as he searches for his seat throughout the vast passenger compartment.

"Masseur, are you all right?" another flight attendant asks him with concern.

"Couldn't be better," he assures her, with an inscrutable grin before succumbing to another series of coughs.

What is good? What is evil? Humans, Adam and Eve in particular, purportedly tried to make that distinction long ago and were booted from the Garden of Eden for it and, as a result, now have to wear these damn fig leaves. "Does this fig leaf make me look fat?" Jenna once asked Henri. That's what he loved about her. That's why they married. It made no sense that they should wed — neither being the spousal type — but what else is there to do when two people find the only other person on the planet that shares the same humor, scientific curiosity, material disinterest, primal sexuality, and basic disdain for humanity? One marries it and hopes for the best. One slips a ring over the other's finger and then heads off in the opposite direction. That's what they did anyway.

"Ladies and Gentlemen, the Captain has turned on the seatbelt light. Please take your seats at this time," one unseen flight attendant announces perfunctorily over the plane's PA system.

Henri squeezes in towards his seat; the middle one in the row of five there in the center section. There's a chubby man in the seat next to his, who appears already annoyed that Henri has come to claim his seat — the seat he has already spread his things over.

"Pardon me," Henri says to the man, with a disingenuous smile, secretly wishing he could fart in the man's chubby pink face as he squeezed past.

So, what is evil exactly? Just because Henri devised a plan to horrifically terminate two-thirds of humanity, does that make him bad? Does that make him any less loved by God? If so, are not his actions defensible by the fact he is only doing all this in order to save the world's flora and fauna from the ravenous infection of humanity, and thereby to save humanity from itself? So, doesn't that make him the opposite of evil? He's just a guy trying to save the world, as much for humans as for frogs; when did that become a bad thing?

Henri takes his seat and buckles in.

the momentum of folly

The chubby man beside him plucks the red Tootsie Pop from his mouth and sticks it on the tray before him then bends over to stuff his briefcase under his seat. Henri glances at the Tootsie Pop, thinking to himself, "Oh, this is too easy."

Within a second, Henri has the chubby man's Tootsie Pop in his mouth. Cherry – his favorite. There is a six-year-old sitting just to Henri's left who happens to witness all this with silent alarm. Still enjoying the Tootsie Pop, while the chubby man still struggles obliviously with his briefcase, Henri raises a wry brow for the six-year-old, calmly pulls the Tootsie Pop from his mouth, and places it exactly where he found it, back on the unsuspecting chubby man's tray.

"Jesus H. Christ," the man groans, sitting upright again, out of breath and obviously frustrated by the passenger compartment's cramped quarters, "they outta call this Air *Sardine* instead of Air France!"

Ignoring the chubby man's quip, Henri just winks and smiles at the six-year-old, thus sealing their little secret, then calmly folds his hands, leans back, coughs once, then closes his eyes, content now to let nature, blessed Mother Nature, run its course.

The Nigerian Air 757 sits out on the tarmac, seemingly ready for takeoff. But inside is a different story: the Captain, summoned back into the main compartment, nods and tries to smile to the passengers – predominantly black Africans like himself – as he moves down the aisle towards the coach section. A Ugandan woman in Western attire, steps into his path to vent her frustration:

"We've been sitting here one hour. Take her off the plane!"

"Yes, yes, I'll do whatever I have to to get this plane in the air," the Captain tells her, quite honestly, with two hands placed reassuringly on her shoulders and looking her in the eye until the woman lets him step past her.

Another passenger shouts out, equally as perturbed, from nearby, "We're all going to miss our connections!"

"I know, I know. Nobody likes it when this happens, especially me!" he assures them all, as he continues towards the problem, another ten rows back.

The commotion centers around an aisle seat in row sixty-three, where approximately a dozen passengers hover around the one troublemaker. The Captain pauses to speak with one of his flight attendants before he enters the fray.

"Is it a medical issue?" he asks, discreetly.

The flight attendant shakes her head, "I thinks it's just anxiety, maybe some family problem; she won't say."

The Captain nods, then ever so politely – using gentle words and his flat, outstretched hand – penetrates the layers of the just-curious and the just-trying-to-help, until he at last reaches the nucleus of the consternation. Here another two flight attendants attempt to calm the passenger of concern; one by kneeling in the aisle and holding her hand, the other by massaging her temples when possible. The Captain leans towards the flight attendant holding the problematic passenger's hand and asks in a polite whisper, "Do you know her name?"

The flight attendant nods and whispers back to the Captain, "Jenna; Dr. Jenna Williams. I think she's American."

The Captain nods. Trying to figure out the most effective way to resolve the matter, he squats on his haunches beside the flight attendant and takes over the holding of Jenna's hand. He then speaks directly to her, in the softest voice he can.

"Dr. Williams, I am Capt. Mutumbo. Are you going to be all right?"

A fresh stream of tears trickle down Jenna's cheeks as she contemplates the question briefly. She clenches her eyes tightly but neither nods nor shakes her head, forcing the Captain to try another tack.

"Would you like me to let you get off the plane? It's no problem. Do you have any family or friends here in San Paulo you'd like me to call to come pick you up?"

With her eyes still clenched, Jenna now violently shakes her head.

"So, you would like to stay on board?" the Captain asks, still trying to understand the source of Jenna's apprehension.

Again Jenna says nothing, and neither shakes or nods, but just clenches her face even more tightly and now even begins stomping her feet – once, twice, three times – thrashing about in utter but still cryptic distress.

Himself at a loss, the Captain glances up to the flight attendant attempting to comfort Jenna's head – which Jenna seems to welcome. The flight attendant shrugs back her own sense of confusion over the problem, stating: "She flies a lot; I don't think she's worried about the plane."

The Captain nods, then turns back to Jenna. Searching for words, he finally tells her: "Sometimes I have passengers who are leaving loved ones or family, or even their own children, who they think they will never see again. Is that the case?"

Jenna clenches her face again, still refusing to confirm or deny the guess.

The Captain and flight attendant exchange another glance; they think he's probably stumbled upon the issue here.

"All right, Dr. Williams, I'm going to leave you on the flight –" he begins, eliciting immediate groans from some of the passengers. "I'm going to let you stay on board, but I must warn you, if I have to, I'll turn the plane right around, or drop you off at the nearest airport, because I have many other passengers who need to make connections or get home to loved ones as well. Do you understand?"

Jenna scrunches up her face again but this time manages to force out a nod.

"Good. Now, whatever's the matter – and it's fine to keep it to yourself – just trust that it will pass. I know it must not seem that way now but these things always resolve themselves. You're obviously a very intelligent woman, so I don't have to tell you."

This gets Jenna stomping again, but just once, offering the Captain and crew hope she may be on the way out of her fit.

"Now, do you have any medication with you?"

Jenna shakes her head, still teary, still mute.

"Can I get you something to drink: water, soda, a cocktail, perhaps?"

At the mention of cocktail, Jenna suddenly relaxes as some Pavlovian response suddenly takes over.

"*Cocktail!* Alright, what, scotch?" the Captain asked, hopeful again.

Jenna shakes her head.

"Gin and tonic with lime? – that's my poison," one of the attendants offers.

But Jenna shakes her head again, almost as if they're all playing Twenty Questions or something now.

Someone else, a passenger, tosses out her guess, "Wine?"

To which Jenna shakes her head yet again, prompting the Captain to ask, "Beer?"

At the mere mention of beer, at the mere prospect of holding an ice, cold one right about now – pressing it to her forehead, sipping it down – Jenna goes completely limp; all tension, all worry, all doubt is instantly allowed to flow from her through the fingertips of the attendant massaging her scalp.

"We have Heineken on ice, right? Go get her one, and hurry, please," Jenna can hear the Captain order someone; it doesn't matter whom; salvation is nigh and the salivary response is undeniable. She can almost taste it — no, she *can* taste it. All is right with the universe, or, at least, soon will be.

Five jumbo jets, each filled to capacity — one just now retracting its landing gear, two still banked in their initial turns, all still ascending to their cruising altitudes — fan out over the Atlantic, each heading off to five different parts of the globe, each oblivious to what they have on board.

Atlanta, Georgia

It's another hot one, and all the local radio and television hosts and commentators can seem to talk about is the drought and the freshwater shortages and the raging dispute over water allocations to be shared with Alabama and Florida, and who has the rights to what. It's the same story over in the Sierra Nevada, where lighter than usual snow pack melted more quickly than usual resulting in 60% of normal reservoir levels. The same chatter can be heard in Spain, Australia, sub-Saharan Africa; the same myopic cries for more dams, more pipelines, more desalination plants.

"What the hell's going on?" Stuart finds himself muttering aloud as he spins deftly, on a wheelie again, out the front door of his and Carl's bungalow. "Oil is over $140 per barrel – *again*. Rice sold for $1,600 per metric ton on the Bangkok exchange this morning. There's food rioting now in over forty countries, by people obviously with still enough meat on their bones *to* riot. Over one billion people live on less than one dollar a day and that dollar buys only one-fifth the rice it did a year ago. "How am I supposed to feed my eleven children?" one Haitian man shouted to a CNN reporter, before turning to hurl a Molotov cocktail at the still-earthquake-leveled Governor's palace.

There was a time, and not all that long ago, when Stuart loved nothing more than to smoke a "fattie" and read the newspaper and laugh at all the bizarre goings-on in the world. But now that hobby is just too depressing. He might smoke the fattie, but then he'll have to forego the newspaper. Or he might read the newspaper, but then – shutter to think – he'll have to forego the fattie. And sometimes – more and more lately – he does neither. *Maybe just one bong hit; a tiny one, out of solidarity for the one billion who have to go with less rice today.* That was his rationale this morning, but even that wee little fraction of a buzz slid a magnifying lens over the news and caused it all to overwhelm him. It's obvious, it's plain as day; It's the end of the world as we know it.

the momentum of folly

"Thank God I don't have kids," Stuart muttered as he pulls the front door closed behind him and locks it. Locks it? *When the hell did I start locking the front door?* he now finds himself pondering, staring at the lock and the keys in his hand. *And what does that say about society or the human race in general; when did we have to begin locking things away from our brethren?* he wonders now, leaping immediately to the macro. But as quickly as his mind wanders away, he reels it in again. *Fuck it,* he mutters to himself with the explanation, *It's just the pot,* followed quickly by the injunction: *Must get to work, must find way through maze, must earn cheese.* Such mind control.

Stuart sets the keys onto his computer case resting there in his lap, then spins his wheelchair towards the plywood ramp. This is his favorite part of the day: with just the right exploitation of gravitational acceleration he can coast all the way to the sliding side door of his VW van. But he has to stay on two wheels to make it; that's the trick. If he were to use all four wheels – particularly the tiny, wobbly front ones – there would simply be too much rolling resistance and he'd never make it even down as far as the sidewalk. He balances there between the never-used handrails at the edge of the porch, psyching himself up like a downhill ski racer in the gates. He begins the beeping countdown: *Five, four, three –*

But that's when he sees it: the Fed Ex envelope. It must have fallen off the porch. It's probably that neighborhood cat's fault; it probably pushed the envelope off the porch while trying to rub his scent on it. *Fucking cat!* The envelope is lying in the flower-less flowerbed now, where even the most drought-resistant weeds have uprooted and migrated away in search of water.

"Fuck!" Stuart mutters again, aloud this time. His distress isn't elicited by the envelope's presence having interrupted his favorite-part-of-the-day-coast-to-the-van; rather, it is all due to the present location of the missive – there in the flowerbed beneath the ramp. It means he'll have to wheel himself down to the bottom of the ramp, brake, climb out of his wheelchair, then drag himself across the dead lawn and through the dirt to get to it. Sure, he's done it before. Lots of times: for the mail, the newspaper, other Fed Ex missives. It's not that it is all that difficult a task; it's just that it's degrading. Particularly if the girl next door who just got her drivers' license happens to be skipping out to her mom's car, already fumbling for cigarettes in her purse, clacking chewing gum, and chirping into her cellphone to some equally-disgusted friend, "Ohmygod, the freak next door is doing it again! Gross! — somebody oughta, like, hit him with a shovel and put him outta his misery. Ohmygod!"

But she isn't there, so Stuart coasts down to the bottom of the ramp, and parks.

Probably <u>her</u> fucking cat! Stuart mutters, somehow just now putting it together that the neighborhood cat might just belong to his, *duh*, neighbor.

Tucking his pride aside somewhere with his keys and laptop, Stuart climbs from his wheelchair and begins to drag himself across the dead lawn towards the deader flowerbed. It actually feels good, the exercise. He really should do more of it; particularly swimming, like his neurologist prescribed. But that's even more embarrassing; him with his withered legs, the lifeguards down at the YMCA having to help him out of his wheelchair and into the hoist chair that winches him down into the pool. And then who has to stay with him? The senior lifeguards always assign the gruesome tasks to the newbie lifeguard, just like it's the greenhorn Army grunt who always draws latrine duty. That's just how it is. And now that Stuart has been seeing the girl next door pull her YMCA sweatshirt over her red, one-piece lifeguard bathing suit, up there through her window curtains, well, suffice it to stay, he just can't go to the YMCA pool anymore. That's just how it is.

Halfway across the lawn the thought crosses Stuart's mind to turn back and just leave the Fed Ex package where it is. There's already a good eight, nine, ten sun-yellowed newspapers there; would it really matter all that much if the Fed Ex missive were to join them? Would the world come to a screeching halt?

It might.

Avoiding the dust-dry clumps of cat poop — *I oughta stuff this shit in her mailbox, that's what I oughta do!* — Stuart stretches out his arm from the lawn, across the flowerless-flowerbed-cum-kitty-litter-box, and manages to just pinch the corner of the envelope between his so-very-useless ring finger and so-very-useful middle finger. And in pulling the envelope towards him and turning it over and reading the address label, he sees that it is from Carl, from Alaska.

He ponders the envelope for a moment — feeling the slight bulge caused by the small vial contained therein — pondering what to do next about it; where to take it, how to proceed with the analysis, who to tell, who to trust? Clenching the envelope between his teeth, Stuart begins the crawl back towards his wheelchair.

* * *

CDC National Center for Immunization and Respiratory Diseases, Atlanta, Georgia

―――

The trucks are already beginning to roll in from the outlaying chicken ranches under contract with the CDC to produce fertilized chicken eggs. Some come from Georgia, others from neighboring states; Alabama, Florida, Kentucky, Tennessee. Most of the trucks are the little box-tail types, carrying ten to twenty thousand eggs tops. That's not a lot compared with the numbers the CDC and WHO will ultimately need. This is just the starter batch in which the virus can be grown then shipped worldwide to the pharmaceutical companies under contract to manufacture the vaccine on a much larger scale; Sanofi Pasteur, GlaxoSmithKline, Aventis, Chiron, Aegis, etc. Aventis and Chiron will handle the vaccine production for the United States, which will top 185 million doses this year. This will require 92.5 million fertilized eggs in which to grow the virus, just in the United States. Global production will be handled by half a dozen or so companies in all, with the aggregate goal of producing nearly a billion doses in eight months. That won't happen of course, it never quite does – there's always some hitch, some contamination, some breakdown in the all-too-complicated process – but that's the stated aggregate goal.

The bobtail truck just ahead of Stuart's van is holding up traffic at the EID Lab's entry gate. The driver it seems is in an argument with the entrance gate guards about having to surrender his drivers' license in exchange for a security badge. How many times has Stuart seen this same scene played out? Dozens.

"Give it up, dumbshit!" Stuart shouts at the truck driver, though his voice barely makes it through his windshield. And right about now is when Stuart would back up his shouts by laying on the horn; that is, if his horn worked. But it doesn't, fortunately, so he just pounds his fist against the center of his steering wheel as if it did.

Finally, with a disgusted, abused, capitulating shake of his head the truck driver surrenders his drivers' license to the guard, indignantly snaps the temporary security pass from the gate guard's hand, and drives on into the laboratory compound, thereby allowing Stuart to finally pull up to the gate.

"Hey, Stuart," the guard says, standing just outside his air-conditioned booth.

"Hey, Ernie," Stuart replies, passing his CDC ID through his forever-rolled-down-because-it-too-is-broken driver's side window. "So, what was that guy's problem?"

"Same as usual. They think I'm out to steal their IDs or something."

Stuart nods then, alluding towards the guard booth, facetious asks, "Which reminds me; got any drivers' licenses in there you'd like to sell me?"

"Damn tootin', I do. Which state?" the guard rifts back, before slapping the roof of Stuart's van and telling him, "Ah, get in there and save the world, you knucklehead!"

Stuart smiles and salutes the guard then drives on through the gate, and into the sprawling campus of facilities.

For whatever reason — probably denial, maybe up-yours stubbornness — Stuart has never been one to use a handicapped parking spot. Doesn't even carry the placard to hang in his windshield. And unlike seemingly everyone else he doesn't try to wedge into the next closest parking spot. Who needs that door-denting headache? — even if he were the type who worried about door dents. Quite to the contrary, he seems to always seek out that parking spot far away from everyone else, and rarely the same one if he can help it. But that is all very intentional on his part: routine worries him. He has a theory that repetitive behavior shrinks the mind by pruning off physical synapses in the neuro-pathways, rendering it ever the more narrow. And who's to say he's wrong? Who's to say taking a slightly different route to work, mixing up one's sleep cycle, taking up a new instrument or language, switching to a completely antithetical religion or gender for that matter, isn't good for the mind? It certainly is exercise, after all. And exercise is good, is it not? And that — exercise being the subject now — is exactly why Stuart has never got himself a motorized wheelchair. That, in his mind, is for handicapped people. He's more of a jock, you see; a jock who happens to be confined to a wheelchair but one who also happens to be able to get around better than most Americans, much better. So let Stella, the 270-pound receptionist, have the handicap spot *and* his placard. She needs it. Not him.

And so Stuart is wrestling his wheelchair out the side door of his van, unfolding it with one shake of a strong arm, when he happens to notice the little boxtail truck he followed into the compound is presently backing up to the E.I.D. lab loading dock. Muttering something to himself like, "Haven't rolled through E.I.D. in a while," Stuart plops himself into the wheelchair, pulls his computer case and Fed Ex package onto his lap, then – with one mighty burst of upper body power – heads away in that direction.

An electric forklift extracts a pallet of ten-gross eggs from the rear of the boxtail truck, then, without turning, backs them into the E.I.D. lab's shipping and receiving entrance.

"Hey, Stuart, that a new bumper sticker you're sportin'?" Denise, the shipping & receiving clerk, quips as she registers the arrival of the fertilized eggs on a clipboard.

"You're referring, I'm guessing, to the iridescent green sticker on the back of my wheelchair which boasts the caption *Hemp-Powered* embossed over a plant bearing an uncanny resemblance to a cannabis sativa leaf?" Stuart quips back, as he pushes through the entrance, spinning once on his hind wheels to make facial contact with Denise.

"That's right."

"I have no idea what you're talking about."

"*Uh-huh*," Denise says, skeptically.

"I'm serious. I'm just a crippled kid; people stick things back there and I can't really stop them!" Stuart fabricates.

Denise smiles and shakes her head, and the doors close.

"By the way, I'd sure like to fertilize *your* eggs!" Stuart calls out to her, but only for his own amusement knowing she can't hear him through the now-closed doors.

"Oh, Stuart, that's the single sweetest thing you've ever said to me," a voice calls out from just behind him.

Shocked and embarrassed, Stuart spins forward again to find the Emerging Infectious Disease Facility Manager Ross Corman, pretending to be responding to Stuart's solicitation as he registers the eggs' arrival onto his laptop.

"Uh..." Stuart stumbles, embarrassed.

the momentum of folly

Ross grins before turning back to the forklift driver, regarding the shipment of eggs, "Alright, take these bad boys straight into the inoculation shed. Gotta get them started ASAP."

The forklift driver nods and drives off with the eggs, permitting Stuart the opportunity to explain, "Actually, I wasn't speaking to you."

"No? Well, now I'm offended," Ross ripostes, wryly.

Stuart decides to change the subject: "How long after inoculation are you fixin' to hold onto the eggs?"

"First batch, the full seventy-two hours. The second generation we'll start shipping out to the pharmaceuticals after just sixty, let 'em cook in transit."

"Not wasting any time, are we?"

"2008's vaccine was only 44% effective. By the looks of this one we're gonna have to swap out all three strains to do any better this season."

"*All three?!* Have we ever had to do that before?"

"Nope." Ross casts Stuart an expression conveying both the threat and dread of the uphill battle awaiting them, then turns and simply walks away, the soft sounds of his shoes echoing up the linoleum corridor.

After Ross pushes through the doors at the visible end of the corridor, Stuart hears the transmission whine of the same electric forklift now backing out of the inoculation shed, conveying another load of eggs. The forklift driver, looking over his shoulder to see where he's going, nods to Stuart as he drives past.

Stuart nods back then signs off by shouting out, "Rock on!" to which the forklift driver just shakes his head and keeps driving, moving the eggs on towards the virus incubation rooms.

Sensing an opportunity, what with the driver looking the other way, Stuart gives his wheels as many mighty arm pumps as it takes for him to catch up with the cargo of eggs being pulled by the forklift. Grabbing onto the back of the egg racks with one hand, Stuart allows the forklift to pull him along for long enough to allow him to slyly swipe a single egg from off a rack. And Stuart hangs on there while he inspects the egg, making sure it bears the dated CDC biohazard stamp which confirms it has indeed been injected with the virus. Seeing that it does, Stuart releases his hold on the forklift, allowing his wheelchair to coast to a slow, pirouetting stop.

Alone now in the corridor Stuart tosses the egg triumphantly in the air once and catches it while saying, *Yes!* But it is a premature display of revelry and he knows it. Holding the fertilized, presumably-infected egg in one hand, he picks up the Fed-Ex envelope containing Carl's presumably-infected blood sample in the other. Now all he has to do is figure out how best to compare the two.

Breaking an egg is no big deal. Breaking an egg remotely using robotic arms and then smearing the yolk onto a slide can be a bit more challenging. But Stuart manages, making only a tolerable mess of it. His next big obstacle could also be mindlessly simple were it not for the potentially lethal nature of the samples to be analyzed: he would simply pick up the slide with his fingers and put it on the microscope's table; so simple a task he could do it with one hand while eating a slice of pizza with the other. But that's not how it works with pathogens, especially those of this caliber. As it is, Stuart is a good meter away from the aforementioned slides, separated by two layers of safety glass, and trying to move them about with these damn robotic arms. And he thought his legs were useless! Carefully nudging the slide to the edge of the containment autoclave he manages to pinch a corner of it with the robotic fingers and pick it up. That was the hard part. Now comes the task of setting it on the microscope table and nudging it into place beneath the atomic force microscope, which Stuart manages quite deftly; as one would expect since this, in a nutshell, is what he does here at the CDC, this is his job.

An atomic force microscope, like the electron microscope and other scanning probe microscopes, isn't the type of device one just peers into with a bloodshot eyeball and then focuses with a shaky hand. In fact the name – "scope" – is a bit of a misnomer in that the machine *feels* rather than *looks* at the specimen studied. This *feeling* is done with a silicon nitrate tip and measured with an array of photodiodes monitoring a lazar beam reflected off a cantilever, which together bring resolution down to a fraction of a nanometer, thus enabling mere mortals the ability – nay, the *privilege* – to be able to actually see individual viruses or even individual atoms. As painstakingly slow as the process always seems to be, it's not long before Stuart is looking at the actual virus strand packed and shipped by Carl back at the Shanghai airport.

"*Boom, there it is!*" he mutters, taking only a moment to revel in this extraordinary opportunity to behold a living Bird flu stand adding, "the baddest of the bad." After a nerve-calming breath, Stuart dutifully photographs then labels – "H5N1/Laos/2010" – then logs the strain into his computer.

Next Stuart pulls from the *Do not ship liquids, blood or fluids in this package* Fed Ex envelope the vial of blood drawn by Carl from his own arm in that grungy Anchorage port-a-potty. Then after more considerable preparation and clumsy robotics, Stuart is finally able to gaze upon the other influenza virus, now viewable up on the atomic force microscope's monitor screen and, as well, on the screen of his attached computer — *"And, boom, there it is.* Well, Carl, you definitely have *a* flu. Now let's see how you match up to *the* flu," Stuart mutters to himself.

After similarly photographing, labeling and logging the strain extracted from Carl, Stuart juxtaposes its image split-screen alongside the strain couriered back from the Shanghai Airport on the screen of his laptop. "Now let's see how you match up against that bad boy from Laos." Side-by-side like this, the two virus strands resemble a couple of withered sea horses, looking similar but hardly clones of one another. But then Stuart rotates the image of one, then inverts the image of the other, then slides the image of one over the other, and *voile*, a perfect match of RNA proteins and sheathing appears before his dazed eyes. It will take gene sequencing of both samples to confirm these are indeed the same exact strain of influenza, but for now, *optically*, the match appears all but certain.

Stuart pulls away from the computer screen to ponder the ramifications of his discovery: if genetic sequencing indeed confirms these two samples to be *one in the same*, as they visually appear to be here, and *that* strain is subsequently proven to be *one in the same* with the one that ravaged the Laotian village — as assured by one of the world's top epidemiologists, Dr. Jenna Williams — then it's a logical assumption for Stuart to place Carl's chances of surviving the next few days at barely one-in-three.

"Shit!"

Stuart hastily wheels himself from out of the Atomic Force Microscopy labs, cellphone pinched between his ear and shoulder.

"Dr. Galloway, please," he begs into the phone, urgency greased with just the necessary proportion of respect to cut through the anticipatable hierarchal buffers.

Meanwhile, a couple hundred meters away over on the ground floor of the Administration Building, Dr. Bronwyn Galloway — arms full, laptop slung over her shoulder, obviously headed somewhere in a hurry — is just trying her damn best to leave her office. And as she does, her assistant — whose endless list of job responsibilities includes maintaining those aforementioned hierarchal buffers – is on the other end of the aforementioned phone call with Stuart. The assistant glances up to her boss for direction. Bronwyn shakes her head adamantly, prompting her assistant to reply into the phone:

"I'm sorry, Dr. Galloway is in a meeting. May I take a message?"

"Did I mention this is urgent; really, really, highly, highly, priority-code-red-type- urgent. Is there a number I can – or *you* can – text her?" Stuart pleads.

As the assistant still hesitates, Stuart tries another tact. Speaking in a hushed voice to make it sound as if the information he's about to confide is highly secretive, he cups his hand around his phone and whispers, "Listen, I'm on your guys' side and all, but if it gets out – say, before a Congressional hearing six or so months from now – that Dr. Bronwyn *could've* had the information I'm trying to get to her but her assistant wouldn't take the call…."

Sufficiently threatened by Stuart's unstated implications, the assistant takes a breath for courage, then holds the phone out for Bronwyn to grab, all the while making sure to avert her eyes so as not to catch her boss's subsequent glower.

Almost out the door, Bronwyn rolls her eyes, then mouths to her assistant, *Who is it?*

"I'll try to reach her. Who shall I say is calling, please?" the assistant asks into the phone, cleverly placing Stuart on the speakerphone.

Stuart groans, weary of the routine. "Stuart Chew, in Microscopy." As soon as he replies, Stuart can hear his voice reverberating over the other end of the call, which causes him to immediately realize he's been put on speakerphone.

Meanwhile, on the other end of the call, upon hearing Stuart say his name Bronwyn shakes her head even more adamantly, thus instructing her assistant not to let Stuart know she is in the room to take the call.

It's a complicated game of telephone subterfuge. But Stuart – correctly deducing that the only reason for the assistant to put him on speakerphone would be if Bronwyn was indeed in the same room – quickly shouts out: "Dr. Bronwyn, I really, really need to speak to you!"

Bronwyn shakes her head again and mouths to her assistant, *Tell him I'll call back*, then steps out of the office., the door closing behind her.

The assistant stammers for a bit, but regurgitates the message, "May I have your number so she can return your call?"

"This is bullshit!" Stuart mutters, before shouting through the phone, "Dr. Galloway! Dr. Galloway!..."

Taking Stuart off the speakerphone, the assistant lowers her voice and attempts to interject in an urgent whisper, "Stuart, Stuart, shut up for a minute."

Stuart pauses, "What?"

"Dr. Galloway's headed for the conference room."

It takes Stuart a moment to realize the assistant is helping him. "Thanks!" he whispers back. After hanging up, Stuart immediately begins pumping his wheelchair towards the nearest exit. After pushing out through the lab door, he spins his wheelchair about in order to shout to the security guard posted there. "Hey, Theo, nobody goes into AFM. Seal it off; biohazard tape, armed guard – the whole nine yards. Nobody goes in, got it?"

"Sure, I got it. And if someone asks *why?*" the security guard asks wryly.

"For fucksake, Theo; this is the Emerging Infectious Disease Lab, use your fucking imagination!"

"It *was*."

"Was what?"

"It was the Emerging Infectious Disease lab. Now it's the National Center for Immunization and Respiratory Diseases lab."

"*Fuck!*" Stuart, already outside and pumping down the concrete walkway, shouts in frustration to the heavens.

"Whatever," the security guard grumbles under his breath, but already pulling the spool of red containment tape with the black biohazard logos from the security cabinet. He shakes his head a last time and shuts the cabinet. "What-*ever*."

Bronwyn comes down the main hall of the CCID Administration building with the weight of a thousand things on her mind. Or, perhaps more accurately, 350 *million* things. Any employee that might have had the sheer luck of glancing up from the data they were perusing and spotted *her* before she spotted *them* knew to quickly steer clear of her, or else suffer the likelihood of being delegated with some new, top priority task that would supercede the top priority task they were already working on and surely dash any weekend plans they might have had.

Bronwyn rounds a corner to find Ross, ten steps away and walking towards her at a fast clip. Ross negotiates an abrupt about-face; but not to avoid her like most everyone else, but rather to bring him in lockstep with Bronwyn.

"Morning," Ross says, intentionally avoiding the standard modifier – *good* – for fear of lighting an unnecessary fuse.

True to character, Bronwyn cuts to the chase. "The NIAID will need the very first batch of vaccine so they can begin field tests."

"I've already got a lot of organizations hounding me for that *very first batch*."

"Yeah, well, if we can't get it licensed we lose this race before it even begins."

Bronwyn and Ross approach the double glass doors at the end of the hall which lead into a glass breezeway connecting the CCID Administration building with the National Center for Zoonotic, Vector-Borne, and Enteric Diseases, the NCZVED, building.

"Not that it matters, but where we going?"

Bronwyn alludes straight up ahead towards the double glass doors, answering wryly, "This way."

"Right."

Stuart is outside the glass-enclosed, climate-controlled breezeway, furiously pumping his wheelchair to catch up with Bronwyn and Ross. Unfortunately, the concrete walkway to which he's confined only comes within about twenty meters of the breezeway. So, as a result, from the closest tangent to their path, the best he can do is to attempt to shout to them: "Hey! Dr. Bronwyn! Ross! Over here! Hey!"

But, encased in the double-pane glass as they are, and preoccupied by the urgent details of the work ahead, neither Bronwyn nor Ross hears Stuart's shouts.

So Stuart whistles; and even though it's one of those shrill and very loud fingerless whistles a cowboy on horseback might employ to nudge along a herd of recalcitrant cattle, still Bronwyn and Ross cannot hear it through the glass.

"Goddamnit," Stuart mutters to himself, coasting in his wheelchair, as he watches Bronwyn and Ross pass from the breezeway and on into a side entrance of the massive NCZVED laboratories building. But his defeat proves only temporary. After a bit of pondering about where their ultimate destination might be, he renews his pursuit, redirecting his furious pumpings towards the building's far end.

Bronwyn and Ross pass from the breezeway, through the NCZVED building's interior automated sliding doors and into its main corridor, artery to over forty biosafety labs. They emerge into the corridor in time to intercept Hank, moving from right to left as he rides aboard a slow-moving electric cart, creeping down the polished concrete alerting potential passersby with a beeping warning horn and flashing yellow strobe lights. Hank is seated alongside the NCZVED building's designated driver who has been with the CDC for so long he now looks to be attached to his cart —*one* with his cart, and in more than just the figurative sense. The procession is under the escort of two armed guards; trained CDC guards rather than the wannabe-rent-a-cops or retired Atlanta policemen offered up by most private security firms. All of this precaution is necessary due to the lethal nature of the cargo being conveyed, for latched down in cart's bed is a sturdy, clear Plexiglas case holding racked vials of the centrifuged serum, which happens to be about the most important stuff on the planet right about now.

"Good morning, Dr. Bronwyn, Dr. Ross," the driver says, with characteristic good cheer.

"Morning, Dave," Bronwyn replies, not at all relaxed as she and Ross join the procession's three miles per hour, overly cautious, compliance-dictated crawl down the corridor.

"Care to ride, doctors? Plenty of room," the driver offers, alluding to the open cart's unoccupied naugahyde rear bench.

Bronwyn, mustering a smile, shakes her head, "Thanks, but I foresee a lot of sitting in my near future."

"Alrighty then, I'll try not to leave you in the dust. Hold on to your hats everyone, next stop BSL-4!" the driver announces facetiously, as if he's about to accelerate, which of course he can't.

Ross walks alongside Hank's side of the cart, whispering to Hank as he alludes to the accompanying security detail: "Armed guards?"

"Protocol."

"You Bioterrorism Preparedness guys take this stuff seriously," Ross quips.

"I don't make the rules."

Another CCID technician, Nancy, spots the passing entourage from her office. Though she is in the middle of a phone call, she propels her desk chair partway out into the hall so she can shout after them from the doorway of her office:

"Ross?"

Ross turns, walking backwards as he speaks with the tech, "Nancy?"

Pointing at her telephone, Nancy tells him, "The FDA needs to know when they can expect the virus."

"Jesus! *Tomorrow*; everyone gets it *tomorrow!*"

"*Jesus*, I'll tell them!" Nancy snaps back, in a sarcastically annoyed way as she rolls back into her office.

"Whoa, everybody snappin' at one another; must be some hot stuff ridin' with us here, eh, Dr. Hank?" the driver asks.

"That's how we have to treat it anyway," Hank replies.

"So how many doses of vaccine should we shoot for?" Ross asks Bronwyn.

"Ideally?" Bronwyn asks back.

"How 'bout we start with *realistically?*"

"As lethal as this thing seems to be, there's no reason to suspect it's migrated outside of its initial village."

"Ergo, the minimum run; ten million doses?" Hank asks.

"But if it *has* spread beyond that initial village?" Ross presses Bronwyn.

"Worst case scenario; Southeast Asia is a busy, crowded, highly-interactive region with not much in the way of public health monitoring or control. So if it gets a foothold there we can expect it to spread fairly quickly around the globe."

"How quick is *fairly quickly?*" the driver asks.

Bronwyn shrugs, "There're a lot of variables, but within two to three months pretty much everyone on the planet — ninety to ninety-five percent of them anyway — could come in contact with it."

"And up to seventy percent of them could—," Hank is about to say *die*, until Bronwyn hushes him with a discreet shake of her head.

"Up to seventy percent of 'em could what?" the driver asks.

"Could get sick enough to miss work," Hank invents.

"Damn, that sure could rattle the already-rattled economy!" the driver reels.

"Exactly."

Ross begins to do the math: "So, what are we're talkin'? — between one and two billion doses to establish an effective herd immunity…"

Bronwyn nods, "Sounds about right."

"Two billion fertile eggs!" Ross says, his mind already reeling in anticipation of the logistics.

"That's one helluva omelet!" the driver remarks.

"No one's asking you to eat it," Ross quips, already wishing he could take the words back, for fear the driver would take it as a jab at his obesity.

"Whether two billion or just ten million, it doesn't change our work load any; whether it has breached that initial village or not, our job right now is simply to grow the virus. As we're doing that, we have to decide — in conjunction with the WHO — which other two influenza strains to include in the vaccine, then make up the prototype vaccine and get it out to the various federal and international licensing agencies ASAP so they can approve it ASAP. Then, as the reports from epidemiologists out in the field begin trickling in, apprising us as to how far and fast the virus is spreading, then it's up to the WHO and us to determine how many doses to license the various pharmaceuticals to start producing."

The driver nods then asks, "How long does that take?"

"From right now — the day we first receive the strain — to the point where there's enough vaccine stockpiled and packaged and ready to begin administering worldwide? — we're talkin' a minimum six to eight months," Hank says.

"So, six months, but the virus can spread in just two to three months, how's that work? How can you stop it?" the driver asks.

"Yeah, well, that's where strategizing takes place," Ross steps in. "First the WHO will focus its immunization campaign just around that initial village and any probable hotspots near there through which infected persons were likely to have passed; adjacent hub villages, as well as any Southeast Asian cities with train stations and airports and harbors and such — stage one. Stage two: next, as more dosages become available, immunization efforts will not only broaden within the affected countries, but will also spread out across other nations and continents in an effort stay in front of the pandemic. In the case of the United States, we — this being the CDC's turf— will issue a *strong advisory* rather than the typical come-on-in-and-get-your-shots recommendation."

"Like back in seventy-six, if you remember – " Hank begins.

"Sure, the the *first* swine flu," the driver says.

"Right. What happened then was, fearing a deadly outbreak, President Ford managed to get 180 of the U.S.'s 240 million citizens to get vaccinated. We were shooting for 100% immunization but as it was — long story short — we got enough to establish an effective herd immunity so that, had it proved to be a lethal strain – which fortunately it didn't – we would've been covered."

"Herd immunity you called it?"

"Right. It's basically the same strategy firefighters employ when they set back fires in a forest so that an otherwise raging forest fire won't have the fuel to continue to burn," Bronwyn elaborates. "Get enough people immunized and the virus mathematically can't spread."

"I see. But what's with all them eggs?" the driver asks no one in particular.

"That's where we grow the virus from which we make the vaccine. Just like in human cells, the virus thrives inside eggs."

"*Fertilized* eggs, where cell division is occurring," Hank adds.

"So, eleven days after fertilization, we inject as many eggs as we think we'll need. We then separate the eggs into three big batches, injecting each with a different strain. Then, as these respective viruses begin to grow in the egg white part of the egg, we then inject a high-yielding donor strain. Somewhere around this point the embryo becomes infected and the virus multiplies. After a few days of incubation, the eggs are cracked opened with machines and the virus is extracted then purified then chemically inactivated then, *voile*, we have the basic components for the vaccine."

"And it takes between one or two eggs to get a single dose of vaccine," Ross adds.

"But, by that stage, the ball is in the pharmaceuticals' side of the court. We just get them the virus; they're the ones who have to then make the millions or, in this case, *billions* of vaccine doses."

"Wow, sounds like a logistical nightmare," the driver exclaims.

Hank nods, "That's why we pay 'em the big bucks."

"Then pray they don't screw up," Ross adds.

The procession passes through a set of swinging double doors and into the wing of the building housing the BSL-4 labs. Herein the seriousness of their work becomes apparent. Monkeys screech from their cages, and virus-killing ultraviolet strobe lights blink from the ceilings. Bronwyn hates this place. She remembers, early in her CDC career, it used to exhilarate her to come in here. But now, as the odds of an accident seemingly become greater each time she does – in the same way that a Russian Roulette hobby eventually catches up with its enthusiasts – she would be content never to have to come past those monkey cages ever again, gladly spending the remainder of her CDC days in the Administration Building – behind her desk and moving paper. She has two kids after all. After a calming breath, she turns to Ross and asks, "Which lab?"

"D – I have it prepped," Ross replies, nodding past the sealed-glass, security-locked doors label A, B, and C, another thirty meters down the hall.

"Well, I only foresee one itty-bitty potential snag," the driver says.

"Yeah, what's that?" Bronwyn asks, as she checks her watch, barely interested in what the driver has to say.

"Well, like you said, you need two or three billion chicken eggs, right?"

"That's right."

"And they ain't easy to come by even in normal times, right?"

Bronwyn is already getting a sickly knot in her stomach, as if becoming aware of some gross miscalculation she may have made, or of some obvious detail she may have overlooked.

Ross doesn't quite see it yet so encourages the driver to continue, "What about it?"

"Well, whenever there's a big flu outbreak, don't they always kill all the chickens first?"

Hank feels it now; that same knot in his stomach. He glances over to Bronwyn, who returns his troubled glance, as the driver continues.

"Like didn't they have to kill all the chickens in Hong Kong a few years back?"

"1997," Hank avers.

"Yeah. Millions of 'em, right? Every single goddamned chicken and duck they had, if I recall. Same thing in, where was it? Ceylon?"

"Thailand," Ross corrects him, as now Ross feels that same knot in the stomach as his colleagues. Funny, how fear spreads much like a virus. If only there was a vaccine for *it*. Ross now turns towards both Hank and Bronwyn, all suddenly bound by the same unspoken code; not to panic, not to say anything, not to spread the fear.

The driver, oblivious of the concern he's ignited, elaborates upon the *snag* as he sees it: "Whatever. Here's my point: if this thing really does grow into a pandemic, and they have to kill most all the chickens the world around, right? –where we gonna get those billions of fertilized eggs? Know what I mean?"

"The farms we contract with all take special precautions against viral infections. That's part of the reason their names and locations are all classified," Hank assures the driver.

"So they, like, try to maintain sterile conditions, is what you're saying?"

"That's right; all post 9/11 precautions to protect against acts of bioterrorism."

"Bioterrorism? – gimme a break!" the driver laughs, "Hundreds of thousands of chickens, serviced by underpaid, potentially virus-coughing immigrant workers, with wild birds flying overhead poopin' and peein' on the *sterile* rooftops and grounds?"

Hank releases a deep sigh, but says nothing.

"Well, good luck with *that!*" the driver adds with a sarcastic chuckle.

He's got a point; a big, fat, good point, but Bronwyn doesn't want to tell him he does. Last thing the CDC needs is some uneducated employee spreading panic about how the coming pandemic is unavoidable, unstoppable. So, instead, she just gives him some patented reply: she's working on it right now. It will dismiss his concerns as somewhat simplistic, while being careful not to be derogatory. She'll simply try to assure him that, if they can't use eggs – because there aren't any – well then, they'll just switch to the MKC method. *The what?* he'll ask. *The Mammalian Kidney Cells method; a cell-based rather than egg-based way of producing influenza vaccine. Sometimes called TC for Tissue Cells, or CB for Cell-based; but, suffice it to say, it's how we currently make polio vaccines. It's really a better method than eggs anyway; for any number of reasons ranging from natural impurities within the eggs or the presence of antibiotics or sterility problems, or sometimes people just have allergic reaction to the egg albumin within the vaccine. There's also the fact that sometimes emerging endemic viruses just don't grow in eggs, and that can be a big problem if it happens to be a particularly nasty strain. CB also allows us to grow more virus more quickly, especially in the event of an egg shortage, much as you elucidated.* There, that would be a good way to dismiss his theory without humiliating him; just sandwich it in the middle of her explanation then move quickly on, making sure to both flatter and confuse him by mixing in plenty of esoteric scientific jargon: *Lastly, viruses grown in cell culture don't have the variants we find in egg culture, thus tend to be more antigenically representative of the wild virus – more like a clone rather than a twin – resulting in a more effective vaccine. So, you see, there's nothing new about this. In fact, we've been working on cell-based vaccines since the mid-nineties, we just haven't made the switch yet because it'll cost a little more initially; you know, to retool and all....*

the momentum of folly

That, anyway, is what Bronwyn is *about* to tell the driver to assuage his concern about any hypothetical sudden shortage of eggs halting vaccine production. And most of what she would be saying is true, though, the fact of the matter is, if this *is* the killer strain they worry it might be, and it *does*, as predicted, spread rapidly around the planet, they *would* have to kill most all the chickens and ducks in the world, which *would* virtually halt vaccine production. Add to that the fact that cell-based production – though tried and true and undoubtedly the wave of the future – simply could not be phased in quickly enough to produce even a fraction of the vaccine quantities needed to quell this imminent pandemic. That's the worrisome truth she'd prefer to keep from him, and she'll do so through some deft misinformation. And that's exactly what she's about to do when a violent noise suddenly interrupts her. It's a repetitive pounding noise, and it seems to be emanating from the large, double-pane window just off to their right. The guards draw their 9mm Glock pistols and take aim – one dropping to a knee, the other taking cover behind a wall corner – as they all, scientists and driver included, all yank about suddenly, reflexively turning towards the source of the ruckus....

But it's only Stuart. He's the one causing the ruckus. He's the one doing the pounding. He's got his wheelchair parked just outside the tempered glass window and is furiously beating on it with his fist while shouting – though nearly inaudibly through the double-paned safety glass – at the top of his lungs: "Dr. Bronwyn! Dr. Bronwyn!"

Bronwyn motions for the guards to put away their guns, sighing heavily, "It's alright; he's one of us."

"You sure?" one of the guards asks, no doubt conflicted by the fact Stuart – what with his scrawny beard and long, unkempt hair – fits the terrorist profile pretty spot on.

"Yeah, you sure?" Ross adds, unable to resist the quip.

And Hank smiles, but Bronwyn doesn't think it's so funny.

"I'm not proposing we whack him per se; just that, you know, we retain it as an option," Ross continues, ever so wryly.

Bronwyn rolls her eyes, then repeats her orders to the guards with their still-drawn and aimed side arms, "Put 'em away now!"

Outside, Stuart continues to pound and shout, *"Dr. Bronwyn!"*

"What?" she shouts back, already annoyed.

"Carl has it!"

"Who?"

"Carl Sims; he's infected and he doesn't know it!"

"*Infected?* With the H5N1 virus?" Hank asks Bronwyn.

Bronwyn shakes her head, "I assume that's what he means."

"But we knew that, didn't we?"

"We *feared* it, but we didn't *know*."

"But now you're positive?"

"Yeah! Well, I haven't sequenced the genes yet, but everything else points to a perfect match."

Ross, Hank and Bronwyn pass around some worried glances, then Ross turns and shouts back through the glass to Stuart, "So, where is he?"

In response, Stuart holds out his arms and shrugs.

"This isn't good," Hank mutters, aside to Bronwyn and Ross.

"No," Bronwyn confirms, with a slow, heavy sigh. "No, it isn't."

WHO Infectious Disease Facility, Sao Paulo, Brazil

Carl's eyes open. He finds himself staring at the same ceiling as before. But, unlike last time, this time he knows instantly exactly where he is – The Slammer. With the lab so dimly-lighted – still by just the machinery lights and the purple UV strobe flashes every ten seconds – and there being no windows to let in sun or moon light, and the fact that he was sedated, it's really impossible for him to determine how long he has been unconscious. Three hours? Three days? Either is just as likely, though the fact that his hospital gown is damp and reeks of urine suggests the latter might be closer to the truth. Repulsed, Carl tries to sit up, and that's when he remembers his arm.

"*Fuck!*"

Still broken.

"Fucking Henri!" Carl shouts out to the empty lab at the top-of-the-lungs.

Wincing from the throbbing pain, Carl lies back down again, takes a deep breath, then calmly attempts to collect himself – to regroup. "Okay, so now what?" he asks himself, licking his parched lips as he thinks it over for a few seconds. Deciding, at least, on an initial course of action, he supports his broken right arm with his left, sits up again, swings his feet over one side of the bed, then stands – all in one painful but mercifully quick motion. The agony is such he would be fully justified to scream again, but what good would it do? *Now* was all about trying to detach himself from the pain – somehow. He had seen this sort of bravado before in sports and war films and whatnot, and all of its associative phrases – *Suck it up!*, *Be one with the pain!*, etc. – but he didn't know if it was really possible. But now was certainly a good time to try.

Almost as an effort to try to get his mind off the throbbing in his elbow, Carl begins to walk the perimeter of his small, Plexiglas enclosure; changing directions on a whim, trying to peer out into the darkness even if he's not sure what he's looking for. He even, if only for old times' sake, tests the hatch door:

yep, still locked. Moving on and arriving at the water cooler he fills a small paper cup and drinks it as he takes inventory of all he's seen both inside and just outside the Slammer cell: overhead air ducts, a couple of wall grommets through which protruded heavy rubber gloves for handling "hot" viruses, lights, those UV strobes, various power cords and cables strewn across the floor, the table around which the scientists sat, the telephone some three meters beyond the Plexiglas, computers, the bed gurney, the old school keypad-less, rotary dial-less intercom telephone thingy by the bed, the I.V. rack, hell, even this water cooler stand and bottle atop it.... a long list for such a sparsely accoutered space. Here was all this stuff but again he didn't know if any of it, or any combination of it, could really be used to break out of here. Sure, the media culture within which he grew up always provided its heroes with some clever means of escape; but they were brilliant and fictional, whereas this was, well, *reality* for one thing. And people died in reality. And some died stupidly. And some met with painfully protracted demises. And some suffered their way through all of the above.

Carl finishes his water, crumples the little paper cup then, just as he is about to mindlessly drop it into the wastebasket set beside the cooler, he pauses. Feeling a bit like the last person alive – like the Omega Man – he stares at the wastebasket; struck by the surrealism of this innate-or-learned desire-or-need to maintain order. It's a moment he could spend eternity pondering, but he knows he doesn't have the time. So, he drops the crumpled paper cup into the wastebasket then issues himself a little pep talk:

"Let's try to stay focused here, Carl."

Glazing out to the telephone set atop the table, Carl finds himself wondering if it is just an internal intercom-type line, like the phone here with him within the Slammer, or if it might have an outside line. No way of telling. He then happens to notice one data cable snaking its way across part of the lab floor between the table's legs, then back around again, hugging the outside of the Slammer wall just outside the Plexiglas.

"If I could just get a hold of that..." he begins, before the obvious question arises: *But how?*

Suddenly, he remembers something. Turning, he quickly walks the nine or ten steps it takes to bisect the Slammer's octagon-shaped floor and bring him to the opposite wall. And there he confronts the thick rubber – perhaps polyurethane or even Kevlar reinforced – gloves protruding through the wall grommets. The gloves reach inward towards a sterile, seemingly never used autoclave. After staring at the gloves for just long enough to mentally test a hypothesis, Carl shoves the autoclave out of the way, its test tubes and beakers rattling but not breaking inside as it rolls off across the floor. Carl then steps closer to the gloves and pauses again, any plan he might be formulating obviously still in its infancy. He narrows his focus to the glove to his left; the one a scientist accessing the gloves from the other side of the Plexiglas would stick his or her *right* hand into. With his *left* hand – his good arm – Carl gently reaches out to the glove's blue protruding fingertips with his own fingertips. Carefully touching each of his fingertips with the corresponding fingertips of the glove, Carl gently pushes his hand forward, towards the wall grommet, effectively inverting the glove inside-out as he pushes his hand into it. Soon his shoulder is all the way up to the Plexiglas wall, with his arm protruding its entire length into the outlying lab. However successful this effort might be, at least one problem persists: he still cannot reach anything; not the stool on wheels less than two meters away, not that desk stacked with humming machinery, and certainly not the data cable snaking just inches below his most strained reach. Hence, all this warrants another frustrated and resounding expletive:

"*Fuck!*"

Carl extracts his arm, leaving its glove protruding, inverted and stiffly, on the lab's side of the Plexiglas wall. More time to think. Plenty of time. Too much time. And yet, ironically, not enough. An inkling causes him to shift his attention to the other glove, the one to his right still protruding towards him into the Slammer. After just a bit of pondering, he crosses back to the autoclave, opens it up, then grabs a clear beaker. Holding it out at arm's length, he drops it to the floor, hoping it will break. But, instead, it just bounces. He picks up another and tries smashing it, but it too fails to break. "Plastic, of course." Looking about the interior of the Slammer, Carl can find nothing that might be considered fragile or even remotely sharp. He assumes this was an intentional measure designed to keep captive patients from killing themselves before whatever nasty pathogen they had could accomplish the deed for them. Better to slash one's wrist than die over a period of days or weeks of some painful hemorrhaging pox, went the ratiocination the designers of the cell were obviously trying to thwart.

the momentum of folly

What would Jesus do? Jesus would *roll away the stone* and somehow magically extricate himself from this cell, but that didn't seem like a realistic option here to Carl. That's why it is often times more pragmatic to ask: *What would an animal do?* – particularly a species with extraordinary survival skills, say, a rat or a coyote. Whether or not this is the right question to ask, within seconds it has Carl taking his teeth to the glove's thick rubber in a desperate attempt to chew his way out. Verily, it's a solution neither very scientific nor otherwise flattering to the human ego but, as Carl convinced himself, *Hey, whatever works.*

Knowing he will need a hole large enough to stick something bigger than his hand through, Carl skips trying to gnaw at the glove's fingertip and goes straight for the forearm portion. And he's at it for several minutes – gnashing the six-mil rubber-Kevlar-polyurethane between his incisors and bicuspids long past the point when his jaw muscles first began to ache – before he finally is able to break through. The striking of tooth against tooth, even chipping the enamel of his upper bicuspid, never felt so good. And once Carl feels it, he pulls his teeth off the task and sets his fingernails to it. And after a few nigh-finger-breaking minutes more, he is finally able to just squeeze the tip of his index finger through the chewed-through rupture in the glove. Pulling his finger from the rupture, air immediately begins rushing into the negatively pressurized Slammer cell, making a low-pitched whistling sound as it flows through the breach in the rubber. Almost immediately alarms begin sounding throughout the lab, accompanied by whirling, flashing yellow warning lights; all obviously set off by the subtle change in air pressure detected, no doubt, by sensors located throughout the lab. And the subsequent din might be deafening were the alarms within the Slammer cell but, fortunately for Carl, they are all located out in the main lab and the halls and offices extending outwards from there, thus the noise comes to his ears more or less muffled by the Plexiglas walls of his enclosure. But the relative quiet proves only temporary as emergency air pumps mounted just overhead automatically switch on; a default measure to keep the air pressure within the cell lower than that of the lab, sucking the presumably infected air away through a series of ultraviolet light and chlorine mist and hepa-filtration systems before it is eventually released from the building.

The noise all makes perfect, logical sense to Carl, he just wishes he didn't have to listen to it. Remembering the box of cotton balls on the bottom rack of the wheeled cart over by his bed, Carl crosses back to it, pulls out a couple of the balls, scrunches them between his fingers and forces one into each ear channel. If there is indeed any resulting noise mitigation offered up by the cotton plugs Carl is barely aware of it, but maybe, just maybe, they will help keep him sane.

On the bed is the sling Jenna fashioned for him. Carl slips it over his head and squirms into it. With his fractured elbow now effectively immobilized with the weight off of the shoulder, it is almost possible to forget the arm was ever broken. This is good. Heading back toward the gnawed glove, Carl spots the wheeled stool. Realizing that it could come in handy as well, Carl hooks the stool with a foot, then flings it ahead of him. It rolls until it bumps into the Plexiglas wall just below the wall grommets. Arriving there, Carl settles onto the stool, takes a weary but determined breath, lifts the limp rubber glove back up to his tired, aching, still-throbbing jaw… and resumes gnawing.

Santa Monica Boulevard, Los Angeles, California

Cliché; that's how it feels to be Latina and pregnant to Angela. She had never wanted it for herself, at least not yet. But here she was; sitting in her SUV in the parking lot just across the street from the Planned Parenthood clinic. A Latina, in Los Angeles, pregnant – how cliché.

She should have had the abortion while she was still at the CDC, then it would have been covered by her insurance. But there just wasn't time. She also thought – she *assumed* – that Aegis offered a health insurance package, but quickly learned she was wrong about that. "Insurance?" her immediate boss laughed when she asked him on Monday, "Insurance is *s-o-o-o* last year!" He quipped, though absolutely serious. Last year Aegis *did* provide health insurance for its 11,000 employees, but not anymore. Erland Zwissler, the CEO, was positioning the company for a buy-out. Of course he knew this was cruel; back in those heady, booming eighties he had promised his employees health and pension, even a workplace gym and weekly massage – all the *bennies* – only to yank them each away. But this is how business is done these days. He had also stripped the company down to a "lean and mean" 4,800, bought out the older employees with early retirement packages, and replaced every two of them with one new hireree now coined "independent contractors" to whom he didn't have to promise health or pension benefits, or overtime pay or even lunch breaks. Why, he didn't even have to fuss with their taxes; how good is that? He had done this because, the fact of the matter was, he was one of the only CEOs of a large pharmaceutical company who wasn't yet a billionaire, and it was becoming, well, embarrassing. "$990 million," that was what his accountants had him at last quarter: "Close, but no cigar." So, you see, he kind of had to yank the bennies. Besides, if *he* didn't strip down Aegis someone else *would*. They'd jump in via hostile takeover and reap the booty themselves. There were a lot of these hedge fund vultures out there. It didn't take much intelligence, just a stiff spine and a calloused heart. So, why shouldn't Erland do it himself? There was no reason. He had gone over the figures with his accountants in private and discovered it was possible — though this was the very high-end guesstimate — it was possible for him to personally make $7 billion off the sale. *Seven billion!* That would catapult him 1,125 notches forward on the Forbes Richest People List. So, why shouldn't he do it? Isn't that what life is all about — winning? Hey, you have to break a few eggs to make an omelet, right? And, as it just so happened, Angela was one of those *eggs*; and an independently contracted, uninsured and unmarried pregnant Latina egg at that.

Outside Angela's windshield, up the sidewalk along Santa Monica Boulevard, a foursome of Latina mothers push their tiny-wheeled strollers containing their most recent spawn, with toddlers and two, three, even four preschoolers in tow. All the kids are dressed nicely and seem well-behaved, though Angela knows it's just a matter of time before a calculable percentage of them join gangs and start getting their prison tattoos — the requisite teardrops on a cheek representative of each incarceration. There's just no way around it; given the poverty, the lack of opportunity, and the real threat these kids will face as they move into their adolescence. Mere survival will force them into gangs, and the gang ethos almost inevitably will lead to time in the joint, in the big house, in the pokey. The basic problem is the fact that youth is exploited by our workplace. Kids will always be paid minimum wage and minimum wage will always be far below what is minimally necessary to get by in this society. As a result, not surprisingly, crime is the only option for just about any kid hoping to pursue the American dream — the bling, the crib, the ride with the low-profile wheels.... What's this mean for the successful business owner? It means that despite having *efficientized* their payroll — working their employees just less than the weekly minimum which would require them to pay overtime or health or pension benefits — and despite having personally reaped tens of millions in bonuses for so doing, they have created a society in which their employees despise them. Case in point: Angela's brother, the "black sheep" one. Between his last two incarcerations an uncle had gotten him a job at Home Depot. He was there four months and doing okay, making $9.75 an hour when word trickled down that their CEO was given the boot after just a six-year ride in the saddle. His punishment? — $210 million in cash and stock options, plus a $20 million severance package, plus $32 million in retirement benefits presumably because who can retire on just $210 million? Angela's brother's fellow employees were so pissed-off that day they basically went on strike by staying on permanent break, managers included. To his credit, Angela's brother kept on working, kind of. His was the only checkout aisle open. Problem was, he had called all his friends and told them to come in and fill their shopping carts and he would take care of them. And he did: they would push past his register with radial arm saws and compressors and boxes upon boxes of tile, and he would only charge them for a toilet plunger. That was his *fuck* *y*ou to the *System* – to back-dated stock options and insider trading and golden parachutes – the toilet plunger. He got caught of course, which is why he's back in prison now, permanently this time since that was his third "strike." The point being: that's not a stable business model. Are CEOs more happy today, in this era where they make 400 times what their average employee brings home, than they were back in 1961 when that disparity was only *twelve*? Doubtful. Somewhere in this blind pursuit of wealth within this system of unfettered free enterprise, not only has the societal destabilization wrought by economic disparity been overlooked, but so too has the fact that making obscene amounts of money at the expense of their underpaid, uninsured employees does not make the average CEO particularly proud of him or herself – especially when they have to live in fear of their resentful underlings. Entry level employees at General Motors are making almost half what they did two decades ago, and have had their health and pensions stripped from their "benefits" packages, all this while their Vice Chairman of Global Product Development – who literally crushed their EV1 electric car division in favor of their Hummer line – personally owns two private jets and helicopters; due compensation, it seems, for helping drive GM stock down to a fifty-eight-year low until a government bailout went into effect. *Privatize reward, socialize risk*: this is the corporate zeitgeist being saluted across America and people wonder why there's voter resentment, why there's employee shrinkage, why there's inner city crime, why society is crumbling. Well, suffice it to say, the chickens – be they black, white, yellow, or brown – have come home to roost.

And prison, that's where a lot of the *take back California* talk is mumbled; *La Reconquista* – the Reconquest. Take back North America. *It's easy; all we need to do is keep having more babies than them. Then they'll be mowing* our *lawns, Homs.* That's the talk, not just in prison, but also at Cinco de Mayo celebrations, or at birthday parties in the park. *La Reconquista.* She's already been to the Mexican stores down on Olvera Street in the El Pueblo de Los Angeles district. She's been in the touristy bodegas whose store *fronts* are set up for gringos while their *back* rooms cater to a different reality; to *La Raza* – the Race. For in those back rooms hang the T-shirts and bumper stickers and banners proclaiming their inevitable victory: "Brown is the New White," "We're the Majority," *"Si, se puede!* – Yes, We Can!"

La Reconquista; at parties, over beers it's the subject of rejoice for her people but, as it might be for her as well except for the disturbing fact she doesn't feel part of "her" people any longer. She has studied the human genome; she knows *all* people are *her* people. She knows everyone here in North America is an immigrant, and that everyone worldwide is an emigrant out of Africa. And if she had to chose which sub-group she would care to call *her* people, she certainly would not let slight variations in skin or hair color dictate that for her. Nor would she allow some arbitrarily learned cultural trait, such as the language she happened to speak at home or the religion within which she was brought up, be the determinant criteria for who *her* people were. Where would be the free choice in that? So, as a result, *her* people – the ones she most cared to hang with, to drink beers or play ultimate Frisbee or watch TV in pajamas or race naked down the beach at midnight under a full moon and, eventually and especially, to build a family with – were those who *thought* like her, those who shared her ideologies and values, those who understood the world and its problems and held as a personal goal to help it get back on its feet. Thus, *her* people are the ones back in the CDC labs, or back in college. *Her* people now are the educated masses – White, Indian, Black, Asian, Latino, what have you. *Her* people are now those looking forward towards the bleak and challenging future and trying their damnedest to fix it. Most simply put: *her* people are part of the solution and not part of the problem. *La Reconquista*: that's no victory for Latinos, not by Angela's thinking, not in the long term anyway. That's taking a continent by overpopulating it then planting a triumphal flag in the heap of polluted rubble left over. It's the classic Pyrrhic victory wherein everyone loses. She knows the numbers: 306 million in North America today, 15% or 46,750,000 of them "non-white Latino"; 434 to 518 million in North America by 2050, 29% or 137,250,000 of them non-white Latino; and maybe a billion by 2100, with well over half of them – more than all the other races combined – non-white Latino. And it's all because of immigration and total fertility rates: Hispanics 2.977 births per woman, Blacks 2.398, Native Americans 2.114, Asians

& Pacific Islanders 1.919, Whites 1.826. A Brown America? That isn't what worries Angela. *It's the environment, stupid!* – that's what worries her. That's what worries everyone with more than a modicum of intelligence and concern. What if she *were* to have this child; what would North America look like by 2050 when he or she is closing in on forty? Will it be sustainably pristine or an overpopulated squalor? Learning from Carl what he learned from his father, Angela knows the sustainable population of the U.S. is 150 million; less than half what it is today. And when her child is her age the U.S. population will be over three times that carrying capacity. *What the fuck are we doing?* Angela catches herself asking, shaking her head as she watches the tiny-wheeled strollers push by. A little more than a decade ago Mexico bestowed their coveted *Mother of the Year Award* on a woman just because she managed to plop out twenty-four children. *What the fuck are we doing?* But Angela knows this *yearning* isn't unique to her people; a Palestinian man is on record for having fathered sixty-seven children, and is currently in search of wife number nine to help him spread his seed further. *What the fuck are we doing?* A dirt-poor South African man with twenty-two kids, after having won their national lottery, rejoiced that now his children can have big, happy families too. *What the fuck are we doing?* And, of course, there's the story of that pathetic California woman, supposedly educated, who even though she was unwed and unemployed and on food stamps and state assistance and already had six children under the age of eight, was allowed to undergo in-vitro fertilization and promptly spawned octuplets. *What the fuck are we doing?!*

Angela takes a breath and shakes her head. There's an image that haunts her whenever she imagines the future of North America: it's of that squalid creek flowing just beneath her and Carl's Tijuana motel room window and the kids that were playing out there in the sewage. Wouldn't it be nice if there were one-third as many kids and they all had pure and wild streams in which to splash about? Wouldn't it be nice if her child had a *less*-crowded rather than *more*-crowded world? Wouldn't it be nice to have genuine optimism for the future? – *real* hope rather than the patronizing image of the shining city on the mountain conjured and spewed by politicians every election cycle, and swallowed by the naive? Wouldn't it be nice if the world actually were getting better?

One of the mamacitas passing along the sidewalk outside Angela's windshield seems almost to read Angela's mind. For, sans any provocation, she turns and stares at Angela and, just for an instant, the two lock eyes. Angela is rattled by the event, by this brief happenstance – this peering into one another's souls. *How old could she be?* Angela wonders. *Fifteen? – if that.* Angela suspects she knows how the girl's pregnancy happened. It's the same old story: making out with her first boyfriend in junior high school, one thing led to that other, and – sans birth control, of course – *wham, bam, thank you, ma'am*, they're pregnant. Abort it? Hell no! For, far from something to be embarrassed about or to regret, this pregnancy is a step up in the young girl's life. Now her life has purpose. Now she has someone who will cling to her unconditionally through thick and thin. Besides, her similarly uneducated friends and sisters all seem so happy for her; just as she does for them when they too get pregnant even if they are all being a bit disingenuous. "Congratulations!" they all say, even though they each know it was a mistake and most of the time secretly wish it had never happened. But, hey, it's spilled milk now, it's water under the bridge, it's sperm in the ol' egg. And that's the cycle of poverty out here in the ever-expanding barrio: get knocked-up, drop out of school, work minimum wage jobs, live in overcrowded homes, beget more uneducated kids, and on and on. But look closely at that beaten-down, worn-out, sphere of a grandmother pushing that other stroller. She probably isn't much over forty but she's educated; talkin' School of Hard Knocks educated. So don't expect her to smile when you tell her you're pregnant: she's got seven kids of her own somewhere, twenty-one grandchildren, three great grandchildren and untold more on the way, and her life has only gotten harder through it all. Fulfillment? Screw that! – she would gladly exchange all the fulfillment in the world for one full night's sleep and the weekend off from having to clean houses and change diapers. And she'd gladly advise any of the teenagers who cared to listen all about how they *should* conduct their lives. What would she say? She would tell them what her grandmother told *her* and what she wished *she* had done: Get on birth control, chica, stay in school, travel, date, take your time, have fun, but, above all, *wait* – wait until you're at least thirty before having kids, and then have just two! *Sí*, she'd give 'em an earful, but she knows they would all just think she was a bitter, old-fashioned fool, just as she did her grandmother. So she doesn't bother. She just smiles disingenuously when they tell her they're pregnant. She smiles and bites her tongue and silently laments the extra hardship to be endured.

Angela knows the cycle-of-poverty trap first hand, even if her family mostly escaped it. Her parents had the Catholic handful of five kids, but the last one –

the only one younger than Angela – died in birth, taking the mom's uterus with it. So, now there were four; two girls and two boys, one of whom she suspects might be gay – or just smart – because he seems to have no intention of getting married or spawning and, perhaps not coincidentally, he seems to be the only one doing all right. The others? Her oldest brother – the gangster, in and out of jail since age nineteen, the prison tear tattoos, et al, you've seen him – he brags he has at least four kids by different mothers but that would take DNA testing to determine for certain and who would pay for that? Angela's sister: three kids and pregnant again, with a nice enough husband who works endless hours as a bagel store manager for his 28k, which keeps them hovering just above poverty level down in Austin where they were all raised. Being avid church-goers they took umbrage to Angela's offer to pay for a vasectomy after their second child; such umbrage they went and named their third *Angel* – after her. And now they don't speak. Four stupid, poverty-bound children; that's what Angela foresees for them, and that's exactly what she had promised herself she would avoid. Yet, here she is: another pregnant Latina. How cliché.

Out across Santa Monica Boulevard, on the other side of the busy street, there's the predictable flank of anti-abortion, "Pro-Life" protesters with their placards and photos of fetuses and pamphlets and Biblical excerpts. Tireless. Just doing God's work. Just clamoring to get into heaven. Angela dreads the confrontation. She has the clinic's number on her cell phone. They told her just to call and they would have some of their volunteers escort her across the street and through the gauntlet of Pro-lifers – shouting *Murderer!* and *You're going to Hell!* and *Abortion stops another beating heart!* – but she dreads it anyway. How did abortion get politicized? That's what she would like to know. She glances down at her phone. She's about to call the clinic, but there's that one bewildering saved message she wants to listen to yet again, so she replays it. There's no voice on the message; just a strange hammering sound – loud, hard, and maybe angry. The Caller ID shows the number coming from the 907 area code. Alaska. She doesn't know anyone in Alaska, that's the most bewildering part. Wrong number? Some toddler randomly dialing as the babysitter makes out with her boyfriend? Then again, after the 907 the number begins with another 9. Doesn't that mean it originated from a public phone booth? Angela had heard that somewhere, some time ago, but she really doesn't even know if it's true. And that hammering, with the clanging and all; it sounds almost like someone beating against one of those big, old, metal public telephones. Probably with a crowbar. Probably some junkie trying to break it open to get at the booty of coins. There's a lot of meth up in Alaska, that's probably it. Meth, pharmaceuticals, quarters, billions of dollars; two ends of the same stick – the same crowbar. Erland is using a figurative crowbar, and a technically legal one, to get at his billions, and he probably won't get jail time for it, but how much different are the two crimes really?

Those are the thoughts swirling, twister-like, through Angela's mind as she stares down at her cell phone... when suddenly it rings. She nearly jumps out of her seat, even though it's not all that unlikely an occurrence. She checks the caller I.D. The call is coming in from her immediate boss at Aegis Pharmaceuticals – Doug. She hasn't slept with him yet. Not sure if she will, though he's certainly laid the offer out there. It depends on what she stands to get in the bargain. But it's him calling so she feels obligated to answer.

"Angela Varella," Angela says calmly, professionally into her phone.

"Hey, Angela, it's Doug."

"Hey. What's up?"

"We have a... *development*. I need you back in here, ASAP like."

"Alright. Is two hours soon enough?"

"Let me put it this way: In two hours I'll already have your replacement working on it."

Although he's joking, Angela knows his humor is just the sugar coating of the truth. With the phone still pressed to her ear, she stares out her windshield wondering how her world became so complicated so quickly,

WHO Infectious Disease Facility, Sao Paulo, Brazil

Blood now trickles from Carl's gums and down his chin as he takes the gnawed rubber glove from his very sore jaws. Inspecting his work, he sees he has chewed about a third the way around the glove's forearm with some threads of the glove's Kevlar reinforcement still defiantly resisting. In an attempt to rip the hole wider still, Carl tucks three fingers from each hand into the rupture and begins to pull them apart, only to have this *seemed-like-a-good-idea-at-the-time* effort immediately thwarted by the subsequent bolt of pain that shoots down from his fractured elbow. Forced to rethink his strategy, Carl gets off the stool and kicks it away, then sits on the floor with his back supported by the Plexiglas wall. Lifting his right leg above him and engaging it with the glove, he wedges as many of his toes as he can into the hole, then crams as many fingers as he can of his good hand in there as well. After pausing to rest and to double check his strategy, Carl begins pushing and tugging his toes and fingers in opposite direction. And though the Kevlar strands slice into his skin to the point where he begins to bleed from several stress points, the reinforcing threads do begin to pop, one by one. It's a slow and painful process exasperated by the fact he is still working at half-strength, if that, due to the influenza. He pauses again to catch his breath and let the pain subside for a bit. Coming around to the conclusion the task won't get done unless he perseveres, he gets back at it, applying even more muscle to it this time and slowly but surely managing to tear the hole in the glove incrementally wider.

After some minutes of this, Carl takes another break to check on his progress. The size of the hole now is such that the air pumps remain on constantly, rather than kicking on and off intermittently whenever the respective air pressures within the lab and Slammer differ significantly. Though this means more incessantly annoying noise, it is also a tangible confirmation of progress and thus a good sign.

the momentum of folly

Encouraged, Carl now sticks his left foot into the glove to see if it will fit through the rupture. It does, even permitting his ankle to pass through without much effort. Ripping off that ridiculous hospital gown and hopping up onto his right leg, he begins pushing his left leg through the grommet, inverting the glove out into the lab as he does. His calf slips through the rupture without much resistance, as does his knee, but his upper leg is another story, his thigh muscles being what they are. For the first time he finds himself wishing he had done *fewer* leg squats and lunges and presses rather than more, and wishing as well he had followed up those countless workouts with a diet soda rather than with his usual protein smoothies. But it is what it is and all he can do now is try to force his leg further through the rupture despite the extremely snug fit, with the hope he can shove his leg through farther than he could his arm. If by so doing he can extend his reach then, with any luck at all, he might just be able to stretch his toes all the way down to the lab floor. That's the goal; to get his toes to the floor in order to grab that data cable and carefully lift it back up and through the wall grommet and into the cell so he can then hopefully tug on it with his one good arm and eventually pull the table — the table with the telephone on it — around the perimeter of the octagonal cell and, *eventually, carefully, hopefully*, right on up to the torn-open wall grommet, so he can then reach through and pull the phone's receiver into the Slammer cell and simply use the phone to call for help. That's the goal. Ah, but that only poses yet another problem: even if the unlikely were to happen and all that worked, whom would he call? — the CDC's main number? *"You have reached the Centers for Disease Control, please listen carefully before making your selection as our menu has changed…"* The CCID? *"You have reached the Coordinating Center for Infectious Diseases, please listen carefully before making your selection as our menu has changed…."* The NCIRD? *"You have reached the National Center for Immunization and Respiratory Diseases, please listen carefully before making your selection as our menu has changed…."* Bronwyn's direct line? — sure, if he knew her extension. Sure, if her assistant let the call through. Stuart? Angela again? The Brazilian equivalent of 9-1-1? — what ever that might be, assuming there is one. So many options and yet the reality is his leg is still wedged in the glove, with his knee shoved not four inches past the hole and his toes another six inches — *six hopeless inches* — above the floor and that *all-so-vital-to-this-otherwise-passable-escape-plan* data cable. Talk about counting chickens before they hatch: does the phone even have an outside line? He doesn't know. Talk about placing the cart before the horse: if he can't reach the cable with his toes can he even pull his leg back out? He doesn't know that either, but, if he can't, wouldn't it all make for a dandy caption for this year's Darwin Award? – "Dumbshit who jumped the Alaskan influenza quarantine found buck naked and starved to death in Brazilian infectious disease confinement cell after getting leg stuck in autoclave grommet." Verily it would. But he can't worry about epitaphs now. Now he just has to persevere. Now he just has to persist in forcing his leg through that Kevlar-reinforced rupture and hope for the best, and pray against the worst. That's about all he can do at this point – *try*.

Lubrication; it has carried humanity a long way since the Stone Age and ought not to be overlooked here. At least that's what Carl is thinking now that his thigh is meeting dry resistance from the rubber tightly cuffing his skin. *And what better lubrication than mucousy spit?* That's another thing he is thinking. Fortunately for him he seems to have plenty of both; the *mucous* coming courtesy of the influenza virus still raging through his system, souvenir from that unnamed Laotian village. And the *spit* – seemingly endless units of it – attributable to the hydrating intravenous saline solution dripped into his arm for the however many hours or days he has laid here unconscious since Jenna and her nerd pals skipped out. Lots of mucous and spit; yes, fortunate indeed. Capitalizing on this bounty, Carl poises his mouth just above his stuck left leg, hacks up a sinus-full of snot and allows it to drool from his lips, ever so majestically, to his thigh. Once the spittle makes contact with his skin, he rubs it between the chaffing rubber and leg with the fingers of his good arm. And it works; once again in the annals of human history lubrication proves to be a good thing, for even though the gnawed-out rubber is still improbably tight around his thigh he is nonetheless able to shove his leg a few inches further through the hole to the point where he can now feel the cool polished concrete floor with the very tips of his toes. How much more of this tourniquet-like grip on his thigh can he take before the constricted blood flow to his lower leg leads to irreparable cell damage; fifteen, ten, five minutes? That's another concern sticking like a burr in his brain as he sweeps his toes blindly about the floor in search of that snaking data cable. *Blindly*, yes, and probably for the better, for if he *could* see his foot right now what color might it be? Pale white? Cyanic blue? Gangrenous green? One of those shades very likely, so it's probably for the best he can't see foot. Ignorance might not be bliss, but it can be helpful in situations such as these.

the momentum of folly

Ah! There it is! He can feel it with just the tip of his big toe! The data cable! And now he's got it between that big toe and that next one, whatever that next toe is called. *Index toe?* He doesn't know its name even though it just might save his life here. And now those two toes have managed to grip the cable securely enough to lift it off the floor. He's pulling it up, lifting it ever so gently towards the wall grommet. *No way this is going to work*, Carl is thinking to himself. Talk about *The Power of Positive Thinking*, talk about *The Little Engine that Could*; Carl, in his self-deprecating way, has no choice but to apply reverse psychology to this effort because there's no doubt in his mind it will fail. *No fucking way.* That's just how he is wired. It's his way of handling every challenge: by taunting success. That way if failure happens, there's no surprise or disappointment. *PhD? No way I could ever do that! Relationship with Angela? Phffft – you're dreamin' dude!* Of course he will fail; he *always* fails, that's the lot of the loser after all. But if he *succeeds…* well, so much the sweeter, no one expected that. Zero expectations equal zero disappointment. The power of *negative* thinking; the key to success. Pessimism: the new optimism.

This reverse psychology is an especially vital frame of mind to cling dearly to now that Carl's toes have the data cable still pinched between them and all the way up to the wall grommet, for entertaining even the faintest wisp of hope, only to fail, could sink him into a spiraling tailspin of hopelessness from which he might never recover. *Of course, I'm going to drop it; it's just a matter of time. No reason to get excited, failure is certain:* That's Carl's mantra as he now sticks his left arm into the other glove already protruding into the lab. But as his left hand slides so easily into the inverted right-handed glove, and with it he is just as easily able to grab hold of the data cable from his less-reliable toes, he can't help but taste the bittersweet tingle of hope – incipient, premature hope, true, but hope nonetheless!

"I should've taken yoga with Angela,' Carl mutters as he awkwardly contorts himself, trying to hold on to the data cable with his good arm while simultaneously struggling to extricate his leg from the other glove. Of course, as he pulls his leg back through the grommet, the glove it is stuck within comes along with it. As a result, for several awkward moments at least, he looks like some gangly bug caught in a sticky web. But eventually, after a desperate frenzy of yanks and cursing and hopping about on the other leg, the glove peels from stuck limb, releasing it in its entirety – thigh, calve, ankle, et al – from the grommet and allowing the sole of his foot to settle, at long last, back down onto the Slammer's cool, polished concrete floor again. This comes as equal relief to both the nearly strangulated, just emancipated leg as to the other – the hopping, balancing right one – bearing the brunt of this weighty drama the whole time. Now with both feet on the Slammer floor all seems relatively right in Carl's world again. All except for one possible glitch: namely, although his left hand has a firm grip on the cable, there appears no way he can pull it through and into the Slammer, since that hand is in the intact glove. His only hope – and his heart sinks as this realization comes to him – his only hope is try to stick his broken right arm in and through the ruptured gnawed-out glove, grab hold of the cable with it, and pull the cable back through the rupture. The prospect of the pain of doing this proves to be great incentive for trying to think of some other solution – *any* other solution – only problem is, none comes to mind. Realizing also that his stalling is only postponing the inevitable, Carl takes one of his courage-mustering breaths and begins to lift his arm from the sling.

The pain is very easy for Carl to describe, for it feels like someone is slowly stabbing a hot knife in between the joints of his elbow. Yes, that's it exactly, but it is a pain he will have to tolerate for a while still as he fumbles the hand of his injured arm through the gnawed hole and crams it down the full length of the glove. And as his elbow straightens as his arm extends, the pain seems to only magnify. In an attempt to cope with the sheer agony of it all Carl does what he can to mentally detach himself from the moment-to-moment physical details of the effort. Whistling seems to work; desperate little airy whistles. And when whistling fails to numb the spikes of the pain, good ol' fashioned cussing and swearing seems to serve him fairly well, or well enough anyway to bide sufficient time and distraction to allow his trembling right hand to force itself all the way down the sleeve of its glove, out the gnawed-out hole at its end of it, and *eventually* in actual physical contact with the data cable. With his left hand he tries to stuff the cable into his right hand but the pain causes the fingers of the latter to behave almost as if they are freezing, rendering efforts to grasp hold of the cable ultimately futile. This leads him to the next best option; looping the cable around and around the wrist of right hand and tying it off with an excessive number of half and full hitches, all in a desperate attempt to make the broken hand incapable of dropping the cable even if it chose to. With this now the situation, Carl begins to retract his right arm, pulling it *and* the cable tied to

the momentum of folly

it back towards him. And this would work – in theory anyway – so long as his bicep were functioning properly. *Ah*, but that's the problem; his bicep – rather, his whole damn arm – simply *isn't* functioning properly, thanks to the break in its elbow and all its subsequent stabbing pain.

"*Fuckin' Henri! Jerk-ass, motherfuckin', frog-eating Henri. . . .*" That's how Carl copes with the pain as he resorts to simply walking backwards, one painful step at a time, away from the wall in order to pull the data cable through the grommet. And the strategy works of course – such a simple plan, how could it not? – managing to extricate both his helpless broken arm and his unable-to-help good arm from their respective gloves in the process. As the first few inches of data cable become visible as the right hand drags it through the rupture, Carl wastes no time in grabbing hold of it with his good arm and unhitching it from the wrist of his broken arm. Making sure to maintain a firm grip on the cable, Carl turns his focus back across the Slammer and through its opposite wall and towards the table with the phone on it. *Now, if I pull on the cable, what will really happen?*, he asks himself, trying his damnedest to visualize every ramification of his proposed action. But it all seems to check out: if he pulls on the data cable – based on the fact it snakes so ideally around the nearest leg of the table – the table et al should just come bumping and sliding around the Slammer's octagon walls and inevitably to the autoclave grommets. It's simple physics, right? What could go wrong? The only unknown, the only foreseeable glitch in this plan depends on how securely – or not – the opposite end of the cable is anchored to the wall-full of equipment to which it connects. But that's an unknowable unknown; that much Carl knows. If he tugs on the cable and it simply unplugs itself, well, then he's shit-out-of-luck, he's up Shit Creek without a paddle, he's stuck in the Slammer for the rest of his days eating one big, fat shit sandwich and hoping those Darwin Award headlines aren't too embarrassing up there in whatever afterlife might await him.

Taking a deep breath then releasing it while muttering an expletive – *Shit* – meant to suppress any waxing hope, Carl begins to gently pull on the cable. The first few arm-length tugs effortlessly draw the slack from the snaking cable. The next tug meets resistance as the cable tightens around the table leg and lifts from the floor. So far so good. And the next after that successfully moves the table a few tantalizing inches. Fortunately the table is of the cheap, lightweight variety purchased, likely, right out of the Ikea catalogue, which is fine by him.

Carl pulls again, then again, making sure not to tug too hard so not to jerk on the cable. The table, obedient to the forces acting upon it, rounds the first 135° corner of the octagon-shaped Slammer wall. Three more to go. And three more arm-length tugs successfully pull the table along the next three or so meters of Plexiglas wall and to the next corner. Were it a square-shaped cell, Carl suspects the friction of the table rounding the corner might prove too great for the cable's anchor to handle. But, as it is, the octagon configuration, with its negotiable vertices, almost ideally suits this escape scenario. A circular enclosure would be better but, hey, beggars can't be choosers. Providing further fuel for optimism is the intuitive understanding that each subsequent corner the table makes it around means less resistance and, thereby, less chance the cable will rip loose from whatever equipment it is anchored to. And there goes another corner: just two more to go and the table and its telephone should be within reach. It's getting easier but Carl is careful still not to give in to the temptation to tug any harder. Three more pulls and another corner is negotiated. Right about now it strikes Carl that this is getting kind of fun; the challenge of it all – outright exhilarating even! Its easy-does-it strategy is kind of like reeling in a trophy fish, but with so much more at stake. Three more gentle pulls bring the table to the final corner. And all is proceeding smoothly even if the data cable's angle of refraction around the table leg is straightening out some, meaning the table is no longer being held to the Plexiglas wall and is beginning to drift away, but only by a few inches. No big deal.

But then something unforeseen happens: the telephone's cord tightens as its own slack is drawn out. Noticing the problem, Carl pauses to mull it over. He gives the cable a gentle pull – just four inches or so – and the table slides towards him accordingly but not the telephone. Instead it drags across the tabletop all of those four inches, coming to rest less than a foot from the table's far edge. The problem is obvious: if Carl doesn't pull the table any closer the phone remains safe and sound atop the table but still some two meters out of reach. But if he *does* pull it closer the phone is dragged from the table and falls to the floor, maybe disconnected, maybe broken, maybe not, but maybe a wee bit closer. There's really no way to calculate the outcome, as pure random luck seems to hold the cards here. Carl finds himself at reason's end: it having carried him along as far as it could. And now there seems nothing he can do but take a senseless leap of faith. Hence, in a recklessly sudden move that surprises even him — spawn, no doubt, from the sheer stress and frustration of the situation — he gives the data cable a forceful yank. The resultant tightening of the cable flings the lightweight table across the lab floor, sliding it some ten meters off to Carl's left where it crashes against an eye wash station. It also happens to spin about the computer server to which it had been connected, ripping the cable from its input mooring and causing all the power indicator lights on all of the sundry monitors and equipment on that wall of the lab to go black. Then, of course, there's the *other* ramification of the rash action — and, suffice it to say, it doesn't help Carl's disposition much that this one was somewhat predicted — the telephone, now rests on its side out on the lab floor, with its receiver, connected by that old-fashioned type of coiled three-wire cable, sprawled out even further away. Attempting to assess the exact hopelessness of his predicament, Carl gazes out at the wall of dark, power-deprived equipment, then down at the seemingly lifeless and out-of-reach telephone. As if to compound his frustration, the overhead vent blowers kick on again — rattling, squeaking, deafening. The situation is indeed dire, and Carl quantifies it as such with one last, heavy sigh.

Exhausted, defeated, Carl walks back to the hospital bed, sits his butt on the edge, braces his bad elbow with his good arm, swings his legs around and onto the bed, then lies back down. If he is going to survive this flu bug — even if it's not the lethal strain — he is going to need rest, that much he knows; maybe another day or two. There seems to be plenty of saline bags stacked over there in the cabinet to keep him hydrated and to replenish his electrolytes; that's all he really needs for now. *How long's it been since I've eaten?* he wonders. *Alaska? No. Did I touch anything on the plane? Don't recall. Shit, I better be careful here. I could drink the saline right out of the bags but that wouldn't be as efficient as hooking myself back up to the I.V. rack.*

Carl is lying on his back staring up at the stainless steel I.V. rack when the idea hits him. He pauses for a few seconds to think it through, to fully imagine it, to weigh its validity. Convinced either that it might just work or simply that he has no choice, Carl bolts upright, swings his legs onto the floor again, then grabs hold of the I.V. stand. Lifting it up, he studies the rack's hooked upper end, then the expandable two-meter length vertical rod, then, lastly, the four-legged stand that holds it upright. Hopping from the bed he begins searching about for something to help him remove the I.V. stand's legs. Reasoning that the bed is the most immoveable object of the cell's otherwise portable furnishings,

Carl locks the brakes on each of the bed's wheels. His next order of business is to pass the stand's upper end through the bed frame. That done, he pauses to prepare himself for an all-or-nothing event, then yanks on the stand as hard and quickly as he can — once, twice, three, four, five, six, no sense stopping, seven, eight, nine times. And nine proves to be the deciding effort, the magic number, for with that ninth and final yank the I.V. stand's legs and the lone bolt holding it are efficiently dismembered from the rest of the stand. And Carl sighs with relief; a wistful, cautious sigh; a sigh which connotes a certain cognizance of the fact that one tiny success, or even a string of them, does not a victory make.

Now virtually ignoring his broken arm, Carl walks the two-meter stainless rod back over to the wall grommets. He slides the stand's hooked end — the upper end designed to support the IV bags, et al — through the right-side grommet hole, passing it without a hitch on through the hole in the gnawed-out glove. Holding the rod steady with the hand of his injured right arm, he then slips his left hand back into the intact grommet glove then takes over control of the rod with it. His next item of business is to carefully allow the rod to slide through his left hand until he is holding it by its broken end, this minor feat earning him a two-meter extension to his reach with which he is just able to hook the phone's hand-piece receiver and pull it most of the way towards him. With the main part of the phone's cord already stretched to its limit, Carl's only hope is to pull slack from the receiver's coiled cord enough to bring it all the way to his hand. And he almost makes it — lifting the receiver off the floor with the I.V. stand's hook and pulling it to within a foot of the stretching fingertips of his right hand — before the cord's elasticity yanks the receiver off the rod's hook and flings it to the floor again and sliding past the main part of the phone.

It's a setback for sure; a defeat which could either be taken as decisive or minor depending upon how Carl chooses to take it. Opting to simply not let it bother him — and thereby exhibiting a level of objectivity and maturity and survivability hitherto unknown to even him — Carl extends the rod's hooked end right back out into the lab, past the main part of the phone, and successfully snags the coiled cord again. Cautious this time not to repeat his mistake, Carl pulls on the cord just a few inches at a time, effectively dragging the receiver along the floor and back towards him again, but careful to pull it only as far as the point where the hand receiver will rest by itself and not be snapped away again by the cord's elasticity. That done, he extends the rod's hooked end back to the main body of the telephone again and carefully turns the heavy black bulk of it towards him. When Carl first sees the phone's dial he feels that wash of intimidation one often encounters when confronting a *new* technology; but here is an *old*, anachronistic technology, engendering within him that same, what is it? Malaise? Inadequacy? Fear? He has never used a dial-up phone before – *Hell, he has never even used an abacus!* –- and that unfamiliarity spawns trepidation. *Analog: will it even connect with the modern digital world?* Reasoning he has nothing to lose by trying – he's seen it done in old movies after all – Carl extends the hook towards the finger holes in the dial. Not sure how to place an international call from Brazil, Carl decides to try the same 0-1-1 he used in Tijuana, to be followed by the "country code" for the United States, to be followed by an area code, then local phone number. All in all this is a lot to manage with a two-meter long rod, through an arm grommet, trying to see through the Plexiglas wall that is only fogging more and more with the condensation of each labored breath he takes. *Fuck! – as if this weren't challenging enough!* And if he screws up, misdialing just one digit, well, he'll have to start all over again. And that's only *if* this phone connects to an outside line.

Carl extends the rod at the absolute full reach of his left arm towards the phone dial. Though he's holding the rod as steady as he can, the hooked end dances all over the finger holes, reminding Carl of an unsteady hummingbird hovering before a flower on a very windy day. Finally he is able to stick the hook into the last hole, marked "0." That done he begins slowly to drag the finger hole clockwise around the dial until it reaches the stop. That done, he pulls the rod back an inch and allows the dial to spin back to its starting position. One digit down, fourteen to go; surely people have surmounted Everest with less effort! With his nose and face smushed against the fogged-up Plexiglas, Carl then reaches for the hole marked with the number "1." The hook bobs above the hole – that hummingbird again – trying to steady itself, trying to find that nectar of life….

* * *

1414 Peach Lane, Atlanta, Georgia

The bong gurgles. Smoke tumbles in the cylindrical translucent purple plastic chamber for a few languid seconds, not a care in the world, until being violently sucked out – *vacuumed out by lungs of steel!* It's quiet here in the kitchen, about all that can be heard, aside from the bonging, is the faint overflow from headphones of the otherwise blaring music being pumped into Stuart's ears – local boys made good REM – as well as Stuart's drumming along to the beat with his index fingers on the kitchen table's edge and his occasionally spirited joining-in for the chorus:

> *"It's the end of the world as we know it,*
> *It's the end of the world as we know it,*
> *It's the end of the world as we know it,*
> *And I feel fine...."*

Yes, it is quiet enough that even the girl next door just might be able to hear Stuart's just-started-to-ring telephone as she heads out the door for her car. But not Stuart. Not with those damn headphones on. The only hope of him realizing his phone is ringing is that he might *see* it, it being of the type whose handset flashes with incoming calls. But what with the phone hidden as it is, on the kitchen table but obscured behind so many boxes of cereal and the comics section of the Atlanta Sun newspaper – and his focus being so lazar-like tuned to the "Jumble" puzzle he is working – there's not much chance of that happening.

Muttering the Jumble's final puzzle solution's clue to himself – *"What goes up must come down,"* – Stuart reaches for the raisin bran, inadvertently knocking the box over in the process. When the box smacks down against the table top Stuart happens to notice the concentric rings rattle across the surface of the milk in his cereal-less bowl. With his senses already magnified by the morning's first bong hit he marvels as the minute waves of milk ripple from the rim of the bowl inward then gradually dissipate, seismographically registering the minute impact

the momentum of folly

of the cereal box – or so he thinks. But just as he is priding himself on understanding the source of the disturbance in his bowl of milk, Stuart sees it happen again – the concentric rings rippling across the milky surface – but this time with no falling cereal box or other obvious impetus. And again, the rippling lasts for a few seconds then dissipate… only to begin anew after another few seconds!

"Now, here's a *real* puzzle!" Stuart mutters, as he folds aside the newspaper. What could be causing this subtle rattling of the table? – an earthquake? No, an earthquake – disregarding how rare they are in this part of the North American – would not register with such a phased pattern. Nor would an explosion. No, the source would have to be mechanical, but what? A diesel motor – say from a bus or truck – rumbling just outside? Possibly, but that wouldn't explain the interruption; the few seconds of on-again, off-again calm between the phases of agitation. A passing siren? That could be it, though it's hard to imagine a siren would carry the bass necessary to create the vibrations. *Ah*, thumping rap music! The girl next door must be dating some new guy and her parents aren't home and he's marking his territory by cranking his car stereo and letting it spew outwards for all the neighborhood to enjoy.

"That must be it; rap music."

Confident now that he has deduced the true source of the concentric-milk-ring-causing, table-vibrating disturbance, Stuart can't help but feel a bit smug as he peels off his headphones in order to confirm his hypothesis. But as he removes them, he is confronted with a humbling surprise: there is no rap, or music of any sort, to be heard!

"Fuckin' A," Stuart mutters, even more befuddled than he was just the moment before.

With his earphones now down around his neck, Stuart turns off his own music in order to better devote himself to discovering the source of the enigmatic disturbances causing his cereal bowl to vibrate so. Still staring at the bowl – the surface of the milk now maddeningly calm – Stuart is just about to accept defeat when the answering machine across the kitchen clicks on, playing out it's droll, outgoing message, voiced by Stuart, to whomever might be calling:

"Uh, so, like, Stu and Carl are, like, not here, right? So, like, um, just whatever. Kno'whad'I'm sayin'?"

And in less time than it takes for the out-going message to play, Stuart solves the mystery of the enigmatic seismographic rippling across his bowl of milk; it was his ringing landline telephone. Quickly lifting up cereal box after cereal box positioned around him, he eventually discovers the cordless telephone handset hidden behind the box of Kashi.

"Another mystery solved," Stuart smugly congratulates himself, as he reaches again for the fallen box of raisin bran, which is just when a sudden rush of noise begins to spew from the answering machine. And even though the machine is across the kitchen the incoming message is shrill and harsh and loud all at the same time, creating a haunting mix of rushing wind, alarms, and distant, barely discernable shouts. The irritating cacophony of noise causes Stuart to winch, then bark out to the imagined caller:

"Fuckin' A, dude. Use a phone much?"

Sao Paulo. Carl has his face crammed into the right-side grommet hole and is shouting, at the very top of his lungs, through the gnawed-out glove and down to the phone receiver resting on the floor of the lab.

"Stuart, are you there? It's me — Carl! Pick up!"

Although his voice needs only to carry a mere meter or so, under the noisy circumstances — the in-rushing air, the ventilator pump motors, the lab alarms — it's something of the magnitude of a miracle he can be heard at all.

"Stuart, pick up the fucking phone!"

Atlanta. Unfortunately, from Stuart's end, the phone call — with all its extraneous noise — sounds more like an in-coming fax than a desperate plea from a fellow human, roommate or other. And so he merely shakes his head in pity as he refills his bowl with raisin bran, then shouts back to the phone, "Dude, like, time to switch wireless companies."

Carl pauses: he thinks he may have heard something — a tiny voice perhaps — seep from the phone receiver laying down there on the Slammer's floor, but he cannot be certain. He interrupts his own shouting to stick his ear in the grommet to better listen. But, even straining, he cannot hear anything over all the ambient din on his end. Frustrated, he looks about at the sources of all the noise around him. There's not much he can do about the alarms, not unless he can escape the Slammer cell and locate the shut-off. Then there's the in-rushing wind coming through the gnawed-through glove, coming in at the clip and noise

the momentum of folly

level of a roaring shop vac. And even though it's the least of the three noises, if he were to, say, tie off the hole in the glove to allow the cell to return to a negative air pressure, well, then he wouldn't have anyway to shout through to the phone receiver. So, no real point in that. The third source, and a substantial contributor to the cacophony, is coming from the dual exhaust vent pumps. Carl looks up towards them, each mounted beyond reach above the Plexiglas ceiling and above their respective grated vents, either capable of handling the ventilation task should the other fail. Reasoning that by somehow disabling the vent pumps might be his best bet and quieting at least some of the noise, Carl climbs up onto the bed, stands, then reaches up with his good arm to see if he can pull off one of the grates. But no; even hanging from it, the grate will not break free of the vent frame.

But then another idea comes to Carl; this one as destructive as it is desperate. Climbing off the bed, he crosses to the wall where he leaned the stainless steel I.V. rack rod. Grabbing the rod, he returns to the bed, hops back atop it, then pauses again to think this new plan through. But he's tired of thinking: he's thought hard all his life so far and look where it's got him; trapped quite probably indefinitely in a remote cell with something akin to a life-threatening illness – stuck between the quintessential "rock and a hard place." Hence, rather than investing much energy in thinking this one through, *again* he just acts. And in doing so, with one mighty thrust he shoves the stainless rod up through the slats in the steel grates of one of the vents. Instantly that ventilation pump's fan blade strikes the rod and yanks it violently from Carl's one-handed grip, whacking him once upside the head in the process.

"Fuck!" Carl shouts, as if it might help. He feels the side of his head, and the bump already forming there, and the blood already beginning to trickle. Diagnosing the injury as really not so bad, he returns his attention to the rod, now hanging just beside him from the ceiling grate. For the moment it seems to be effectively jamming the exhaust fan, the only problem being that the ventilator's jammed and straining motor makes an even louder more irritating noise. But, thankfully, this lasts only until something, probably a circuit breaker within the unit, clicks off and shuts the power to the motor down completely.

"This is good. This is good," Carl mutters to himself, beginning to feel that giddy pulse of optimism yet again.

This leaves just one of the two exhaust vents still running. To fix this — by again breaking it — Carl tries to yank the rod free of the disabled vent, but, tug as might — even to the point of hanging his full weight from the rod and bouncing — there's no extricating it from the twisted and entangled vent blades.

"Well, that sucks," he mutters. And though he's only trying to humor himself — that a vacuum pump might *suck* — his quip gives him an idea. Sticking his hand up to the remaining working vent, he feels the powerful suction it creates as it pulls the air from the Slammer cell. Looking about for something he might be able to use, Carl spots the bed pillow. Reaching down and grabbing it, he then raises the pillow to the vent. This works even better than he anticipated as, even before he brings the pillow in contact with the vent, the suction from its powerful motor yanks the pillow from Carl's hand and sucks it fast against the grate. And though the motor keeps running, the pillow effectively muffles the noise as the ventilation pump seems to attempt to smother itself.

Encouraged, Carl hops from the bed and rushes back to the gnawed-out grommet. Now the ambient noise is a fraction what it had been, especially now that the inrushing wind through the ruptured glove has been effectively neutralized. As a result, now when he sticks his head in the grommet, his face is met with only a gentle incoming breeze rather than the deafening, shopvac-esque torrent as before. With the extraneous noises reduced so, Carl shouts again through the grommet and down towards the phone receiver: "Stuart! Stuart, it's me, Carl! Can you hear me? Are you there?"

Stuart wheels himself back across the kitchen with the phone's handset on his lap. Well aware of his tendency of keeping the handset on the table for days at a time he suspects it might be losing its charge again. That could even be the reason he couldn't hear the caller. This happens occasionally; the handset battery dying. Chalk it up to forgetfulness. Chalk it up to too many bong hits. He really should cut back a bit. Carl challenged him to quit completely; vowing he'd do it if Stuart did. But that only lasted three days, until Stuart caved to his vices again. Carl, he could take it or leave it, but Stuart, well, it's his crutch. And now Stuart is thinking about Carl again. He wishes he wouldn't but it's hard not to, especially with a houseful of Carl's stuff around: the ratty couch, the blender for protein smoothies and margaritas, the framed picture of Carl and Angela — both naked but for body paint and faux fur — Stuart snapped of them at Burning Man a couple years back.... Verily, through the mere presence of his stuff Carl himself is, ipso facto, present. No getting around that. It's been forty-eight hours since the phone call from Alaska, and Stuart knows there's a damn good chance — *a seventy percent chance* — Carl might well be dead. Nevertheless, without solid evidence of it, Stuart would rather not entertain the possibility of his roommate's demise. "No news is good news," Stuart mutters to himself, and not for the first time, as he lifts the handset back up towards its charging base. And that's exactly when he hears Carl's barely audible, mouse-like squeak of a voice come through the phone:

"Stu, it's me — Carl! Pick up! Can you hear me? Pick up!"

Suddenly aware that it's his dear roommate on the other end of this so-very-frail-connection Stuart pulls the handset back from its charging base, presses the "Talk" button, then wedges it between his ear and shoulder as he spins his wheelchair back towards the table and nonchalantly answers, "Hey, C-man. What's crackin', cracker? I've been worried sick about you."

From Carl's end, strain as he might, he can only just barely hear Stuart's voice, but not make out anything he says.

"Stu, I can barely hear you. You're going to have to shout."

"Ah'ight," Stuart replies, but still too quietly.

"What?" Carl shouts back.

"Alright; shout, got it," Stuart now yells back while wheeling across the creaky, worn-wood floor and into their tiny living room, coasting to a habitual stop in front of the big front window — prime vantage point for watching the neighbor's daughter's comings and goings.

"Good. I could hear that," Carl shouts back.

"Well, you might not want to hear *this*; I've got some bad news," Stuart begins, finding it awkward to be both loud and sensitive at the same time. Right about then, the girl next-door pops out of her side screen door, already in her red lifeguard one-piece swimsuit and a T-shirt. Just ten meters away with the bungalow windows and front door wide open, she probably hears everything Stuart is shouting. "The blood you sent from Alaska — you know, *your* blood — it tested positive to the Laotian strain."

Carl couldn't quite hear Stuart. "I did what?"

"You tested positive!" Stuart screams back.

Reaching for her car door, the girl next door overhears Stuart's shouting, and somehow it confirms everything she and her girlfriends had always suspected about the two weird guys – the Odd Couple, as they called them – living next to her. She shivers from the perverted imagery conjured by this new data; the kind of cute nerd with his greasy, ever-leering paraplegic roommate. *Gross! What-ever!* – she seems to be thinking as she throws herself into her VW bug, backs down the driveway as quickly as possible, and – in less time than it takes Stuart to sigh – squeals off down the street.

"I don't have it," Carl shouts back.

"Yeah, you *do*. H5N1/Carl, H5N1/Laos; Bird flu, Bird flu; I ran the tests myself!"

Carl reels again, mulling over all the circumstantial little things he knows to be true in an effort to assure himself he cannot possibly have the Bird flu. He can't accept that; the whole mortality thing. Besides, Dr. Jenna risked her life for his. Or did she? And then it hits him again; her *accidental* sticking him with the needle in China, and her casual, *"Oops."*

"Carl, you there?" Stuart asks again.

"Stuart, she jabbed me with a needle when we were still in China," Carl shouts, as he tries to make sense of a still-fuzzy, still-forming theory.

"She did what? I can't hear you all that well."

"She stuck me with a sterile syringe – " And then it dawns on him, "She *vaccinated* me!"

"Vaccinated you for what?"

"She tried to pass it off as an accident, but I really think she was vaccinating me against H5N1!"

"And why would she do that?"

"So any antigen test would make it look like I caught Bird flu."

Stuart shakes his head, "Dude, denial is one of your most endearing traits and all but I'm tellin' ya, whatever you've got matched up with the Laotian strain. You've gotta get back here and rest and hydrate and take your Flintstone vitamins and all that shit, ASAP!"

"Stuart, shut up and listen, alright? She vaccinated me for Bird flu *before* we got the call of the outbreak in Laos; well before we left China."

"So?"

the momentum of folly

"So, she needed me to test positive for H5N1, because she wanted us to think that that's what the Laotian strain was – Bird flu!"

"But that's what it tested out to be."

"Only because she switched the samples on me at the Shanghai Airport. The strain we sent back from China is bogus, as is my own blood sample."

"Nothing bogus about H5N1, man."

"I know, but I think the strain I witnessed in Laos is worse; maybe far worse."

"Worse than Bird flu?" Stuart asks, skeptically. "Like, what could that be?"

"I don't know. Maybe some other avian subtype."

"So, you've got your hemagglutinin threes, fives, and sevens, each with nine possible neuraminidase combinations; so, twenty-seven to chose from."

"And all the H3s are all pretty mild."

"As are the H5s with the exception of Bird flu."

"That leaves just hemagglutinin sevens."

"Like, say, H7N7?" Stuart posits, clearly troubled by the prospect.

Carl shrugs, "Certainly highly virulent yet never shown to have made the interspecies leap to humans."

"Unless –" Stuart begins, warming to Carl's line of reasoning.

"Unless something up in the Arctic caused it to mutate – "

"Via our aforementioned golden triangle –"

Carl nods, "Migratory birds, dogs, seals, whatever –"

"… just enough to make it highly contagious to humans –"

"… and possibly even more lethal –"

"… and, ergo, your perfect pathogen. All new and improved."

"That or simply altogether *new*."

Clearly overwhelmed by the flood of Carl's conspiracy theories, Stuart pulls back to attempt to make sense of it all: "Okay, and why again would she do all that? All this subterfuge – vaccinating you for H5N1, all while knowing she's about to march you into a hot zone of H7N7 – "

"Or something altogether new," Carl reminds Stuart.

"Right. Whatever. Point is: what's the point of her doing that?"

"To tie up the CDC and WHO's resources working on the wrong strain – "

"Sending them into full-production on the H5N1 vaccine?"

"Right, while they spread the *real* virus."

"Wow, okay, so running with this wild hypothesis: how do suppose *they* plan to do this? — spread the *real* bad-boy strain, I mean."

"I'm not sure. All I know is they all infected themselves with it, I'm guessing, like, a day or so ago. I don't know exactly — I've been pretty grogged-out."

"And this is the same *they* you were wanking about last time; you know, on your flight to Alaska?"

"Yeah — same *they*."

"And you say they gave the real virus to *themselves?*"

"Yeah. I watched them do it."

"Man, that's hardcore," Stuart reels, incredulous. "Wait, so where are you anyway?"

"In an L-5 Slammer."

"L-5? But the only Level-Five lab is the WHO's in Sao Paulo, Brazil!" Stuart shouts back skeptically, certain Carl must be mistaken.

"That's right," Carl shouts back glumly, as he gazes about his confines.

"Fuckin' A," Stuart reels, "I'm jealous!"

"Well, don't be. I'm trapped in here."

"But if you don't have the lethal strain, why won't they let you out?"

"No one's here. They split. The place is deserted."

"They *splat*, or maybe *splitted*," Stuart attempts to correct Carl, only to puzzle himself in the process.

"Stu, could you *focus* a bit here?"

"Right. Okay. So you're like, what; stuck in the Slammer cell all by yourself?"

"Exactly."

"So, what are you going to do?"

"*So*, I need *you* to get me out."

"*Me?* What, can't you get out of there?" Stuart shouts, suddenly paralyzed by the mere hint of responsibility.

"What part of *locked-in* don't you understand?"

"I'm just saying this is some serious shit to throw on me!"

"Yeah, well, I'm sorry, alright? But it's not like I have any choice here."

Stuart takes a breath, trying to suppress the panic attack he feels coming on. He has to fight through this. "Alright. *Fuck!* Alright, what d'ya need?" He asks, turning away from the window, and wheeling over to his computer. Parking there, he slips on his headset, which he jacks into the phone.

"There are five scientists behind this."

"*Five?* Jesus. How do you know?"

"She introduced me to each one of them."

"Dr. Jenna did?"

"Yeah. They were all here."

Stuart shakes his head, "This just gets weirder and weirder,"

"Wait 'til you hear who they are."

"Googleable?"

"Definitely."

Stuart opens his computer browser. "Alright, hit me on."

"Okay, first up, Jenna's ex-husband; Dr. Henri LaFond. L, a, f, o, n, d. He's done most of his work out of Oxford."

Stuart already has a Wikipedia entry pulled up and is reading from it, "Boom, here he is: Professor of Biology and Biogenetics, Oxford. Born: Chamonix, France. U.C. Berkeley, PhD in Biogenetics."

"That's where he met Dr. Jenna."

"Looks like he works mostly with amphibians. Thesis entitled: *Anran Demise and Extinction*. Cliché, wouldn't you say?"

"How so?" Carl asks, puzzled..

"*French* guy, working with *frogs?*" Stuart replies, wryly.

"Whatever. I think he's the ringleader; maybe he *and* Jenna."

"*Ahhh*, I hear sharing hobbies is the secret to a strong marriage," Stuart quips glibly, before stumbling upon something else in Henri's bio: "Oh, this is interesting...."

"What's that?" Carl shouts, not quite able to hear over the din.

"Your friend Henri is also part of that Influenza Genome Sequencing Project."

"But he's not a virologist."

"Nor a geneticist; that's what makes it so interesting."

Carl ponders the new data. "Do you think it's possible he and Dr. Jenna may have tinkered with the strain?"

"*Weaponized* it – in TV disaster show parlance."

"Maybe trying to make it more virulent or stable?"

"It's more than new and improved, it's *weaponized!*" Stuart quips, unable to resist a comic riff before turning serious again. "I don't know, but it's certainly possible; heard of *sheathing?*"

"No."

"Suffice it to say, researchers have successfully *sheathed* certain Pox and Ebola viruses within the proteins of other, innocuous strains, permitting them to slip through the immune system and into the cell undetected."

"This shit is *real?*" Carl asks incredulously.

"Not only is it real, but it's also potentially dangerous. You won't find any of the Pox sheathing data anywhere online. You have to dig for it."

Even though Stuart gilds his confirmation with humor, it nonetheless sends a shiver up Carl's spine. "So, if they've tinkered with this flu virus — found or manufactured some new lethal strain and sheathed it in the proteins of a more common strain —

"Like concealing moonshine in a can of Mountain Dew."

"Then again, unlike Pox or Ebola, influenza generally kills *because* it triggers a hefty immune response, in which case you might *want* it to be recognizable," Carl says, thinking aloud but getting nowhere.

"I think we may be wandering too far off into hypothetical oblivion here for our own good. Rather than trying to second guess what they *may* have done, let's adopt the Rumsfeldian strategy and begin with the *known unknowns.*"

"The perps."

"Exactly. Who else was there?" Stuart shouts back.

As much as Carl's brain feels like some amorphous sea sponge soaked in morphine, he does his best to squeeze it for any droplets of recollection. "All right, there was a Latino professor guy... try Perez; Fernando Perez, I think. University of Lima, Peru. Not sure what field. Economics maybe."

One step ahead of Carl on this one, Stuart reads from his screen: "Political Economics of Natural Resources, to be precise. Another mover and shaker: Professor Fernando Xavier Perez won a Guggenheim for a little something he called Worldwide Aquifer Depletion and Arable Land Loss. Obviously another glass-half-empty sort. Who else you got?"

"There was a Japanese guy — older than the others."

"Not much help, buddy."

"Wait, he's a climatologist, I think. Try Nobel laureates."

"Well, that should narrow the field," Stuart smirks, as he refines his search with the qualifiers *climatology* and *Nobel Prize* and almost immediately gets a result. "Whoa, okay: Professor Hiro Nakayama, Tokyo University –"

"That's him!"

"… shared that group 2007 Nobel for his work with the International Panel on Climate Change for his tracking CO_2 levels in Arctic core ice, *blah, blah, blah.*"

"That's definitely him," Carl replies through the grommet. He shifts position, kneeling now to take the weight off his feet as he calls out the last name. "Alright, one more: a Dr. Singh, University of Bombay –"

Even with the long distance delay, Stuart cuts Carl short. "Alyesha?"

"What?"

"Professor/doctor *Alyesha* Singh, Marine Science Institute, U.C. Santa Barbara, and another Guggenheimer; tracked large marine predator declines and extinctions."

"Could be; I'm not sure."

"Itty-bitty thing. Wears a sari most of the time, until it practically melts off of her after being tossed in the pool at Faculty Club bacchanalias."

"You *know* her?"

"She was at UCSB same time we were. I was a graduate T.A. for her Micro Marine Organisms course, back when it looked like dichlorococus might be the answer to CO_2 absorption; back in those heady days of optimism. You don't remember her?" Stuart asks incredulously.

"Vaguely."

"Damn, she was only like my default whack-off fantasy. And you would've known why if you'd've seen her climb out of that pool at the Faculty Club – clingy, wet sari, nipples erect – into the silvery light of the full moon," Stuart recalls, with a pining sigh. "Oh, what a vision; her smiling, ever so shyly, right at me…"

"C'mon, Stu, try to focus!"

"I *am* trying to focus, but you keep trying to interrupt me."

"Stuart, please!" Carl begs, trying to steer Stuart back to the present.

"Alright, alright; was that the last of them?"

"That I met anyway."

"Well, that's quite the eclectic group of conspirators you've compiled. And they were all there, when – yesterday?"

"Give or take a day."

"You don't know?"

"I've been unconscious; they've kept me on morphine!"

"Lucky. So, then where'd they go?"

"That's what we need to find out."

"I hope you're not asking me to break international law and hack into Dr. Singh's credit card account on the slim hope I just might still remember her PIN number as clearly as I do the sight of her climbing out of that pool," Stuart says sarcastically, buying himself time as he enters the string of digits necessary to do just that.

"Of course not."

"Sounds like you are."

"Stu, just get the names to Bronwyn. If she decides the threat is legitimate I'm sure she can get Homeland Security or whoever on it," Carl pleads, exasperated by Stuart's apparent inability to take the matter seriously.

"Yeah, and in just a month or three she'll finally be granted the FISA authorization permitting us to look into each of their respective flight itineraries."

"Stuart, c'mon, this is serious."

Dr. Singh's airline itinerary pops up on Stuart's computer screen.

"Uh-oh. Um, dude, we've got a problem here."

"I'm well aware of that." "No, I mean a big, *big* problem," Stuart responds, with uncharacteristic gravity, which Carl immediately senses.

"Why, what did you find?"

Stuart begins reading the flight itinerary: "Singh, Dr. Alyesha, Air India flight 1221 to Jakarta, continuing on to Dhaka, Calcutta, New Delhi, Mumbai. One night's layover then Garuda flight 5055, Mumbai to Amman, Islamabad, Karachi, Katmandu, Bangkok, Singapore, and Sydney. All that in just one week."

"Booked solid for her entire contagious period," Carl mutters, the ramifications of the multiple flights not lost on him.

Remembering something else – "Oh, shit!" – Stuart pushes away from his computer and rolls over to the pile of junk mail heaped just inside the front door.

"What is it?"

"I saw something –" Stuart begins to say as he rifles through the pile, soon excavating a UCSB Alumni newsletter. "Here it is…." Opening the newsletter, he flips to a page with a photo of Dr. Alyesha Singh then reads the accompanying article. "Dr. Alyesha Singh will be discussing *The Promise of Dichloracacos and CO_2 Absorption* in her upcoming Southern Asian lecture series of the same title commencing — well, how 'bout that? — commencing *tomorrow*."

"She's on a lecture tour?" Carl asks, already worried.

"So it seems." Stuart rolls back to his computer with the newsletter to check the lecture dates against Dr. Singh's flight itinerary. "She's not even pausing to sleep."

"What about the others?"

"I can't think of a way to access their travel itineraries. I would need some social security numbers or PINs or something."

Carl pulls his head away from the grommet to think. As an idea comes to him, he shouts it back towards the phone to Stuart.

"Forget their flights; just do a search of the science lecture circuits. Maybe the others have tours going on too."

"*Duh*," Stuart replies with a self-deprecating slap of the forehead as he begins typing furiously away again. "Trying Henri LaFond…" He drums on his knee as he impatiently awaits a result to pop up on his computer screen. "Bammo. *The Sixth Mass Extinction Event: It's not just about frogs anymore.* Medal of Science recipient Dr. Henri LaFond discusses Earth's present ecological collapse. Paris, London, Istanbul, Rome, Madrid, Prague, Moscow. Boom goes London, boom Par-ree —"

"Sounds like the same m.o."

Stuart nods as he continues singing the Randy Newman song, "… More room for you, more room for me…"

"What about Nakayama?"

Stuart searches the Internet for lectures to be given by Hiro Nakayama. "Bingo: I.P.C.C. Member and Nobel Prize winner Dr. Hiro Nakayama to lecture on CO_2 and irreversible climate change. Tokyo, Bangkok, Seoul, Manila, Shanghai, Beijing."

"How frequent are his lectures?"

"June twenty-fifth, June twenty-sixth, June twenty-sixth again, June twenty-seventh.…"

"So, no more than a day apart."

"With some *twice* a day."

"Crowded jet, lecture, crowded jet, lecture…"

"Man, these be some serious type A-ers you stumbled upon," Stuart notes as he types in another name.

"What about Perez?"

"I'm one step ahead of you, buddy-bud, per usual," Stuart says as his search pulls up a similar lecture schedule: "Mexico City, Bogotá, Buenos Aires, Guatemala City, Quito, Santiago, Lima, Havana, Caracas, Montevideo, La Paz."

Carl reels as the scale and thoroughness of the scientists' endeavor becomes apparent to him for the first time. "So what about our dear Dr. Jenna?" he asks, shouting back through the grommet to the phone.

Stuart enters a quick search for Dr. Jenna William's lectures. Then, as her calendar pops up on his computer screen, he takes a deep breath and sighs, "Same-shit; Nairobi, Cairo, Addis Aduba, Kharrhi, Johannesburg, Lagos. Sensing a pattern here?"

"What do you mean?"

"Perez, South America. Nakayama, Asia. Singh, Southeast Asia. LaFond, Europe. Dr. Jenna, Africa…."

Carl nods, as the dots connect. "Each is taking out their ethnic homeland."

"Yep. Kinda touching, ain't it."

"So, who's got *North* America?"

Stuart rolls away from his computer, pops a wheelie in his chair and spins — *to think* — but as no answer comes is forced to concede, "Good question."

As Carl ponders the same conundrum the lab's lights begin to flicker then go out completely. He snaps his focus over to the bank of machinery in time to see all their tiny power indicator lights go dark. And, simultaneous with that, the overhead exhaust vent suddenly shuts down, causing Carl's noise-muffling pillow to drop from the ceiling. What with the outage and the subsequent termination of all the sundry electronic machinery, the cell and surrounding laboratory now becomes a chamber of utter silence. And of utter *darkness* as well, though this lasts only until battery powered, strategically placed, emergency backup lights begin switching on — each one announced by a loud *clank* — in most every corner of the lab. Similar but distant *clanks* can then be heard as other emergency lights come on in the adjoining corridor just outside the lab.

Already accustomed to having to shout over the mechanical din and listen attentively in order to converse with Carl, Stuart is now troubled by the sudden silence coming from the Brazilian end of the phone connection. "Carl? You still there?" he calls out worriedly.

Due to the fact that the Slammer's old-fashioned phone carries its own low voltage power source, wholly independent of the facility's and fed to it through its frail transmission wires, it ends up it is the only electronic, non-battery powered device still working. And working well, as it turns out, with Carl now able to easily hear Stuart's voice squeaking out of the hand piece.

"Yeah, still here," Carl calls back, with more ease than before, to Stuart.

"What happened? Why can I hear you now?"

Already testing another theory: Carl crosses the cell to its hatch door, calling out as he does, "The power's out."

"Just there in the lab or the whole facility?"

Rather than shouting back to phone again, Carl instead gives the hatch door a gentle push. As expected, the now powerless magnetic lock offers no resistance allowing the door to swing freely open. Carl steps through the hatch then walks over to the phone, picking up its receiver with his good hand.

"Impossible to say just yet," he replies, now using a normal voice.

"Whoa, I can hear you perfectly!" Stuart remarks, perplexed.

"Because I'm out of the Slammer cell."

"How?"

"The power outage."

"Ah, electro-magnetic locks; stands to reason. So, why's the phone working?"

"Don't know. It's one of those old school types; must have its own power source," Carl answers, cradling the handset between his ear and shoulder as he picks up the phone's bulky main body with his good arm again and begins to wander about the lab.

Stuart nods, already understanding. "Which tells us it's just the facility's power that has gone down." Stuart's face now twists in confusion once again. "Which makes no sense at all."

"Why's that?" Carl asks, now crossing to the door leading from the lab. He peeks through the door's wire reinforced Plexiglas window and out down the building's main corridor, lighted every twenty meters or so with more emergency backup lights.

"C'mon, we're talkin' the only Level Five facility in the *world*; it should have backup generators up the whazoo!" Stuart answers, then ponders it all a bit more before opining: "Somethin' ain't right about this."

Carl gives the door a push, and it too swings open. He pauses at the threshold, hesitant to step through. "Maybe they *want* me to escape."

Stuart rolls his eyes. "If that were the case, then why'd they bother to lock you up in the first place?"

"Maybe *I'm* the one that's supposed to carry the virus back to North America."

"But you're not infected, right?"

Carl, uncertain of anything at this point, says nothing.

"I mean, we thought you were — at least I did — but then you did a bang-up job of convincing me otherwise, right?" Stuart continues, exasperated by the uncertainty of it all. "Isn't that where we stand? — you not infected?"

"Yeah, well, now I'm not so sure."

"Jesus!" Stuart groans.

"Well, think about it: first they needed a scapegoat, now they need a carrier."

"An *unwitting* carrier?"

"It explains why they didn't kill me when they had the chance."

"So, what is it? They know you're infected, but at the same time know that you think you're *not*, which is why they're willing to let you just walk out of there confident you'll just, what? — stupidly hop aboard a commercial flight and unknowingly float the virus back to the States and begin spreading it around up here? And that's these evil geniuses' grand plan for North America?" Stuart asks, not even trying to mask his skepticism.

"Something like that."

"That's fuckin' paranoidically moronic!"

"Maybe. But it's the only thing that makes sense."

Like any good scientist, Stuart steps away from his position in order to give the argument the critical distance needed for objectivity. And after investing much thought on the matter, he concedes, "All right, maybe you *are* an integral component of their plan. I'll grant you that."

"Thank you," Carl says, facetiously.

"Then again, what with them passing through so many international airports, and coming in contact with so many travelers headed to or through the

U.S., maybe they've surmised the pandemic's establishing itself here is inevitable – regardless of your participation."

"That stands to reason as well," Carl admits.

"Though having you as the lone renegade carrier *would* make for a tidy headline, and certainly simplify the finger-pointing."

"And it would all be too late by the time the truth caught up."

Stuart sighs, and shakes his head. "So, what do you want me to do?"

At the end of the phone's cord, Carl makes his way back into the lab. "Try to find out exactly which flights they're on. Tell Bronwyn and Hank so they can quarantine those planes before they reach their destinations."

"But they took off, when, like yesterday we think, right? So they could well be on their second or third flights by now!"

"Then those flights will have to be quarantined too, as well as every flight every one of their co-passengers took afterwards."

Stuart is already feeling overwhelmed by the task. "Well, I think I speak for the entire epidemiological community when I say *fuuuuck!*"

"While you're at it, book me a seat on the next flight back to Atlanta."

"A *commercial* flight?"

"It's the quickest way."

"You're high!"

"Stu, I need to get back ASAP so we can isolate the strain and get started on a vaccine; it's the only hope for stopping this thing!"

"Maybe, but no one's gonna let you on a commercial flight, fucking doofus."

Stuart's point gives Carl pause. "They don't have to know."

"Don't tell the airline you're infected?" Stuart asked incredulously.

Carl nods, "Just have them quarantine the plane when we land."

"Then allow me to rephrase what I just said: *I'm* not going to let you onto a commercial flight."

"But –"

"No. Shut the fuck up. Sixty-six to seventy percent mortality rate, Carl. Two out of three of your co-passengers will die if it's the lethal strain."

"It's collateral damage."

"No, it's *bullshit*, that's what it is! Jesus, didn't we just have this conversation when you were en route to Alaska?"

"Maybe we can scare up a private plane."

"What about this don't you understand? You're a probable carrier of one of the most deadly viruses in the history; any contact with the outside world might push us past any hope for containment. Get it? – you're exactly where you need to stay. You can't leave there!"

Despite the perfect logic of Stuart's argument, Carl resists it. "So, what am I supposed to do; wait here to see if I die or not?" he asks.

The question is too direct: Stuart, for perhaps the first time in his life, is utterly speechless. Several awkward moments of heavy silence pass as both roommates, on their respective parts of the globe, ponder the bleak conclusion of their reasoning: Carl must stay put, to die if that's how the dice roll out.

Meandering aimlessly about the lab, Carl crosses over to a wall lined with several metal cabinets. Not having a clue what he might be looking for, he opens the first cabinet – surgical gloves, smocks, facemasks, etc. – then the next – sundry wound care bandages and antiseptics – then finally the third – wherein hangs one, lone biosafety suit. Carl pauses, staring at it for a beat as he tries to imagine its applicability to his quandary.

"I can wear a suit."

"You can wear a fucking *tux*, they're still not going to let you on a plane," Stuart retorts, misunderstanding Carl.

"No; a *biosafety* suit."

"Oh. Right and, what, they're going to just let you walk onto the plane and sit your scary ass down between the crying kid and the pregnant lady?" Stuart scoffs.

"Maybe they can sneak me on before general boarding; let me sit on one of those flight attendant jump seats in back."

Stuart is shaking his head. "I don't know, I don't see it happening. No airline would take that risk. You asking them to allow a guy with a figurative bomb onto the plane just because he promises he won't light the fuse. Besides, what if it turns out you're *not* infected? We jump through all these hoops only to get you back here to discover we still don't have the right strain. Huh? What then?"

All Carl knows is that he doesn't have the answer. He crosses back to the table where the scientists infected themselves one by one. Mesmerized he gazes down at the thermos and its intentionally spilled puddle of coagulating blood and chunks of lung tissue. In a way, the worst part is his not knowing if he is infected with the lethal strain of the virus. He'd almost rather know he had the lethal strain than *not know* he didn't have it. At least that is how he feels right now; right now it's the uncertainty that is killing him.

"Besides," Stuart, ever the voice of reason, continues, "the Spanish flu killed people in as few as ten hours after infection; the *healthiest* people — middle of the Bell Curve folk just like you — and yet, here you are, three, four, five days after your initial exposure and you seem to be getting along fine. Would you agree; are you feeling better?"

Carl thinks about it: he *is* ambulatory now; Stuart is certainly right about that. He feels his forehead: no indication of fever, or sore throat, or coughing, but that could just all be because of the morphine. But even so, if his immune system is still fighting off the viral infection, he should at least be sweating. Quite to the contrary, for the first time in weeks — seemingly for as long as he, in his delirium, can remember — he *isn't* sweating. This could mean one of two things: either he's nearly over this nasty flu bout, or his beaten-down immune system has completely exhausted itself of its ability to fight the infection off any longer, and it's now just a matter of time before he fully succumbs.

"Stu?" Carl says, reigniting conversation as he continues to ponder the puddle of lung tissue and coagulated blood on the table.

"Yeah," Stu replies, face in his hands, physically and emotionally exhausted.

"How long can influenza survive at room temperature?"

"What're we talkin' — airborne? The virus itself is actually pretty fragile. If someone sneezes it can only hang in the air for something like an hour or so before it starts to break down."

Carl is still staring down at the tipped thermos. Picking it up and gently swirling it he finds there's still a few ounces of blood and lung tissue in it.

"How about in a blood sample?"

"Longer; days, maybe a week — depends."

Carl takes a deep breath, beginning to formulate a plan. "What about in live blood or living tissue?" he asks, now picking up a glass pipette from the table.

"Completely different story: easily a week or two, *indefinitely* maybe so long as it is supplied with uninfected cells in which to replicate itself."

As Stuart speaks, Carl places one end of the pipette in his mouth and the other down into the thermos. Using it as a straw, he begins to carefully suck on it until he has drawn a few milliliters of the ruddy, lethal soup up the tube, but making sure to stop an inch or so before it reaches his lips. Pulling the pipette from his mouth, Carl quickly caps the top end with his thumb in order to suspend the bloody fluid in the tube with the vacuum created by the airtight seal.

Meanwhile, back in the Atlanta bungalow, the disturbing line of questioning coupled with the protracted silence coming from Carl's end of the phone has Stuart beginning to worry again what exactly what his roommate is up to. "Uh, so, like, why do you ask?" he asks tentatively.

Reticent to explain his thought processes, Carl ignores Stuart's question, and instead simply tilts back his head and drains the pipette's contents directly into one of his nostrils, the unnatural act causing him to cough and snort violently.

Stuart listens worriedly from his end of the phone line. "Carl, what are you doing? You'd tell me if it was anything really, really stupid right, roomie?"

Still ignoring Stuart's question, Carl inhales quickly through his nose, sniffling the fluid deeper into his sinuses. Once settled, he then draws up another pipette full of the ruddy fluid from the thermos and does the same thing to his other nostril. Again he chokes and coughs then quickly snorts the fluid and tissue chunks up and into his sinuses, soon feeling them trickling down the back of his throat.

"Carl, please explain this awful feeling I have in the pit of my stomach," Stuart says, pleading for an explanation.

But again Carl dodges the question.

"Stu, I need you to do something."

"You mean, you need me to do something *else*."

Now that the seriousness of his situation has escalated dramatically, Carl ignores Stu's quip, instead stating simply: "Call Angela, tell her what's going on…"

"Yeah? – *I* don't even know what's going on!" Stuart scoffs angrily.

"Call Angela and tell her I'm willing to trade her company a portion of the Laotian strain in exchange for secured, private jet transport back to Atlanta."

Stuart pauses, clearly skeptical of the implications of Carl's proposal. "You want to give Aegis Pharmaceuticals first crack at the vaccine?"

"It's not a matter of my *wanting* to; we need to get this strain back to the CDC as quickly as possible. Aegis's CEO will smell the potential windfall in this; I'm sure he'll find a way to get me out of here fast," Carl replies, matter-of-factly.

"But isn't that kind of like dealing with the Devil?"

"I don't see that we have a choice."

* * *

A rarely-if-ever-opened metal security door squeaks and groans on dry, rarely-if-ever-lubricated hinges as it is pushed open — slowly and with considerable effort — from the inside. It's a plain, dirty, off-white door in a vast, plain, dirty, off-white, windowless, construction block wall; the kind found on the backside of some shopping mall somewhere — anywhere. Anytown, USA. Anytown, Planet Earth. But the security door is eventually pushed open enough to reveal… Carl — the pushing force — now sporting the WHO biosafety suit he found hanging inside the Level Five lab. Like stepping from a darkened movie theatre out into the way-too-harsh midday glare, he squints painfully, reeling from the stark contrast between the interior darkness and the exterior's wash of sunlight. As he tries to pry his eyes open from the mere slits they are, he takes a step away from the building, releasing the door. He feels lightheaded. Maybe it's just the sunlight, the first in quite some time. Maybe it's the days upon days of morphine. Maybe it's the weeks of being sick — exacerbated by the one, two, three, who knows how many different strains of influenza coursing through his body. Whatever the cause of his lightheadedness, the result is that the outside world feels very, very surreal to him. And this feeling is only underscored as he hears the sudden *whooomph!* as the spring-hinged security door pulls itself closed behind him. He spins about as quickly as he can, only to find the handle-less, self-locking security door already shut and sealed and appearing as if it hasn't been opened in years, if ever. Didn't he just pass through it? — already Carl can't be certain, such is the *surreality* of it all. But of one thing he *is* certain; he is now locked out of the deserted building, a realization he verbalizes all in one pithy little sentence:

"Well, this sucks."

Supporting his broken arm with his still useful one, Carl turns a slow, pirouetting gaze-about; a 360° reconnaissance of his present location. Based on what he sees, he appears to be on the flat, third story roof of the sprawling, split-level, four-story WHO facility. And judging by the sizeable expanse of smooth concrete with the giant, fluorescent yellow "H" on it, he's found the building's heliport and, thus, quite by luck, is precisely where he was trying to get himself.

His eyes adjusting to the sunlight better now, his lightheadedness abating some, he walks out to the edge of the roof and looks down. Down there, he sees the facility's vast and empty parking lot, as well as the similarly deserted walkways connecting the complex's many buildings. The dearth of any signs of other human life has him feeling like the Omega Man; every boy's dream in fantasy, but in reality not much fun. Lifting his gaze to the horizon, he finds the facility virtually surrounded by slashed and burned rainforest, marooned within a logged wilderness temporarily spared from further development only because of the current global economic crisis. Off in the distance — in a direction that appears to be east, but is impossible for Carl to ascertain due to the directly overhead position of the sun — he can make out the brown haze that implies civilization. Probably Brazilia, he assumes, if memory of the lab's location serves him at all.

Off to one side of the helipad, Carl notices a lonely concrete bench. It too strikes him as surreal; why is it made of concrete? Why is it here at all? Has anyone ever sat on it? Those are some of the questions that swim through his brain as he — the boy in the bubble — stares at the bench. With nothing to do but wait for his ride, Car walks over to the bench, turns his butt towards it, then sits.

University of South Africa, College of Agriculture and Environmental Sciences.

It's standing-room-only in the "Unisa" lecture hall, packed with post grads, teachers, and the just plain curious. They applaud respectfully then settle into their seats as they welcome their guest speaker to the podium. To them, Dr. Jenna Williams embodies the triumphant story of a local African girl who made good; Nobel laureate, world-renowned epidemiologist, all the pioneering research in RNA-based viruses, et al. It doesn't seem to matter to them she was born up in Zaire and not in South Africa, nor that her parents were both American. It's not a national thing, or even a continental patriotism that has them rooting for her. Rather, it's just the fact that she is black; black like most of them, and thereby of more obvious African roots than most guest lecturers who come to speak here; black and yet has managed to rise to the fore of her field. If she can do it, they all can. She is a role model, a confirmation their aspirations are attainable after all. And so they applaud.

Upon hearing the College of Agriculture and Environmental Sciences President's warm introduction and the subsequent applause, Jenna crosses from the darkened wings out to center stage. There she first shakes hands with the President, then receives an unexpected hug, which seems to stimulate the audience up a notch in their clapping. It's all very embarrassing for Jenna. She has risen, whether deservedly or not, to pop star status and it doesn't suit her. *Why do people gush and fawn over others just because they are, for whatever reason, famous?* — that's a question Jenna has pondered but kept to herself ever since winning the Nobel. Sure, the praise was flattering at first but now, on this first lecture of her current tour, she is beyond embarrassed by it all. Truth be told, she is outright shamed by the praise. *If they only knew!* — is what she is thinking, her conscience pounding like a migraine, as she steps up to the podium. Yet, despite all the guilt and shame and

the momentum of folly

embarrassment, she musters a smile and some nods to acknowledge and settle the gushing audience's applause but still all the while is thinking, *If they only knew.*

"Thank you.... Thanks.... Thank you very much. You are very kind; *too* kind!" she tells them, with a bit of a stuffed up nose. Those in the front row or two might notice the beads of perspiration on her brow, or even hear her sniffling as she pulls away from the lectern mike. But there's no cause for concern: who hasn't had a cold?

"Thank you, it's wonderful to be back here. It's good to be home," she tells them, with perhaps unwarranted emotion, except for the inexplicable fact that she feels it too – this African homecoming. She then pulls away from the microphone to sneeze discreetly off to one side. This prompts her to switch on the large but quiet, oscillating floor fan set up just behind her. It was in her lecture contract – in all of them, in fact. It was the one curious stipulation which she explained away with an innocuous statement about how stagnant, stuffy air – common in over-crowded lecture halls – can make her feel faint. The College had no reason to question her request, however odd; anything to make the "star" feel comfortable. As the fan's blades began churning the air, pushing it past Jenna and out over the audience, swinging its aim from the left side of the room to the right side then methodically back again, Jenna returns to the lectern microphone. Alluding to the fan behind her with a casual nod, she quips:

"My biggest fan."

Her trite play on words elicit a smattering of laughter from her naïve audience, each and every one of them oblivious of the *real* reason for the fan. The laughter, that's another thing about fame; the slightest, dumbest joke gets a response. There's a King Midas-esque aspect to this phenomenon that makes her skin crawl, but she can't worry about that now; she has bigger fish to fry.

Centers for Disease Control, Atlanta, Georgia.

Bronwyn sits at the conference table, silent, fuming. She is revealing herself to be the kind of person who, under extreme conditions of stress, becomes angry at bad news; one of those who tend to blame the messenger, an idiosyncrasy which bodes none too well for Stuart, sitting just across the table from her.

"*The wrong strain,*" she says, or asks; or maybe it's a request for confirmation even though she certainly does not need it, as she heard him clearly the first time. It really doesn't matter which. The point is she is repeating what Stuart has just broken to her but with such downplayed, acidic seething that he is already wishing he hadn't told her, even if possibly billions of lives depended upon this trickling flow of data from him to her.

Stuart squirms in his wheelchair. Somehow, throughout the decades of sitting in it, he never felt as uncomfortable as right now. An awkward nod precedes his reply: "Yeah, well, we think so," he confirms, about as meekly as a human can. Oh, how he wishes he did not have to be here. Oh, how he wishes he could run. If somehow he were given the ability, he would run away and run forever, the stresses of the CDC, the anger of his confinement, the woes of all humanity – all of it, the wind at his back. But it seems he can't; reality being the cruel, cold, unfair motherfucker that it is.

Hank, sitting to Bronwyn's left, is the next to jump onto the *blame train*. But his rage comes as no surprise; it has always been there, right on top of his skin like a festering melanoma. And it seems Stuart, albeit for reasons inexplicable, has forever been his primary irritant.

"*He thinks so,*" Hank begins, repeating Stuart's last works with passive/aggressive disdain. Ostensibly Hank is addressing the others at the table but, no mistaking here, his wrath is directed right back at Stuart. "One hundred and twenty million injected, fertile, possibly *ruined* eggs later, and he *thinks* we're working with the wrong strain!"

"It's not like I've been sitting on this. I just fucking found it out too!" Stuart retorts, angry enough to convey to the others that, if they need a scapegoat, they should look elsewhere.

"It's alright, Stuart —" Ross begins, proving himself to be the counter-balancing angel to Hank's devil, sitting just off Bronwyn's right shoulder.

"No, it's *not* alright. Carl and I have been busting our asses to figure this out and you treat me like some kind of —"

"Stoner?" Hank interjects, with a very intentional jab.

Stuart glares at Hank. *If looks could kill….*

"So, where is Carl now?" Ross asks, not attempting to dispel the tension so much as merely trying to glean more information.

"He's coming," Stuart replies.

"Bringing the *real* strain with him?" Bronwyn asks, hopefully.

Stuart hesitates. "Yeah, well, we think so."

Hank groans and throws up his hands. And it's not just him who is visibly disappointed by Stuart's uncertainty, for, from all around the table — of which there might be three representatives from each of the six branches of the CDC present — a collective, groaning, conveyance of frustration can be heard. Stuart watches as heads shake and drop into their hands, mourning all the funds and effort and time squandered on producing the vaccine with the wrong strain. His visual sweep around the table eventually brings him back to Hank, still glaring at him.

"Alright, fuck it!" Stuart says, fed up with it all. Opening his leather satchel, he begins stuffing all his papers and documentation into it with haphazard disdain. He pauses, "No, fuck all of *you*!" Reversing his actions, he now begins yanking his various papers and printouts back *out* of his satchel then angrily flings them randomly about the table towards the others. "Here're the names of the scientists we think might be behind this." Stuart grabs another handful of printouts and flings them in another direction, "And here're their lecture tour dates, *we think*, and locations, *we think*, and probable flights, *we think*, and whatnot." And yet another handful of papers is pulled out and flung in yet another direction, "And here's a bunch of other shit for you all to roll around in. So, if you really want to get to the bottom of this and possibly even try to contain this outbreak — you know, like, *do your jobs* — I suggest you make an effort to find out exactly which flights these people are on and start quarantining anyone and everyone that has flown with them, then maybe start emailing or faxing or getting on the phone with whoever you think might give a shit because, frankly, I don't anymore!" And with that fit of anger and air of finality, Stuart pushes away from the table, spins, and thrusts himself towards the nearest exit.

"Stuart…" Bronwyn calls out to him.

"Save it!" he shouts back, without even turning to face her – his boss.

"Stuart!…" she shouts again.

"No, no; can't fire me, 'cause *I quit!*" he shouts back over his shoulder as he fumbles his way out through the door and out into the relatively fresh air of the hall.

Bronwyn waits a beat, shares a quick glance with Hank, then shouts out after Stuart one last time, and just before the door closes:

"… good job!"

Somewhere over India.

It is a routine flight, Calcutta to New Delhi, aboard a creaky Boeing 777. The captain is taking a nap; justified as much by the nearly errorless record of auto-pilot devices as by the numerous studies on his profession being overworked by management well beyond what is considered safe. The co-pilot could be doing the same but has instead opted to squander his autopilot time gazing down to the reddish wasteland slipping 30,000' beneath their wings. As subterfuge he's holding the recent issue of an American pop magazine just for when the cute flight attendant brings in his tea. He knows it will pique her interest. He knows she'll beg him to let her read it and that could be a bargaining chip – for dinner or drinks or who knows? – once the crew reaches their layover in New Delhi. So, he holds the magazine open on his lap even though his real interest is in the geography passing beneath them. Even though he grew up somewhere down there, he still finds it hard to believe such desolation can sustain life; barren, red wasteland – might as well be the surface of Mars. Now Bangladesh – all green and watery – that place at least looked habitable when they flew over it on the way from Dhaka to Calcutta, which is no doubt why it now has one of the highest population densities in the world; 170 million in an area one-fifth the size of Texas. India, on the other hand, most of it anyway, looks a lot *like* Texas; not down there on the ground, of course, but from up here – from the air. Similar also to Texas, vis-à-vis the border it shares with Mexico, is the new fence separating India from Bangladesh, built to protect India from the anticipated inrush of Bangladeshi immigrants. But it's not the usual illegal immigrants India is worried about – not the kind seeking better paying jobs, et al – but rather the first wave of *climate refugees*, folks merely seeking dry ground on which to live. And there will be a lot of them, possibly one hundred million, since half of Bangladesh's total land mass lies at an elevation within one meter of the current sea level. Yes, it certainly will be interesting times once climate change raises sea levels that mere one meter and floods the Bangladeshis out of their low-lying

the momentum of folly

Ganges-Bramaputra Delta, chopping in half the total area of their already soggy nation. This, obviously, will double Bangladesh's already exorbitant 2,800 per square mile population density, subjecting their huddled masses to the winds and waves of polluted cyclones whipping in from the Indian ocean on one side, while the border fence traps them in on the other. Good times. And yet here — beneath the airliner's wings right now — is arid, seemingly uninhabitable India. The co-pilot gazes out wondering where the 1.3 billion of his fellow countrymen actually live. He recalls once when he was young, eight maybe, an American came through his neighborhood in Lucknow. The American held a rally, gave out candy and brochures, put up a banner. And even though his father and some of the other men from his village promptly tore the banner down and burned it claiming the event was undoubtedly a Pakistani Muslim plot to eventually outpopulate the Hindis, the co-pilot still remembers it clearly. He even remembers the hand-painted banner: "For us. For them. For it. Just two children. Just two billion. We can live with that."

A hard-to-ignore *ping!* emanates from the Boeing's onboard computer yanking the co-pilot from his reminiscence and apprizing him of an urgent email.

"What is it?" the captain asks, without even lifting his cap from his dozing eyes.

The co-pilot hesitates, not sure he's reading the order right, not sure if it's genuine.

"We're to change destination."

"To *where?*"

"Diego Garcia."

"Diego Garcia? The U.S. Naval Support Facility?" the captain asks, now sitting upright and blinking the sleep from his eyes — clearly bewildered.

"That's what it says."

Hoping the email is just some mistake or glitch, the captain taps on the computer screen as he asks the co-pilot, "Is it your birthday?"

"No."

"You getting married tomorrow or something like that?"

"What, you think it's a prank?" the co-pilot asks, a slight tremble in his voice.

The captain shrugs as he slips on his headphones. "I don't know. If there was a problem at Delhi I would think they'd simply reroute us to Lucknow or

Jaipur; not dispatch us to a remote island in the ocean." He then takes up his radio handset and speaks into it:

"This is Air India 1221 requesting confirmation of orders for flight redirection. Over." The captain waits a few seconds before repeating his effort: "Repeat: this is Air India 1221 requesting confirmation of orders for flight redirection. Over."

"Uh, sir?" the co-pilot initiates timidly.

"What?"

"I think there's our *confirmation*," the co-pilot continues, now directing the captain to the two Sukhoi-39 Indian Air Force fighter jets rising to within ten meters of either of the Boeing airliner's wingtips.

After exchanging a troubled glance with the co-pilot, the captain sighs deeply and nods, "Switching off autopilot."

Back somewhere with the huddled masses in the coach section of the 777, Dr. Alyesha Singh finally ends a long paroxysm of coughs with a mucousy discharge into her already snot-soaked handkerchief.

The sari-wearing woman seated beside — one of those who have been with the flight ever since it boarded way back in Brasilia — scowls her dark, bagged eyes at Alyesha not even trying to conceal her irritation. She's got four restless kids with her. She hasn't slept in over twenty hours. She certainly doesn't need some uppity, worldly, erudite, childless *sister* coughing incessantly in her ear. Hell no, she'll stuff that little waif of a woman in the overhead compartment if she has to; Big Mama needs her sleep!

"Sorry," Alyesha tells the woman, apologizing for much more than is obvious. And though the woman turns back to her reading, the heat from her ire, especially as she shakes her head, still can be felt.

Suddenly the plane banks steeply to the left, indicating an unplanned change of direction, from its former north by northwest bearing to something that feels like due south judging by the swing of the sun across the plane's fuselage. Glancing out her high-side window, Alyesha looks up the full length of the 777's right wing and sees the escorting Sukhoi-39 floating along beside them there. The fighter pilot turns towards her, and for an inexplicable moment the two exchange a stare. Does he know who he is looking at? Does the fighter pilot know *she* is the reason he has been dispatched to intercept this commercial plane? Alyesha tries to calm herself, certain it is only her overactive paranoia that is making this wild assumption. But, then again, it is not such a stretch of the imagination. After all, the fact they have singled out *her* plane tells her the authorities have somehow learned of the plot. And if they indeed have learned of the plot, they probably know who she and her cohorts are, and would certainly be privy to the airline's seating arrangement. Hence, that fighter pilot out there could indeed know who she is. In light of that, it's certainly no stretch to assume they have orders to shoot down the flight. That would be the prudent thing to do. A stitch in time saves nine. They are probably just waiting until they can nudge the plane over a sparsely populated region to do so. Then again, the virus would survive the plummet to Earth and thereafter spread easily to the impoverished villagers below who came to comb through the wreckage for wallets and jewelry and gold fillings and such. Hence, the-powers-that-be behind this interception are probably just waiting until they can steer the 777 over open ocean before they shoot it down. It refueled in Biac so the plane could probably make it well out over India's southern tip, well past Sri Lanka even. *That must be the plan: shoot us down over open, uninhabited saltwater,* Alyesha surmises to herself, *That would be the only logical way to nip the viral threat in the bud.*

Alyesha takes a nervous breath then crunches some vague numbers: *Dhaka, Calcutta; if enough sufficiently-infected passengers deboarded there — say, a hundred in each — and managed to slip away before quarantines went up — well, then, maybe just maybe there is hope yet for humanity.*

Narita International Airport, Tokyo, Japan

Dr. Nakayama sweats from a high fever as he tows his one small carry-on suitcase up a busy corridor. Pausing at a water fountain, he fishes a one-dose packet of aspirin from his shirt pocket, which he then tries futilely to tear open with his fingers. It's his joints that are the problem; they are too stiff to grip the packet. The pain is intense. He knows this is a good sign, however; that it is an indication the influenza is in full grip of his system. Clenching a corner of the packet with his teeth he is finally able to tear it open and extricate the two aspirin tablets sealed therein. Tilting his head back, he drops the aspirins on the back of his tongue, then leans over the water fountain, takes a long sip, raises his head again, tilts it back, swallows, and the little pills slide dutifully down on their little water ride to oblivion. Being mere *palliatives* as opposed to actual *medicine*, the aspirin will reduce the fever, swelling and general pain of the infection without stymieing the spread of the virus through his system. And this is a good thing.

Behind him, Dr. Nakayama becomes aware of a commotion brewing. Ironically, it is not the random din of chaos that piques his curiosity, but the rhythmic, out-of-place beat of *order*. Turning towards the commotion he sees the source; a small, particularly well-trained squadron — but of what exactly, he does not know, *police?* — jogging lock-step down the airport corridor. And it is not the assault rifles they are toting that trouble him about the scene, but rather the fact that each is bedecked in a crisp, white biosafety suit. This tells him something. This drops a sick feeling into his already queasy stomach. The team divides; some beginning to seal off the corridor to prevent any more passengers from entering, the rest heading off to the individual departure gates to make sure none of the corralled passengers slip down the gangway tunnels and into the awaiting planes.

Three other policemen — plain clothed but sporting bacterial facemasks — are making their way down the center of the corridor. The middle of the three holds a clipboard that the other two check repeatedly as they study the faces of each passenger they pass. Dr. Nakayama, still forty meters from this oncoming trio, can only assume the clipboard has his picture on it. And so, knowing there's no escape, he looks about for a seat upon which to sit. His goal is to blend into the crowd, to look as inconspicuous as possible. Should he find a seat that faces him *away* from the police scrutiny, or one that faces them *directly* in the hope that such boldness will convey innocence? Or should he strike a noncommittal profile and pray they just pass him by? Never one who was very good at deceit, he finds a seat that presents his backside to the police. That done, he removes his glasses and quickly wipes the sweat from his face and finger combs his hair all in an attempt to disguise his trademark lab-rat appearance. Without his glasses the bank of windows – which would bring those with normal eyesight a clear scene of the comings and goings of sundry aircraft – present to him only a muddled blur of moving shapes and colors, like staring through an automobile windshield in a downpour. Vertical shadows pass from side to side, which Dr. Nakayama assumes must be the silhouettes of fellow passengers. He feels alienated from them, estranged, though he doesn't know the reason for this, as he's never felt quite like this before. Is it just because of his poor eyesight, or is there a sense of betrayal that has slipped in between him and them? He is trying to kill them after all; for their own ultimate good granted, but murder nonetheless. This puts them on the side of good, and he on the side of evil; could that be it?

He can hear the murmurs of the three policemen approaching from behind. And something about it – perhaps a combination of his blind vulnerability and his exposed neck – makes it feel as if a samurai executioner is sidling towards him, sword in hand.

One of them calls out his name in Japanese: "Dr. Nakayama?" But he ignores the entreaty, pretending they have the wrong guy, hoping they will just mosey along.

He recalls reading somewhere that the decapitated head is fully conscious for some thirty seconds after being severed from the body. It drops and rolls and gazes about and tries to maintain a sense of calm about the incident, a modicum of dignity. Sometimes the moving lips try to impart one last pearl of wisdom but, cruelly, the lack of oxygen makes it appear as if they are merely gasping for air, like the mouth of a fish pulled onto the deck of a boat. And then there's the decapitated head's bulging eyes: no matter how calm and collected the mind therein might be, its eyes make it look terrified of the oncoming mystery, terrified of slipping forever into that void of neither darkness nor light nor time. And these combined – the terror struck eyes, the mute but flapping lips – only make the desperate decapitated head look *silly* rather than wisened and thus becomes the last, indefensible slap in the face of an otherwise prideful being.

    He can hear the laughter of children somewhere. He searches the muddled blur for their images. There, over by the window; there are their shadows; playing tag by the looks of it, as he once played as a child himself! *Oh, where did those days go? Oh, oh, where did those days go?*

Falkland Islands, Royal Air Force Base

A Taca 737 sits quarantined in a desolate corner of an already remote airstrip. An inexperienced pair of Argentine reserves, fitted into HAZMAT suits and respirators, heed the instructions of a World Heath Organization Infectious Disease containment specialist as they install air scrubber filters to the plane's cabin exhaust ports. Another pair of WHO specialists advise the twenty or so more reserves guarding the plane's perimeter, some of whom are armed and posted as sentries around the encompassing loop of red biohazard tape, while the others erect a tall, chain-link containment fence.

But inside the plane the chain of command is decidedly different, with the WHO specialist apparently the least significant component of the military SWAT squad — outfitted in chemical warfare suits and following the short barrels of their various assault weapons — storming its way down the single aisle. Sure, there are the predictable outbursts from crying children and hysterical shrieks from elderly women who lost loved ones to such brutish tactics back in the Peron days but, for the most part, the passengers remain calm.

If the architects of this plane-storming mission knew their subject a wee bit better, they would know that even a single, armed soldier would be an excessive use of force. But they didn't so they don't. Instead all they know is they are searching for one member of *"... a hitherto unknown covert cell of radical ideologues bent on the mass destruction of billions of innocents by viral attack,"* which therefore, in the not-so-nuanced paradigm of counterterrorism, clearly warrants *overwhelming force* tactics.

Like their Japanese counterpart, this SWAT unit consults a photograph of their target as they thrust forward, with meticulous haste, row by row through the cabin. In short order they arrive at row 28, seat B of which is conspicuously empty in the otherwise full plane. Regarding the vacant seat, the unit commander speaks in calm but succinct Spanish to the woman sitting in 28C:

"Where is the man who was sitting here?"

the momentum of folly

The terrified woman shakes her head – conveying the universal *No se* response.

Proving to be somewhat short-tempered, the unit commander rips the clipboard from his subordinate's hand, then holds it up so all the passengers seated nearby can get a good look at the photograph on it as he shouts threateningly, "This man is a terrorist. His goal is to kill you. Where... is... he?"

Sans hesitation the boy sitting in 28A – the one who already knows he wants to fly Cobra attack helicopters for the Argentine Army, he's got all the posters in his room – answers the request, *"En el baño!"* pointing behind him to the plane's rear lavatory.

"Gracias, señor," the commander tells the boy, treating him with the respect of a peer, a comrade in this global war on terror. And though the boy only nods back – the universal *De nada* – inwardly he beams, gushing with pride.

The commander motions for his unit to proceed down the aisle. And they do, moving at a crisp pace until they reach the locked and "Occupied" restroom door. One of the commandos looks back to the commander for the next order. Receiving the *proceed* nod, the commando then quickly pounds a fist twice against the door before quickly pulling back into a defensible crouching position behind his XM8 compact assault rifle, and shouting, "Argentine Army, open up!"

Several seconds of silence pass, before the unit commander steps past his commandos to take his turn knocking on the restroom door.

"Professor Fernando Perez, abierto la puerta, por favor." He waits a few beats, then barks again through the closed door, "Doctor Perez?"

After again receiving no response, he nods to his go-to commando. Instantly heeding the order, the commando surges forward and abruptly kicks in the frail door with the heel of his jungle boot, the door's lock quickly snapping though the folding door itself yields only partially. It's not that it is particularly sturdy – far from it – rather there seems to be something blocking it from opening completely. Two commandos now apply themselves to the task of kicking and pushing on the door, until finally they get it fully opened.

A little girl seated nearby is the first of the craning passengers to steal a glimpse past the commandos and into the cramped lavatory; the first to see in and, hence, and not surprisingly, the first to let out a horrified scream.

Now it's the WHO field agent's time to move forward. With urgent but patient repetition, she calls out "Excusé, excusé. Step back, por favor. Excusé!"

as she wends her way through the wad of rubbernecking passengers and even the curious commandos. "Excusé, excusé. Step back, por favor. Excusé!" she repeats yet again, until she squeezes through to the fore. Shouldering past the commander and his last commando she finally is able to see into the lavatory stall. Now she understands what is eliciting all the fuss, for there in the stall is a most troubling sight indeed; it's the unnaturally crumpled corpse of Professor Perez, made even more horrific by his unnaturally cyanotic lips and ears and fingertips, and unnaturally dark, almost black skin, and unnaturally blue, oxygen-deprived blood flowing from his very *intentionally* self-slashed wrists.

The WHO agent and SWAT commander exchange a troubled look; nothing more to be said.

Belozersky Institute of Physico-Chemical Biology, Lomonosov Moscow University.

Henrî LaFond is standing – at least he thinks he is standing – eyes clenched closed, clearly disoriented, it's difficult to tell. Feeling like he is going to pass out any moment he decides he might have a better chance remaining conscious if he opens his eyes. So he does. The glare; it's not the sun, is it? – no, artificial light; some sort of spotlight, key and fill. Regardless, the glare nearly knocks him over. Fortunately he is leaning against something. What is it? Oh, yes; a podium. It's supporting most of his weight. This is good, he thinks, *in English!* He marvels at the fact he is thinking in English – *the tongue of the oppressor*, as Jenna would call it. It's her fault English has crept into his thoughts; it's all because she refused to speak French at home. It's a good thing they finally went their own ways; it would've never worked out. *Se bon.* That's better; he is thinking in French again. But now he realizes he is shivering, as he had been the whole flight to Moscow. The walk through the subway, that was the hardest. He had ducked the limo driver waiting for him in the airport arrival gate, to use the subway instead reasoning there would be a better chance of exposing the virus to more people there as well to a different strata of the populace – the working class Russians – that was important. Until then it had been all airlines and lectures to the intelligencia: what were they trying to do, wipe out the upper-income, educated masses and drive humanity back a century? He tried to argue that very point with the others but Jenna said the virus would spread to everyone regardless. Didn't matter where they started, just so long as they could maximize intimate contact with others throughout their contagious period. Airlines; perfect. Lectures; the next best thing to orgies. Sweat trickles from his brow and down his face and then finally drips from his chin and onto the pages of notes in front of him, smudging some of them. *Notes?* – lots of notes; pages and pages; printouts, clipped articles, handwritten – where the hell is he? Damn this bug is disorienting!

Looking up, he squints out past the glare of the spotlights, actually using a hand to visor his eyes from the glare. Out there, in the relative darkness, he sees the blank, indistinguishable faces of student after student after student, staring back, like some Biology 1A course for clones. Whatever it is he is talking about, he certainly has their interest. Or maybe it's the fact that he *doesn't* know what he's talking about that intrigues them.

Fuck, is this just like that recurring nightmare, or what? – Henri mutters, feeling the déjà vu of this personal version of the classic student nightmare of taking a final exam for a course never attended. That one. His version, the teacher's version, involves standing before a vast class of students while trying to wing one's way through a course he has just realized he knows nothing about. But this, this isn't a nightmare; far worse, this shit is *real*. This lectern is real. This microphone is real. Those lights are real. And those are real students out there.

Fuck!... Well, at least fuck's a French word.

Clearly his mind in wandering. Thinking he should try to focus a bit here, he decides to try reading verbatim from his notes. He picks up an article – a download he found, who knows where – and, after a few seconds of stretching and narrowing his eyes until he can make out the print font, begins to read:

"One curious but accepted explanation for the rapid decline of frog species – aside from the already postulated causes: habitat loss, UV penetration, outbreaks of the chytrid fungus brought about by climate, etc. – a new reason seems to be the recently observed phenomenon of "gender bending" or spontaneous sex change, when exposed to one of the most commonly-used herbicides, atrazine, used in some eighty countries over the past fifty years. Male African clawed frogs, for instance, *Xenopus laevis*, showed a ten-fold decrease in testosterone levels, bringing them below levels found in normal females."

Sensing a consternation somewhere out there in the darkened lecture hall – doors opening, heads turning, furtive whispers, etc. – Henri pauses. Did he already read from this page or something? He really does not know; hasn't a clue. So, just in case, he flips to the next page down in his pile of notes to begin to read from it instead. But just then some fluid drips onto the page. This time it's not sweat. *What is it?*, he wonders. *Oh, it's blood.* It seems he has a nosebleed. Never one prone to spontaneous nosebleeds in the past Henri is forced to conclude this to be yet another symptom of the virus bitch-slapping its way through his immune system. A sinus bleed-out; this means it's just a matter of hours before his other organs begin hemorrhaging, if they haven't already. And once that happens, it's just a matter of minutes before he internally bleeds to death. *Well, that's just great,* he humors himself, *As if this event weren't nightmarish enough already!*

"Dr. LaFond?" a voice booms out, over the same P.A. system that had been carrying his lecture.

Henri looks up, squinting out into the vacuous darkness for the source of the voice, but cannot locate it. To him, his atheism aside, it sounded a bit too much like *God's* voice. But there, coming down the side aisles in pairs, armed police. KGB? Interpol? Who knows? – but here they come, outfitted in some sort of urban chemical warfare suits, all gas-masked and gunned. *Ah, yes; now it's all beginning to make sense.* And then there are others; no gasmasks or suits, just guns – sharpshooters by the looks of them. There are two or three of these guys at least, and they have taken up positions in the upper corners of the lecture hall; some on one knee, one laying down, each with a long, blue barrel pointed at him.

"Dr. LaFond, please make your way over to the stage wings where a paramedic unit is prepared to transport you."

And then, most curious of all, there seems to be no attempt being made to evacuate the students. At every institution at which Henrî has taught they have had to go through numerous and tedious evacuation drills, but here today, nothing – they seem perfectly content just to let the students watch.

This tells Henri just one thing: they are on to him, the plot has been compromised somehow. They are *perfectly content to let the students watch* because they, no doubt, already have the building under quarantine. No one in here is going anywhere for two weeks at least. He knew they should have killed that Carl Sims punk when they had the chance. But, *no-o-o,* the ex-wife couldn't do it. Irony of ironies; she was willing to commit genocide but not murder.

"Dr. LaFond, the infectious disease unit at the hospital is prepared to begin treating you immediately upon arrival. Dragging this out only wastes precious time."

He has two more flights and lectures he won't be able to make, meaning the chance of his sparking the pandemic has been reduced by at least sixty percent.

the momentum of folly

Oh well, it was just a matter of time anyway. One can only do what one can do. Perhaps his colleagues got further along in their lecture tours. But taking the subway; now that was a brilliant idea. Does he have another trick up his sleeve? How can he maximize his potential here? This will take focus: how can he make lemonade of lemons?

Mustering one swift threatening motion, Henrî thrusts his right hand into the inner breast pocket of his sports coat. This works. Every barrel trained on him was waiting for this. Even though there was nothing in that breast pocket – nothing more than an idle threat, nothing more than a seventy-nine cent ballpoint pen – within the span of two seconds at least six bullets hit his torso. They feel like punches though surprisingly not all that painful.

A firing squad; not so bad. But a cigarette would have made it outright civilized. A cigarette would have made it... delicious.

The force of the impact not only sends Henri falling over backwards but also treats him to a rare visual spectacle. For – illuminated so thoroughly by the spotlights, and back-dropped so ideally by pitch-black darkness of the lecture hall rafters – a spray of his own blood, forced like an aerosol from his torso by the bullets' impact, rises instantaneously and hangs there as a misty cloud above him. Microscopic droplets individually, now collectively gathered into visible fog, the blood is a dark bluish-gray at first but then ever so quickly, like a starcluster firework, explodes into a brilliant crimson. And though this all happens in but a fraction of a second, Henri's scientific mind perfectly understands precisely what is happening; the vaporized blood – initially blue from cyanosis – returns to its familiar bright red coloration once exposed to the room's plentiful oxygen content. Simple really. But as rare as – well, as rare as someone on the very brink of death by oxygen asphyxiation getting shot instead. So rare it's probably never happened before. And this, in fact, is the very last lucid thought that passes through Henri's brain – *Wow, I bet nobody has ever experienced this before!* – as he continues to drop backwards, in complete awe and wonder of the colorful spectacle taking place above him.

For Henri – still falling, still bearing tenuous witness to the last vestiges of this world – this is about as close to a legitimate spiritual experience he would ever allow himself. And that brilliant, misty, cyanic-cum-crimson, vaporous, bloody, virus-infected fog suspended there above him? — why, that's his spirit, his life-force, finally liberated from his body; hanging around only until the room's efficient ventilation system grabs hold of it with its unseen currents and begins to whirl and tumble and disperse it out over and into the unsuspecting spectators. *Voile, mission accomplished!*

Jomo Kenyatta International Airport, Nairobi, Kenya

The small airport terminal's dirty, decaying concrete façade reflects off Jenna's just-a-year-or-two-out-of-fashion sunglasses. Everything was hip once: the airport's stunning Frank Lloyd Wright-esque architecture-on-the-cheap, mirrored white-rimmed sunglasses, world peace, environmentalism, hope. Everything.

With her Cal Bears baseball cap pulled low and daypack slung over one shoulder, Jenna drags along at the very rear of a trail of some eighty other passengers as they make their collective way across the scorching, unbearably-humid tarmac towards an awaiting, engines-screeching, ancient, Nigerian Airlines 727. Jenna is coughing and disoriented, and the nauseous smells of burnt kerosene and diesel finally drop her to one knee and cause her to vomit right there on runway 06/24. As pukes go it's not very productive – a "girlie hurl" as her ex, Henri, would have derisively called it – consisting of barely more than a handful of the white rice she has forced herself to eat over the course of these past couple of sickly days in order to maintain the energy to just keep on going. But, thankfully, between the deafening din of jet turbines and eye-crushing, midday glare, nobody notices her pausing to vomit; and, even if they had, nobody would care.

Still on the one knee, and perhaps wondering in her delirium if this is Lagos or Nairobi or Douala she is defiling, Jenna becomes aware of a pair of sirens-blaring ambulances racing past. She lifts her head just enough to watch as the ambulances pull up to the front of the trickling queue of her co-passengers, intentionally blocking their path to the awaiting Nigerian Airlines 727. Three black, windows-tinted, removable-blue-emergency-lights-flashing, Chevy Suburbans angle in from other directions and similarly skid to a stop up near the front of the queue. And though this is all happening some seventy-five meters up ahead from where Jenna still kneels she can make out the distinctive blue WHO biosafety suits as the teams of medics and guards pile out of the emergency vehicles, and hastily begin corralling the puzzled flock of passengers within an encircling ribbon of red biohazard tape. And, as they are doing this, two airport shuttle buses — empty but for their biosafety-suited drivers — weave past Jenna, heading up to either side of the temporary enclosure.

Like that proverbial unseen fly on the wall, Jenna watches for a bit as the quarantine goes up. And however detached she might be feeling from the emergency happening *way up yonder*, part of her virus-addled mind is still cognizant of the fact she is the reason it is happening at all.

Looking about, Jenna notices that another plane — a turboprop floatplane, parked some 150 meters away in the opposite direction, its image wobbling in the mirage effect rising off the hot tarmac — seems also to be in the process of boarding. After a failed attempt to contemplate the ramifications of such a spontaneous change of plans, Jenna decides to simply *throw caution to the wind*. Clambering unsteadily back to her feet, she slings her daypack back across her shoulder, pulls her cap down tight, and heads off in that direction, trying her best to use the plane as her compass, her navigational star, as she stumbles towards it.

The prop of the right engine is just exploding to life with a pop of blue exhaust, the other dozen or so passengers are already on board, and the co-pilot is in the process of pulling in the cantilevered gangway stepladder by the time Jenna is within earshot of the floatplane. She shouts up to the co-pilot in French, "Wait! Please! One more!" But he — in his crisp, white, short-sleeved shirt, sharp black tie, tightly-cropped, retro Afro, and mirrored aviator sunglasses — shakes his head without so much as even looking at her.

Behind him, in cursive lettering arched across the top the plane's curved hatch door, is the phrase, *"The Nairobi – Lake Victoria Express!"* And something about it — whether it's the soothing down-hominess of the hand-painted lettering, or the familiar red-yellow-green Rasta colors, or the full-circle happenstance of returning to Lake Victoria of all places — *something* causes her to turn back to the co-pilot, and slip into full, pleading-female, anything-you-want mode.

"Please!" she calls up to him, now pulling a handful of Euros from her belt-pack and offering them to him. But again he shakes his mirror sunglasses and resumes pulling in the gangway. *"Please!"* she shouts again, this time pulling off her sunglasses and cap and shaking out her hair in a very unnatural-for-her attempt to convey some vague sexual promise. But again, and this time with obvious pity, he shakes his head and resumes his departure duties.

And now the left engine explodes to life, blowing its cloud of blue smoke past her. She is more desperate than she has ever before in her life been, and, worst still, she knows this. Operating now under the *when-ya-ain't-got-nothin'- ya-got-nothin'-to-lose* credo, she drops to her knees, clasps her hands, and shouts out her final plea — *Please!* — her words, though powered by every last erg of her strength, are nonetheless completely and hopelessly drowned beneath the full-throttle roar of the engines.

But the effort, her resolve, is not lost on the co-pilot. He pauses, sighs, then turns to his right, presumably to ask his pilot if he should let her on board. Aware of the discussion that might be transpiring, Jenna turns towards the cockpit window in time to see the pilot's faint profile leaning forward in his seat to peek back and down to her. She shakes her clasped hands and repeats the mouthed plea to him — *Please!* This last effort seems to do the trick as, a moment later, the pilot mouths something back to the co-pilot, who nods in compliance, then begins to lower the gangway steps back down for her.

Jenna nods a thankful *Merci, merci!*, takes a strength-gathering bite of air, stands with as much strength as she can feign, grabs hold of the gangway rail for support, then pulls her weight over her first weary step aboard.

WHO Infectious Disease Lab, Sao Paulo

These types of aircraft are, no doubt, known to military aficionados or appear in glossy corporate brochures or websites somewhere for spoiled CEOs still looking for toys with which to flaunt their successes, but for Carl the hybrid fixed-wing/twin-tiltrotor, ultra-sleek, dark metallic-gray, Bell-Boeing V-22 Osprey presently corkscrewing from out of the sky is something of pure science fiction. With its rotors now pulled and locked into a vertical position it begins to settle towards the rooftop as would any exceptionally large helicopter, except that it swings its cockpit 180° away from Carl to instead politely present its rear hatch door towards him to abet his entry. Before it even touches down onto the rooftop heliport, its rear hatch ramp lowers to reveal four biosafety-suited guards, all obviously body-built males, and yet another Aegis employee but with decidedly girlish curves. Even without being able to see her face, just by the way she holds herself, Carl can tell it's Angela.

The Osprey lands, keeping its turbines whining at a high rpm for immediate take-off. Carl hesitates before making a move towards the aircraft, checking in with his conscience to see if he's making the right decision. Still not sure he is, he mutters, *Fuck it!* then begins towards the craft nonetheless, leaning forward into the intense wind and ducking his head from the invisible but obviously whirling rotors.

Two of the guards come down the ramp to help him aboard. But Carl, still sporting the WHO biosafety suit, waves them off; he doesn't need their help, and he especially doesn't need them tugging on his broken elbow. As he comes up the ramp, his pace slows involuntarily as he and Angela exchange a wordless glower from behind their respective clear plastic visors, neither quite knowing what the other is thinking, neither wanting to be the first to extend any olive branches. After that short but awkward beat Angela motions for him to sit in any one of the dozen or so plushly-appointed leather seats, all of which face one another in some quasi conference style arrangement. Carl selects a seat at

the momentum of folly

random. After he sits Angela nods to two of the guards, who then settle into the seats on either side of Carl. Even through all their respective protective gear, Angela can see Carl roll his eyes, can sense his frustration, as she settles into the chair directly opposite from his. On either side of Angela's helmet – as too on her suit's left breast, as too on each of the replicant guards' suits, as too on every leather headrest and pillow and cup and blanket and napkin and parachute and any other item imaginable within the cabin, as too both exterior sides of the aircraft – is the Aegis logo; a pseudo-handwritten "A" circumscribed within a circle. Carl knows, of course, that this was the former symbol for the Anarchist movement. But, being anarchists, they, of course, never thought to register the symbol. Hence, as a result, it was available when the Aegis founder/owner/CEO decided he wanted it. And it could only help his company's "visibility" that the symbol was already scrawled and spray-painted on freeway underpasses and abandoned buildings and pre-proto-punk band bass drums everywhere. And so he brashly commandeered it, ripped it off and registered under U.S. copyright protection. And now the circumscribed A legally belongs to Aegis, and he could sue any anarchist who tried to use it. Why, he could have them prosecuted and sent off to jail if he wanted to. But for now, as long as the exposure continues to serve him and his stock price, he'll let them have their rebellious fun, he'll let them vent, he'll let them rage against the machine, because, the more they do, the more it serves *his* machine.

So there's the circumscribed A over Angela's heart; over the breast Carl so loved to fondle. No sense mentioning it though. No sense picking at the scab of her move over to the dark side, he cautions himself; that wound is still too fresh.

"So," Carl begins, opting to break the ice with some good old-fashioned sarcasm, "did'ya ever get that parking ticket taken care of?"

Angela just stares at him. If she heard him she's not letting on, not dignifying the barbed quip with a response. She's beyond that. She's moved on. Or at least she's trying to convince herself that she has.

The turbines roar to full rpm again. The Osprey begins to lift from the concrete rooftop. As hydraulics pull the ramp hatch door up and seal it closed, the passenger cabin becomes surprisingly quiet. At least Carl is surprised: without mentioning it however, he imagines there must be reams or bolts or tons – however they measure that stuff – of soundproofing separating the cabin from the rest of this violently grunting, quivering, implausible beast. Quite a feat of engineering, just to soundproof it, and that's the very least of this craft's extraordinary abilities for, in a matter of seconds, the tiltrotors begin to do their tilt thing, and vertical flight levels out to horizontal. As the craft picks up forward momentum the lift it requires to stay afloat is gradually assumed by the airfoil design of its fixed wings, just beneath which begin to slip the remnant, scraggly tip-tops of the slashed and burned, raped and pillaged jungle canopy.

Angela presses a console button turning on a pair of flat-screen monitors mounted above the seats on opposite sides of the cabin. Another console button pressed summons opaque window screens to slide across and block any sunlight seeping in from outside. As the cabin darkens, Carl becomes aware of the ultraviolet strobe light blasting through the room every few seconds or so. And were his air not being filtered through his biosafety suit's respirator, he has no doubt his nostrils would be burning slightly from a generous concentration of aerosol chlorine. Anything to beat back the bug.

"A jet is en route to meet us in Brasilia," Angela tells Carl, seemingly apologizing for the Osprey.

"What's wrong with this? – seems plenty comfy."

"Comfy is one thing, delivering you quickly to Los Angeles is another."

"*Los Angeles?* The deal was Atlanta."

"Was it," Angela replies dryly, in that way of hers.

"Don't worry, Dr. Sims," a voice calls out to him from either flat screen monitor.

Carl turns towards the screen most convenient for him just as a man in a polo shirt takes a seat in a swivel office chair, which he then turns towards the camera. He's tanned and well-groomed and pushing sixty while looking forty, with a bleached and beguiling smile. This of course the Aegis CEO – or "head honcho," as he likes to call himself – Erland Zwissler. He continues, "... we'll whisk you to L.A. then on back to Atlanta as fast as humanly possible. Certainly faster than anyone else could."

"That's reassuring, but that wasn't the deal," Carl protests.

"The *deal*, yes. Let's see if I can explain this without too much legalese.... How about *tough shit?* Eh? Does that help enlarge the fine print of our aforementioned *deal?* I certainly hope so."

Carl seething, nonetheless nods.

"Good," Erland replies sarcastically, before turning towards Angela. "Angela, dear, sensitive guy that I am, I can't help but feel your friend and I got off on the wrong foot. Could you please introduce us so maybe we can start anew?"

Angela nods. "Carl, this is Erland Zwissler, CEO of Aegis Pharmaceuticals. Mr. Zwissler, this is Dr. Sims of the CDC."

"Much better. I sense a kindred bond already. And might I interject a heart-felt *thank you* for thinking of us when you came to realize you needed transportation."

Carl levels with him, "I figured it would take the CDC days just to start the paperwork."

Erland smiles and nods knowingly. "I suspect we both know what's going on by now: in effect we've been double-crossed. Or, perhaps more accurately: I was double-crossed, you were merely, I don't know, *duped*, I guess is the best way to put it."

"You financed their expedition to Alaska," Carl submits, beginning to connect the dots.

"I did."

"Drs. Williams and LaFond – "

"Yes. Charming couple. Inseparable," Erland quips, hinting he knows something of the two scientists' uniquely strained relationship.

"So, just so I understand: they offered to excavate and exhume the Eskimo mass grave in order to isolate the *real* lethal influenza virus –"

"Right so far. She shared her hypothesis – I guess we could call it her post 2009 Swine flu hypothesis – that whatever had struck those isolated communities back in 1918 had to be something other than H1N1. And, of course, it made a lot of sense."

"… all so you could manufacture the antiviral and have it all packaged and ready for the pandemic you would then initiate."

"Whoa! Please, you make me sound like some villain. *Packaged and ready*, yes. *Pandemic*," Erland is shaking his head, "never part of the arrangement. This whole thing, this wasn't a conspiracy; at least not on my part."

"You never planned to release it?" Carl asks, skeptically.

"I'm a virus *collector*, Dr. Sims. *Be prepared* is my motto."

"You'd make quite a Boy Scout."

"Why, is that their motto *too*? I wonder if they've copyrighted it," Erland muses, revealing his ability to poke fun at himself.

Feeling a need for clarification, Angela attempts to explain her boss's motives to Carl. "Aegis only wanted the antiviral ready in case there was ever an outbreak."

"The *ounce of prevention, pound of cure* thing," Erland interjects.

Angela continues: "Williams and LaFond approached Aegis with the proposal to search for an unknown, possibly avian influenza virus in Eskimo mass graves."

"And I said, *Go for it*. I'll buy, you fly," Erland explains. "Our goal — Aegis's mission statement, if you will — is to stockpile antivirals for all the world's great threats lurking out there in the shadows."

"We've done the same thing with a number of viruses: small pox, ebola..."

"How altruistic," Carl says, sarcastically.

"Well, altruism aside, there's the monetary incentive of getting a jump on the competition," Erland admits.

"The only problem being that it is illegal."

"Well, yeah, there's that. Nonetheless it *is* prudent, I think you would agree."

"As every epidemiologist will tell you, it's just a matter of time before the Eskimo Flu emerged again naturally on its own. So our position is: why not be ready for it?" Angela states, ever so logically.

"But somehow you weren't," Carl posits.

"You're referring to the outbreak in the Laotian village?" Erland asks, then sighs, "Therein lies the double-crossed part. Jenna and Henri were merely supposed to find the virus, isolate it, and bring it back from Alaska. Illegal maybe, but otherwise all on the up-and-up. There was never any mention of testing it. I didn't anticipate that, and I wouldn't have agreed to it. That was monstrous, but then, who could've known what they were actually up to?"

"So you ordered the village to be massacred."

"Of course, though I'd never admit to it in a courtroom."

Seething, Carl turns towards Angela. "And this is the *good guy* you were speaking about?" he says, alluding to Erland.

"Put yourself in my shoes, Dr. Sims; if I *hadn't* most of Southeast Asia would be infected by now!"

"Innocent men, women and children, Angela. Those that didn't die of the disease were shot or burned to death, each and every one. I watched it happen!"

"But it would have spread," Angela says, beginning to tremble as she tries to defend her boss's motives. "There would have been far more suffering."

"But it never would have happened in the first place if he hadn't financed the expedition. That's why we have laws against stockpiling lethal pathogens, because shit happens!"

Sensing Angela's allegiance beginning to erode, Erland changes the subject.

"Dr. Sims, in retrospect I certainly would not have financed their endeavor. That's obvious to us both now. But we are where we are: water under the bridge. About all we can do at this point is to try to minimize the suffering to come."

"Which is why I have to get the virus to Atlanta as quickly as possible in order to get started on the vaccine," Carl interjects.

"*No*," and now Erland has a smirk on his face, "which is why *we* have to get it to *Los Angeles* as quickly as possible in order to get started on the *antiviral*."

Carl glares at Erland.

Sensing the impasse, Erland argues his case further: "Carl, Aegis Pharmaceuticals has lived up to its end of the bargain by providing you with transportation; now it's time for a little *quid pro quo* from you. One liter of blood, please."

On cue, one of the Aegis employees unwraps a needle and sterile sack in preparation of drawing Carl's blood.

Carl stares at Erland, then shakes his head. "I can't do it."

"But we made a deal!" Angela reminds him.

"I said what I had to say in order to get back to the States," Carl confesses.

Angela fumes.

"Carl, unfortunately the world doesn't have time for us to be dicking around like this. We need the blood in order to get started."

Carl again shakes his head. "A liter would cut our first batch of vaccine in half; costing us precious weeks."

"Half a liter then," Erland offers, reluctant but willing to compromise.

"Get real; it takes *months* to generate antivirals from small molecule screens!"

"We've managed to streamline the process some."

Carl holds his stare. "No."

"Really? Even if an antiviral is the only way to save the thousands, if not millions, already infected? – people like you for instance. What is it: sixty-six percent mortality rate? Those aren't good odds."

Involuntary tears begin to well in the corners of Angela's eyes. Similarly her hands *unconsciously* find her slightly swollen belly, just holding it without her even realizing why. One thing about biosafety suits; there's no way to wipe tears away, no way to hide them. One is protected, yet at the same time exposed.

Meanwhile, Carl is still in his locked-eyed stare down with Erland, wholly unaware of any emotional tremors that might be rumbling through Angela. Again Carl turns down Erland's offer with an adamant shake of his head, "This bug is going to spread way too fast. The CDC and WHO are going to need every drop of blood I can give them for vaccine production."

"Millions could die needlessly; virologists, epidemiologists, doctors, nurses among them who might otherwise be helping out," Erland counters.

"And literally *billions* are at greater risk of becoming infected while you're trying to manufacture your antiviral for those relative few who might be able to afford it."

"Fuck you, Carl!" Angela blurts out, surprising both Carl and Erland.

Carl turns towards her. "Fuck *me*? What about *him*? He's the one who's just in it for the money!"

"And if he can save lives while he's at it, what's wrong with that?"

Carl now levels a stare at Angela, "Oh, I get it now; you're getting a piece of the action, right?"

Angela just stares back, reticent to admit to anything.

Carl swings his inquiry back to the flat screen. "So, what does Angela stand to make off the antiviral?"

Erland shrugs. "The same as any Aegis employee who isolates a useful virus for us; it's a percentage of units sold algorithm."

"And if this one goes pandemic?"

Erland hesitates only briefly before acknowledging the ramifications: "If this particular strain does indeed become a pandemic, then you're in the presence of a very *potentially* wealthy woman."

Carl nods, and turns back to Angela, staring accusatory daggers at her. "Mama didn't raise no fool," he says, quoting her from what already seems a lifetime ago.

But Angela only stares back at him with daggers of her own.

"I'm sorry, I couldn't hear that," Erland says, pressing the volume button on his console.

Carl turns back to Erland. "I was just telling your *very potentially wealthy* employee here how sorry I was that she wouldn't be making a dime off the antiviral because there wasn't going to be one."

"No? And why is that?"

"Because I'm not giving you so much as a *drop* of my blood."

"Well, I'm very disappointed to hear that."

Behind Carl, and unbeknownst to him as he speaks with Erland, Angela can be seen removing a compact but weighty fire extinguisher canister from the Osprey's wall. And from Erland's perspective, it's not clear what exactly she is up to until, in a blurry flash, she violently strikes Carl over the head with the fire extinguisher, knocking him out cold.

"Angela, Jesus!" Erland barks from the flat screen, genuinely shocked.

Angela stands, chest heaving, heart pounding, over Carl's crumpled, unconscious body. She looks up at Erland on the screen, unable to account for her actions; it was the involuntary reaction of someone being denied her life-long dream.

Erland seems to read all this in her panicked, apologetic eyes. Trying himself to keep from panicking, he runs his hands through his hair as he tries to figure out what to do about this sudden change of events, this sudden departure from anything defensibly legal. And yet, not one to overlook the opportunity Carl's unconsciousness affords him, Erland rubs his chin nervously then barks a quick order:

"Alright. Jesus, alright.... First: I didn't see that, got it? Everyone clear on that?" he says, already covering his tracks, already trying to wash the blood from his hands in the event of any pursuant litigation.

Angela and her co-workers nod towards their CEO's panicky image on the flat screen. "We're clear on that," Angela confirms, speaking for them all.

"Good. Good. Now, take one unit of blood from him – *one!* Got it? Then at the airport make certain our jet takes him *straight* to Atlanta – *not* to Los Angeles!"

"What about the unit of blood?" Angela asks, confused by the change of plans and obviously concerned about her stake in the antiviral.

"You'll carry it. At the airport in Brasilia we'll find you a direct flight back here to L.A. Shouldn't set us back more than a few hours. Just make sure you *hide* the blood. Last thing we need is some TSA agent confiscating it and pouring it down some drain!"

Angela nods, already thinking of places on her pregnant body to hide the plastic sack of precious blood.

Up on the flatscreens, Erland seems to be gathering his composure again. "I'm hoping the fact that we're bringing Dr. Sims straight to the CDC will mitigate *your* having taken the blood from him *involuntarily* — if it comes up."

"His erratic behavior made us concerned he might be a flight risk," Angela conjures, with a cool shrug of nonchalance. "There was a scuffle..."

"That's good. Whatever; just make sure the culpability stops with *you*. Your reward, your risk. Understand?" Erland narrows his glare directly at Angela, conveying that if there's to be a fall guy, it's going to be her.

Angela nods dutifully. "I understand."

"Alright. Well, then..." Erland says, wrapping up the transmission with a deep, nerve-calming breath and "... Godspeed." And with that the screens go black.

On her own now, Angela looks down at Carl's unconscious heap. She then turns to her similarly nervous co-worker to her right. "Hand me that," she says, alluding to the catheter needle and sack he holds.

All too eager to wash his owns hands of the misdeed, the co-worker passes the kit to Angela. Kneeling beside Carl, Angela rips off the duct tape-like sealant wrapping his wrist, then pulls the glove from Carl's unbroken arm. Next she rolls up the rubbery-plastic sleeve of his cumbersome biosafety suit until she uncovers bare skin, whereupon, sans any hesitation whatsoever, she skillfully inserts the catheter needle into his vein. Carl's dark, but still red blood begins to trickle down the clear plastic tubing in slow, steady pulses. Angela straightens out the tubing to aid the process, positioning the one-liter receptor sack on the floor beneath him to allow gravity to do its part.

The Osprey banks to the right, telling Angela they must be on approach to the airport. She takes a deep, calming breath: it shouldn't be long now.

Centers for Disease Control, Atlanta

Carl opens his eyes, and once again with no idea where he is. He's lying on his back; he knows that much, probably on another gurney in another lab somewhere. He's naked now, or mostly so, with a nasal cannula piping in cool oxygen and a bright operating light glaring down on him, forcing him to squint. There doesn't seem to be anyone around. About all he knows is he's growing tired of this crap. In and out of consciousness, disorienting drugs, sensory deprivation, mysterious aircraft... Who are these people? – the CIA? What are they doing to him? – extraordinary rendition? He tries to raise his head, but finds he's far too weak to lift it off the pillow. Nevertheless, his movement catches the attention of someone standing nearby; someone in a white biosafety suit who had his back turned to Carl and, thus, just kind of blended in with all the similarly sterile equipment.

"Oh, hey, Carl. You're finally awake," a slightly muted voice says, from somewhere within the biosafety suit.

Carl narrows his eyes; the voice is not only friendly but familiar as well, as is the pleasant smile there behind the suit's plastic visor. Both are *very* familiar in fact, but difficult to tuck into context under the circumstances. The face acknowledges Carl's confusion with a knowing grin.

"It's me – Hank."

"Hank..." Carl mutters, happy to see Hank – means he's back at the CDC in Atlanta – but too weak to say much more.

"Yep, good ol' Hank. FYI: I've got a catheter in your arm here to draw some blood..." Hank lifts a half-filled receptor sack for Carl to see, then nods towards Carl's other arm explaining, "Also got saline coming in over there, and a weenie bag you probably know where. So, what I'm sayin' is, no sudden movements, okay?" Hank grins.

A familiar whirring sound pulls Carl's attention to a centrifuge mounted on a lab counter nearby. It is currently spinning down a unit or so of blood –

probably his, Carl assumes – separating the red blood cells from the sera. And there is another centrifuge sitting idle and waiting beside it.

Hank turns a shut-off stopcock on the catheter coming out of Carl's arm, then removes the tube and full sack. "That should do it."

"How much d'ya take?" Carl asks weakly.

"One liter," Hank replies.

Carl licks his dry lips, mustering the strength for another word or two. "Take another."

"*Two?* No, no. Your girlfriend already took one; three would be half your blood, don't want to over-milk the cow."

"*Cow*," Carl repeats, barely able to verbalize the word, eyes closed but, ever so faintly, smiling.

Hank smiles back as he strips any lingering, precious drops of blood down the tube and into the sack. He then carries the sack over to the second centrifuge, carefully pores the blood into it, and turns it on. Finished here for the time being, he calls out to Carl, "You rest up, Elsie. I'll be back in a few," as he pushes out of the lab through the back entrance.

Humored but not yet capable of showing it, Carl merely closes his eyes. He can hear the airtight door close after Hank's departure, then the decontamination shower coming on as Hank rinses the exterior of his biosafety suit in the lab's antechamber before exiting completely. The faint hint of chlorine slips past Carl's nasal cannula. The quiet, metronomic beeping accompanying the UV strobe flashes is audible over the gentle, whirring of the blood centrifuges. These are all sounds and smells and sights that restore a sense of security to Carl. These are the creature comforts of home.

From Carl's perspective, it is impossible to say if that restive little closing of his eyes lasted a minute, or ten, or an hour, or even another day. He doesn't think he slipped into another drug-induced coma – it didn't even feel like he napped – but it's so hard to know anymore. Regardless, what nudged him back to some level of awareness was the gentle alarm that sounds whenever the lab's front entrance is opened; this alarm serving as the gentle reminder to: *Hey, be careful with the germs, the door to the unprotected outside world is open.* Of course, just as with the Level Five lab in Brazil, or the handful of other Level Four labs scattered across the globe, an airtight Plexiglas barrier separates the main lab from the Slammer-esque chamber wherein Carl lay, permitting people to enter the former without having to wear biosafety suits. Despite the Plexiglas, the alarm's subtle beeping seeps through, causing Carl to open his eyes again and lean them towards the main lab. And there he sees Stuart, just then rolling into the lab. Stuart smiles, then propels himself over to the wall-mounted intercom.

"Well, well, well, if it isn't the White Devil," Stuart begins, though not quite sure how much humor Carl's delicate health can take.

Carl shakes his head, closes his eyes again, but manages a smile, and by that Stuart can see his humor, maybe even his presence, is helping.

"So, by my count, you've suffered through three different flu strains in almost as many weeks. At least one of them deadly. Might be a record. Wouldn't be surprised if they bump your pay up another nickel-ninety-five an hour."

Near Stuart, but on Carl's side of the Plexiglas enclosure, one of the two centrifuges stop spinning, drawing Stuart's attention. He wheels himself over to the wall grommet intentionally mounted near the centrifuges. Stuart gazes in at the paused centrifuge and its rack of test tubes with its separated layers of blood; red cells, white cells, and plasma. Sliding his arm into one of the thick rubber-polyurethane gloves mounted within the grommet, Stuart gently lifts one of the test tubes from the centrifuge rack and brings it up to the Plexiglas so he can look at it more closely.

"So, this is the stuff that's going to save the world, eh?"

Carl, closes his eyes again and licks his dry lips, this being as close to nodding as he can manage at the moment.

Still holding the test tube, Stuart lifts his attention to the chlorine-charged decontamination shower positioned just above the centrifuges. Well within his reach is a clearly marked emergency pull chain. One yank of the chain's handle activates the chemical shower in the event of, say, a test tube spill or breakage, the subsequent release of the chlorine hopefully killing or disabling any pathogenic bacteria or virus accidentally released. Lowering his gaze from the emergency pull chain back down to the spun-down rack of blood serum, Stuart begins speaking again, albeit very tentatively. "Ya know, I've been poring over Dr. Jenna's gang's credentials; Guggenheim, Medal of Science, a couple of Nobels...."

Carl opens his eyes again, his concern piqued by the decidedly serious tone Stuart's voice now connotes. After studying Stuart for a few seconds, he takes a breath and musters a response. "What about them?"

the momentum of folly

Stuart hesitates, not sure if he should divulge his recently modified ideology.

"Suffice it to say, I'm beginning to wonder if maybe *we're* not the bad guys here."

Stuart turns towards Carl, the two now sharing the most serious stare down of their friendship, the tense silence exacerbated as the second centrifuge also automatically shuts down. And it does not escape Carl's notice that Stuart is still holding the test tube, nor the fact that he could easily and intentionally drop it then pull the emergency pull chain, thus destroying the virus and along with it any hope of making the vaccine. And this, of course, could, *would* realistically cause most of humanity to die from the then unstoppable pandemic – people of all ethnicities and religious affiliations and class strata, the world 'round. And he could easily make it look like an accident, possibly even an equipment malfunction.

Carl struggles to get a single word of advice to his lips: "Don't."

Stuart hesitates again but then has to ask: "Have you really thought this through?"

The two roommates stare at one another. A protracted moment lumbers past – silent and heavy. But then, slowly, ever so minimally, Carl nods, muttering: "There's a better way."

Stuart continues to stare at Carl, searching for a crack in his certainty. But Carl holds the stare, unwavering.

Suddenly, the open-door-warning alarm begins to beep again as Hank and a trio of CDC techs return to the lab. Capitulating to Carl, and certainly not wanting to have his treacherous thoughts revealed, Stuart furtively slides the test tube back into its centrifuge rack, slips his arm from the wall grommet glove, then calmly backs away from the Plexiglas wall.

Hank is already barking orders as one of the techs begins sealing him back into his biosafety suit, "Alright, both centrifuges have cycled, let's get the serum down to incubation ASAP. We've got us some serious catch-up to play!"

Hank then notices Stuart, and can't resist a passing jab. "Ah, Stuart. I see you've reconsidered your early retirement."

Stuart forces a smile, "What can I say? – without you my life has no meaning."

Hank shakes his head and smiles.

With his techs following, Hank enters the cell through the negatively pressurized hatch door. Crossing to the centrifuges, they begin removing the twenty test tubes from each, then placing them in secure racks within two sturdy, steel and plastic, foam-padded, airtight and light-proof cases.

As Hank and his techs busily prepare the sera for transport, Stuart swings his attention back towards Carl, casting his best friend in the world a somber *I-hope-you're-right* look, before turning his wheelchair towards the door and pushing away.

Hank walks cautiously down a florescent-lighted, linoleum-floored, antiseptic-smelling, subterranean CDC corridor alongside a cart being pushed by one of the techs. He has his hood off but still sports the rest of his biosafety suit, as do the three techs moving with him, all their suits still dripping from the decontamination showers. As a precautionary measure, Hank keeps one hand on one of the airtight, lightproof transport cases carrying the sera. He is doing this, of course, to add yet another degree of security to the rolling procession should any of the *known-to-err* humanoids involved stumble, causing the cart and all to crash into a wall or something, or should some other equally *prone-to-screw-ups* humanoid mindlessly 'round a corner and crash in to them. That could be disastrous; depending, of course, on one's perspective.

Five meters behind Hank and his immediate tech sidekick, the other two techs escort the second cart in the same fashion. They don't speak – nobody speaks – or, if they have to, they keep it to a bare minimum. However mundane this task may be, it is one of the weak links in getting the virus from the field and into vaccine production, so they must keep focused. "This is serious shit," as Hank put it, "one mishap here can set us back months, half a year even, endangering – well, you get the idea." Once they get the sera packaged up and shipped off to the three pharmaceutical companies under contract to manufacture the vaccine, well, then the onus is off of them; they've done their job, the ball's in the other court. Only then can they relax.

World Health Organization, Geneva

It's the conference call heard around the world. Here in the World Health Organization's headquarters in Geneva eighteen GISN epidemiologists and virologists and administrators sit around a conference table as an efficient communications coordinator connects the call with the WHO's four Collaborating Centers – located in the United Kingdom, United States, Japan and Australia – and the three Influenza Reference Laboratories – the Therapeutic Goods Administration (TGA), the Food and Drug Administration's Center for Biologics Evaluation and Research (CBER), and the National Institute for Biological Standards and Control (NIBSC). And soon thereafter the data collected and the strategy devised here in Geneva will be disseminated out to the sundry regulatory agencies, academic libraries, the six pharmaceutical companies responsible for vaccine production this year, and the 118 National Influenza Centers located in eighty-three nations around the globe. Ever since the GISN was formed back in 1952, it's been done basically this way, with slight or gross tweaks, expansions and transmogrifications to the system made each new season as the global community evolves. Once everyone has settled into their seats, the communication coordinator projects her voice towards the speakerphone located at the center of the table.

"Geneva is present and seated. Zero-nine hundred GMT. Good morning, good afternoon, good evening, everyone. Japan, are you there?"

Tokyo. In a similarly ultra-modern conference room, eleven members of the Japanese Collaborating Center sit or stand, some in lab smocks, some in suits as they listen in on the call. One white-smocked epidemiologist with moussed green hair deftly works their speakerphone: "Sixteen-hundred Tokyo time. All team members present."

"Good. United Kingdom, are you on?"

the momentum of folly

Oxford. The UK team is situated in the antique looking, high-ceilinged, polished wood main conference room within the Royal Academy of Science Library, established way back in the days of Sir Halley in the seventeenth century but accoutered, here in these proto-post-human times, with the hippest technological gadgetry. The speakerphone is a perfect example of this interbreeding retrofit between eras past and present; wireless and implanted within the skull of a saber-toothed cat mounted there in the center of the table. The bleary-eyed but nonetheless regal-looking scientist nearest the speakerphone, scratches at his graying beard as he replies: "London present at, let's see..."he checks the time on his iPhone, "...*zero-eight hundred*? For fucksake, that can't be right, can it?"

"It's right," another English accent confirms from somewhere in the background.

"Bloody hell," the first groans, adding, "that aside, we do all seem to be here."

"Very good," the Geneva-based coordinator smiles. "How about Australia?"

All in Geneva wait in silence for Australia to answer. After what seems like a respectable time, the communication coordinator tries again, "Australia, are you there?"

Melbourne. It's a prank the Aussies always like to play, no matter what time the call comes in. They have kazoos and noise-makers and an ABBA CD they crank, and 1,000 ml beakers they clink together near the speakerphone all in an effort to make it sound like they are recklessly partying-down when, in actuality, they are gathered in a rather uninspired second floor office overlooking the harbor herein the University of Melbourne. It's an image thing, you see. One cargo-shorts-and-sandals-sporting virologist feigns a drunken stupor as he slurs into the speakerphone: "Five of the clock Melbourne time, mate, and well into Happy Hour, all of which is to say, this better be important." A chorus of party-hardy cheers arise around him.

"How very *special* you people are," the Geneva-based coordinator quips before addressing the last team: "And last but certainly not least, the United States?"

Atlanta. Bronwyn answers the call from the conference room of the Coordinating Center for Infectious Diseases. Like Hank and Ross and the handful of other heads of the various Centers within Centers here in the Centers for

Disease Control, she sits bleary-eyed at the table back-dropped by the wee-hours darkness laying over the rest of sleeping Atlanta.

"NCIRD of the CCID of the CDC here, zero-three hundred Atlanta time," Bronwyn answers, her decidedly curt and humorless response setting the tone for the rest of the conference call. She's tired and this is serious; that's basically what she is conveying to her giddy, immature colleagues out there: *We're in some deep shit, grow up and deal with it.*

There follows a moment of silence before the conference coordinator responds: "Very good then, to bring you all up to date, the CDC have apparently isolated another influenza subtype – apparently one of dire concern – that has just begun to appear in several cities. Dr. Galloway, can you fill us in?"

"I will try," Bronwyn begins, knowing she won't be making any friends with what she is about to say. She glances at Hank, then at Ross, then turns her chair directly towards the speakerphone in order to address the epidemiological world at large as clearly and concisely as possible: "Some seventy-two hours ago you all were sent a strain of Bird flu which we, at the time, had every reason to believe was responsible for a deadly outbreak in Laos. The initial theory was that the H5N1 strain had finally mutated via antigenic drift to the point where the virus was now fully capable of an interspecies leap from birds to humans, just as we had always feared. But, as it turns out, we were mistaken. In fact, we were intentionally misled."

"*Misled?* By whom?" the Japanese end asks.

Bronwyn takes a breath and sighs wearily, "Details are still a bit blurry at this time but it is beginning to look as if one member of the field reconnaissance team that first encountered the outbreak *intentionally* sent in the wrong virus sample."

"But why?" the Aussie component – in all seriousness now – asks.

"I think we all know *why*," Bronwyn blurts, fatigue causing her to speak when she should be employing restraint, "I suspect we've all – while stuck in traffic, or watching a famine unfold, or standing by powerlessly as specie after specie go extinct – that we've all secretly prayed some magic virus would come along and..."

Hank cuts Bronwyn a *what-the-hell-are-you-saying?* glare. And it works; effectively nudging the bleary-eyed director back on script.

"What I mean is we've all *entertained* the fantasy of *culling the herd* some, and yet we've all managed to keep our wits about us and our priorities straight," Bronwyn adds, bending her response. But now she's got herself stuck in a bit of a trench. She would like to tell them what she and the handful here at the CDC suspect was the objective of the outbreak and the intentional sending back of the wrong strain, et al, but she's not sure she should due to the circumstantial nature of the evidence gathered thus far. Reputations could be tarnished, careers destroyed. But then there's fatigue again, working against her self-restraint. Thus, again, she blurts before thinking:

"It appears — and I caution you, this is all just conjecture at this point — nevertheless it *appears* a handful of scientists purposely isolated and have now intentionally released an avian subtype that is even more virulent."

"More virulent than Bird flu?" a Japanese epidemiologist asks, incredulously.

Bronwyn nods and repeats herself, "Significantly more so."

"Any idea where they got it?" an Aussie asks.

"From what we can gather, they isolated it from an Eskimo village, previously thought to have succumbed to the Spanish flu back in 1918."

"It appears they then field-tested this recovered strain in Laos just over a week ago," Hank adds.

"Then — with the alarming *success* of that test — "

"We're talkin' a mortality rate of between sixty-six and seventy percent!"

"At this point they sent both the WHO and CDC a strain of H5N1, identifying it as the cause of the deadly Laotian outbreak."

"So that we'd pour all of our resources — *exhaust* all of our resources — into manufacturing a vaccine based on the Bird Flu strain?" the British liaison posits.

"So it seems," Bronwyn affirms.

"Have you identified this Eskimo subtype?" a Japanese constituent asks.

"Yes, well, it appears to be the avian H7N7," Hanks explains, "yet considerably *evolved* from any previously isolated strains, to the point where any current vaccine we have for it would likely be wholly ineffective."

"Is there a terrorist organization suspected to be behind this?" The Geneva coordinator asks.

Hank swings his chair toward the speakerphone to answer this one: "Dr. Hank Bruckner of the Coordinating Center for Terrorism Preparedness and

Emergency Response here and, regarding your question: No, we have no reason to believe any known terrorist organizations have anything to do with this event."

"And their objective is, what exactly, simply to kill people?" the member of the Japanese component asks.

"Yes. We think so; a *lot* of people as it happens, maybe even *most* people."

"And why is this not an act of terrorism?" the Geneva coordinator asks.

"Subtle difference. Terrorists kill to invoke fear and political and/or ethnic change, whereas the people behind this decidedly *apolitical* endeavor just seem to want to kill – *indiscriminately*."

"*Indiscriminately* – so, they aren't focusing on any particular race or creed or ideology or nation?" an Aussie asks.

"Correct. In fact, quite to the contrary, they seem to be going to considerable lengths *not* to prejudice their extermination efforts."

"To what end?" the British spokesman asks.

"It seems they are just, well, just trying to save the planet."

"Oh, *that*," the British spokesman lets slip glibly.

"Yes – *that*."

An inadvertent silence follows Hank's confirmation; a palpable and telling silence from every end of the conference call that none, in any corner of the world, dare acknowledge.

Bronwyn takes it upon herself to break the silence, "But again, I caution you all, especially while details are still *blurry*, please keep this, I don't know, *conspiracy theory* just amongst ourselves. Right now the last thing we need is to lose the public's trust in our ability to protect them."

"Seems only prudent," the British spokesman avers.

"Indeed. Now, as was said at the top of this call, we now believe we are in possession of the *correct* strain. It is being packaged and shipped to the FDA for testing and approval, as well as to you all as we speak. So, please, halt whatever work you're doing on the H5N1 strain, notify your manufacturers to destroy and dispose of all eggs injected with this bogus strain –"

"And tell them to start stockpiling eggs anew," the Australian spokesman cuts in, already with a hint of defeat in his voice.

"Yes."

the momentum of folly

"Excuse me, Dr. Galloway, but it is already *July*," the Japanese component says, voicing what each team already knows. "Normally by this time the vaccine is already well into the testing stages —"

"And here we still don't even have the three strains selected!" the Brit adds with similar disapproval.

"No: we *do* now have the three strains —" Bronwyn tries to correct, only to be interrupted again.

"Nevertheless, this is something that is normally well underway in *May!*"

"And I can't speak for *your* chickens," the Aussie grumbles facetiously, "but ours downunder here, when we try to order them to lay more eggs —"

"Six hundred million more!"

"Right, they just kind of give us this *Up yours!* look. It's very unsettling."

Bronwyn, annoyed and exhausted, tries to keep the conference focused: "Look, I'm not saying we'll deliver on time; as far as I'm concerned that's no longer even a realistic goal given the extraordinary circumstances we're dealing with. Sure, it would be nice, but it wouldn't be of much help if we deliver the wrong vaccine, *again*, particularly when we've got a strain as lethal as this one knocking on our doors."

Hank interjects to bolster Bronwyn's argument, "At risk of picking at an old scab, last time we were hasty about getting the vaccine into production – 2004 – we whiffed completely; resulting in barely a fifty percent efficacy. And all three strains had to be swapped out of the vaccine mix the next year."

"We also had only *two* manufacturers producing vaccine that year. We currently have *six*; a correction we sought largely *because* of the problems from that season," the communications coordinator adds defensively.

"So, you're saying 2004 can't happen again?" Hank snips, accusatorily.

"No, I'm merely saying there's less of a chance of it happening due to the lessons learned!"

"Sounds like a classic battle between *a stitch in time saves nine* verses *haste makes waste* philosophies," the Aussie spokesman opines, trying to quell any nascent animosities.

"I'll drink to that," the Brit comments.

After a weary sigh, Bronwyn returns to the conversation, "Regardless of how many manufacturers we throw at this bug – two, six, a *dozen* – the challenge before us is formidable: to retool this late into the season simply may not be possible. There may simply be no way of stopping this pandemic, nor the cataclysmic impact it could *easily* incur. That said, and the two-month late start and half a billion egg deficit aside, at least two of our manufacturers will be using cell-based production methods this year —"

"Hence, no need for eggs for them," the Tokyo delegate adds.

"Right. Unfortunately both are only capable of fairly limited production quantities."

Ross leans towards the speakerphone, "Uh, and there's also one, Aegis Pharmaceuticals, who will presumably have an antiviral ready, albeit in very, very limited doses within our timeframe."

"How can they be working on an antiviral if they don't even have the virus yet?" the coordinator asks.

Hank swaps glances with Ross and Bronwyn. With the tacit agreement they should keep what they know of Aegis's tactics mum for now, he clears his throat then speaks towards the speakerphone, "That's, uh, something we are trying to ascertain as well. Suffice it to say, they *claim* to have the right strain already isolated. This, of course, yet to be verified."

"Verified or not, even the *claim* of having a vaccine all packed and ready for a pandemic as threatening as this could be quite the boost to the value of their stock," the British constituent states.

"Aegis Pharmaceuticals: now are they publicly traded yet?" the Australian end asks.

"No," almost every end of the call answers in unison.

"*Hmm*, too bad no one's watching that one," the Australian contingent quips back, his wry riposte met with hesitant yet welcomed laughter.

As much as Bronwyn appreciates the levity, she understands too well the vital importance of keeping her colleagues on task, and so she ignores the quip in order to quickly steer the discussion back on track, even at the risk of coming off as a bit of a bitch: "People, every second counts here. Waste your own time, but please don't waste mine."

After an uncomfortable silence, the Australian apologizes for his momentary lapse of professionalism, "I'm sorry, Dr. Galloway. Please continue."

"I'm sorry too; haven't had much in the way of sleep for a while." It takes Bronwyn a moment to gather her own thoughts. "Okay, regarding production: even with successful cell-based vaccines and the antiviral, over ninety percent of

the momentum of folly

the vaccine stock will rely on the good old-fashion egg-based method, meaning full production and packaging and FDA licensing will probably not happen until late September rather than early August as we had previously hoped."

"Pushing the release well into October," the Japanese representative notes.

"Which is typically when we begin the vaccinations," Geneva adds.

"Also, just so you know," Ross now interjects, "we're toying with the idea of adding a fourth strain —"

"Two Type A's, two Type B's?" Tokyo asks.

"That's right; like 2009's vaccine, but possibly with am H5N1 component just to cover our bases."

"Cover our *asses*," the Brit corrects.

"Well, them too."

"Mind you, we'll only do this if we determine it is necessary and won't prolong the release date," Hank assures the others.

"Regardless of how many strains we include in the vaccine, we are going to have to be *very* accurate with our initial distributions," the British delegate-cautions. "We'll need to pinpoint the outbreaks and vaccinate around them immediately. Unprecedented monitoring and surveillance is the only way we are going to suppress this outbreak; it's the only way we can keep it from blowing up in our faces."

Another protracted silence follows before the conference coordinator speaks again, this time to wrap up the call: "Well, thank you, everyone, for making yourselves available however inconvenient the hour. Now then, owing to the setbacks from starting production on the wrong strain, we have recalculated our estimates for the total number of global vaccine doses available six months out down from the three hundred million maximum figure now to just under 220 million. That said, if we focus our initial vaccination programs around the emerging hot zones, *and* see what help we can obtain from local governments to suppress travel, it is not mere optimism that suggests we can effectively contain this pathogen. Thank you all again."

"Excuse me," Bronwyn interjects.

The Geneva conference coordinator answers, "Yes, Dr. Galloway?"

"I'd just like to add one last thing."

"Of course."

Bronwyn pauses to search for a way to verbalize exactly what she is feeling. "Doctors, colleagues, all of you: please let there be no mistake here; this *is* the big one. This *is* the outbreak we've feared all along. 2009's Swine flu pandemic hopefully prepared us for this, but — just because we won that battle, largely because that strain ended up much more mild than it could have been — I strongly caution against complacency when setting up against this one. I suggest, once you have that initial batch of vaccine ready, go ahead and inoculate yourselves first — even your family members — because we, the *world*, will need you physically, mentally, and emotionally on the front line if we are going to have any hope of stopping this thing."

Bronwyn's somber assessment and proposal is met with utter silence from all ends of the phone lines. She takes another breath then adds, "I guess that's all I have to say except, you know, good luck and all that."

Sanofi Pasteur Laboratories, Lyon, France

Ten, individually-cupped conveyor belts carry streams of eggs through the sterile warehouse room wherein a hundred surgically-smocked and masked and latex-gloved technicians lift and gently puncture each and every egg, one at a time, with hair-width, stainless steel syringes, pumping a milliliter, if that, of a solution containing the live flu virus through the shell of each egg. The amount injected is just enough to infect the egg white and allow the virus to replicate its RNA therein several thousand fold over the course of the next seventy-two hours, after which time it is ready to be harvested. But today, just now in fact, a call has come in from headquarters, then barked by a P.A. system, then repeated via urgent shouts, in French, from the lab foreman across the vast and noisy room:

"Hold it, everybody! Stop vaccine production immediately. Save any uninfected eggs, destroy all others! I repeat: *all, full, stop!*"

The conveyor belts and their rivers of eggs come to an abrupt halt, causing the facility to fall quiet while giving rise to the troubled murmurs of the hundred or so technicians working herein. At the far end of the room, where the injected/infected eggs are re-racked and stacked onto forklifts, normally then to be transported off to cozy incubation sheds, a pair of lab techs share bewildered glances over their respective masks. It takes a moment but now each realize that everything has changed: what they had just been at full-throttle to *create*, now must switch to full-throttle to destroy. And this they acknowledge with a mere exchange of shrugs, after which time one of the techs climbs into the driver's seat of an electric forklift while the other wheels a stacked tower of some fifteen racks – now a cube of stainless steel framework firmly cradling 13,500 eggs – into position before the forklift. That done, the lift eases forward, gently sliding its forks beneath the rack. The tower of eggs wobbles and teeters but withstands the nudging with nary even a single Humpty Dumpty taking a fall. That done, the assisting lab tech climbs aboard the forklift as the driver slips

the momentum of folly

its transmission into reverse, and begins backing its *injected-with-the-wrong-strain* cargo towards the exit.

The forklift backs out of the injection lab, down a main corridor, out of the virus-growing BSL-3 certified warehouse building, then out into the blustery and rainy afternoon. Under normal conditions they would keep the tower of injected eggs within the main warehouse and just move them into one of the many incubation sheds and there allow the eggs, some fifty million in all, to grow their infections. But today, what with the sudden changes of plans, the transport techs instead direct their embryonic cargo out across the facility's smooth concrete parking lot and towards the entrance of a smallish, seldom-used, building housing a pair of industrial biohazard incinerators. And this will become the fertilized eggs' fate; to be reduced to heaping mounds of gray ash and the putrid waft of sulfur spewed from the incinerator smokestacks.

With over sixty percent of their eggs already infected with the "wrong" strain of influenza, Sanofi Pasteur will have to destroy some thirty million fertilized eggs this way. Could take weeks. Then, of course, they will have to find and purchase another thirty million more to infect with the "correct" strain in order to make up for the mistake. And that could take months. But that is what *must* and *will* happen so that Sanofi Pasteur can make good on its contract promise to deliver one hundred million doses of vaccine this year, twice what it delivered just back in 2008.

And though their techniques may vary or their automation may or may not be as state-of-the-art or volume as large as Sanofi Pasteur, the same basic infected-with-the-wrong-strain egg destruction processes are happening at the other five pharmaceutical companies under contract with the WHO and CDC to produce vaccine this season, be it GlaxoSmithKline or Novartis or CSL Biotherapies of Australia or the newly-relicensed Chiron Corporation – decertified after a 2004 contamination problem – or even MedImmune with its live attenuated influenza vaccine (LAIV) administered via nasal spray. They will each have to start all over. Most of their 300 million doses tossed out while still in the virus-growing stage. Most of their 150 million fertilized chicken eggs destroyed. It's back to square one for each of them.

Centers for Disease Control, Atlanta

This time Carl can feel it coming. For the first time in weeks he can feel himself rising through the layers of sleep towards the gleaming daylight of full consciousness. For the first time since he and Angela had that little episode in Tijuana he is not sick and not medicated, and he relishes it by purposely taking his time *coming to* even as Bronwyn nudges his shoulder again while gently calling out:

"Dr. Sims.... Carl, wakie-wakie...."

When Carl does finally open his eyes, Dr. Galloway's soft-focused smile is the very first thing he sees. She looks beautiful, radiant, angelic even; a sight for sore eyes for sure. Then again, who wouldn't look so to someone emerging from the hell where Carl has wallowed these past few weeks?

"Hey there," she smiles from his bedside, "Welcome back."

Carl smiles back, and kind of nods.

Bronwyn then rolls the four-wheeled stool on which she sits, a few feet and over to a portable desk. With a quick swirl of her finger she "awakens" the laptop computer waiting there on the desk, which she then jacks into a larger flat screen monitor.

Watching her, Carl can't help but notice she is wearing that weird CDC military uniform; a uniform that looks to be an unimaginative knock-off of something between that of the Navy's and Coast Guard's, and is normally kept in the closet until that rare event she has to make some sort of public statement or testimony. All of the CDC "brass" have these uniforms, but none really cares to ever wear them. They'd rather not be reminded that the CDC is a branch of the U.S. Military, but it is, and ironically the branch that arguably protects its citizenry the most. But the fact Bronwyn is presently dressed in her uniform is not the surprising thing to Carl; what *is* surprising is the fact she is not wearing any biosafety gear. None whatsoever. This encourages him. This is a sign of hope. Looking around, he discovers he is in the CDC's own tiny hospital ward, which they fondly call "Sick Bay." Turning back to Bronwyn, he licks his lips to speak, for the first time in God knows how long.

"You're not wearing any protection."

Not taking her eyes off the computer screens, Bronwyn quips, "Excuse me?" – poking fun at Carl's choice of words.

Carl feels the warm flush of embarrassment in his face, then musters a lame attempt to rephrase his observation: "I meant, you know, for the last, I don't know how long now, anyone coming near me was either wearing a biosafety suit or shooting at me."

"Well, I *could* put on a biosafety suit if it would make you feel more comfortable, but there's really no need."

"I never had it?" He asks, chagrined.

"The H7N7? Oh, no, you had it alright; *big time*, in fact."

"And yet I survived."

Bronwyn nods, "Thanks in part, I'm loath to admit, to your girlfriend's antiviral medication, which in turn owes its *complete* thanks to your unorthodox method of conveying the virus. *Intentionally infecting yourself...*" Bronwyn says, shaking her head.

"It was the only way I could keep it alive long enough to get it back intact."

"We figured as much. Ross had the highest praise for your heroics: *ballsy* – he called it," Bronwyn says, with a wry grin.

She then backs her stool slightly off to one side so Carl can see the two screens and the pair of microscopic images she has just pulled up thereupon. "All right, let's break it down for you." Pointing to the larger monitor screen to the left, she begins the deconstruction process: "Over here, screen left, the H5N1 strain Dr. Williams had you courier back to us from China, after leading you to think it was the same strain encountered in Laos."

"Duped."

"Yup." Bronwyn then redirects Carl's attention to the subtlety different-looking strain on the laptop's screen to the right. "Whereas, over here, the real deal: the H7N7 you pulled out of the Eskimo mass grave. Let's pull up the gene sequencing so we can distinguish them a bit better."

After a few adroit strokes of the computer keys, the microscopic images are replaced by RNA genetic sequencing rows of the respective virus strains. As Bronwyn juxtaposes the rows side-by-side on the monitor screen, their differences – albeit subtle – become apparent. She points to the one on top, "Bird flu," then the one on the bottom, "Eskimo flu. Do you see that?"

Carl nods, as the difference between the strains become visibly apparent to him.

"Have you seen any antigenic drift within the virus yet?"

Bronwyn looks at him curiously, "Not yet. Why do you ask?"

"Stuart and I were worried they may have tinkered with the virus; maybe found a way to keep it more stable."

Bronwyn raises her brows. "*That* certainly would be cause for concern. Usually with particularly lethal strains of influenza they fairly quickly mutate back to the mean."

"How's that?"

"Flu generally packs somewhere between a half to one percent mortality rate, right? Any strain that comes around with a higher or lower lethality – given the rapid mutability of the virus – is going to be short lived. That's how the original Spanish Flu pandemic finally ended; it just mutated back to a relatively harmless strain, burned itself out. But if your *buddies* found a way to stabilize it, even for a few months, that could make it devastating," Bronwyn affirms as she shuts down the computer.

Carl nods, but his thoughts are already a few steps ahead. "What strains are you mixing into the trivalent?"

"Well, for a while we considered including four strains but then, as one of the Influenza B's weren't showing up in any of the field tests, we decided to drop it."

"So, two Type A's and one Type B?"

"Right. First of which is clade I influenza A/Vietnam/1203/2004."

Carl nods, "One of last year's H5N1 bird flu components."

"Yes, but not a wild-type this time 'round. Instead we're running with a human isolate via plasmid rescue, with hemagglutinin and neuraminidase genes derived from avirulent egg-adapted A/PR/8/34."

Carl nods. "Sounds prudent. What else?"

"Another blast from the past: Malaysia/2506/2004."

"From the Influenza B/Yamagata lineage?"

Bronwyn smiles, "For someone who disdains lowly flu research, you're getting pretty good at it."

Carl barely acknowledges the compliment. "Leaving us with, last but certainly not least, the trivalent's third component – the H7N7."

Bronwyn already has another grin on her face, "Right, the strain we've since classified as A/Alaska/Sims/2011."

This homage to his efforts catches Carl off his guard. "No way!"

She smiles, "Way."

"Really? – a viral strain named after me?" Carl asks, incredulously.

"Well, you certainly earned it."

Ready for her exit, Bronwyn stands, closes her laptop and tucks it under her arm.

"Regarding my *buddies*, as you call them: any word on where they might be?"

"Yes, as a matter of fact: Nakayama, Perez, Singh, and LaFond – each and all confirmed dead."

Carl is taken aback by the abruptness of this news, but his concerns swing immediately to the lone, unaccounted-for conspirator: "What about Jenna?"

"Dr. Williams? – presumed dead. That's based on numerous eye witnesses reporting on her condition just before she eluded capture in Nairobi."

Carl is surprised by how conflicted he feels about this news. Part of the problem is that it's all so hard to imagine: Dr. Williams, Jenna, *dead?* That feels almost like stating the sun won't rise tomorrow; she seems to Carl *that* indomitable, that much greater than something so mundane as life and death. But Carl keeps his feelings to himself; he bites his tongue, nods, and changes the subject.

"Is it okay for me to go?" he asks, good patient that he is.

"If you're feeling up to it. You're still teeming with antibodies but no longer contagious."

Carl swings his legs off the bed, placing his bare feet on the cool linoleum. He takes a deep breath, fully expecting to have to cough… but doesn't.

* * *

CDC War Room

Though the designation "War Room" conjures images of the clandestine, subterranean, immense innermost cavernous sanctums of the Pentagon or NORAD or even Homeland Security, replete with vast, wall-covering computer displays tracking every evildoer doing evil on it, the War Room here at the CDC is nothing more than a modest-sized auditorium – formerly known as Auditorium A, to be precise – retrofitted with just enough of the latest technologies to warrant the aforementioned designation. This all came together back in early 2003 in an urgent effort to track and attack the latest bug – SARS. In all the retrofit cost a little over $7 million, over half of which was generously donated by private persons and companies. Before then smaller versions of war rooms were thrown together willy-nilly whenever the need arose and where ever the CDC could find room for a few more chairs, a map of the world, and a coffee machine. Back then it was a common joke around the CDC that the reason they didn't have a *real* war room was because they fought *real* wars, unlike the *hypothetical* wars the Pentagon *hypothetically* waged with multi-billion dollar weapons they never used against *hypothetical*, paper tiger foes that came and went like the seasons. *We need new supersonic stealth bombers and bombs and nuclear subs and Star Wars satellites and UAVs and tanks and everything else we can dream up because we don't need the smoking gun to be a mushroom cloud!* That is the military-industrial complex's rant anyway. And it always seemed to work; the Pentagon never seemed to have funding problems, even in spite of the fact that a "mushroom cloud" has never claimed even a single American's life *ever,* whereas influenza alone snuffs out some 36,000 a year. Go figure.

But now the CDC *does* have its war room so, even if the whole thing *did* cost less than a single Predator drone, the employees here can stop their whining. Of course, even the most state of the art technologies have a way of becoming obsolete in a blink of an eye; hence, ever since that initial outlay and bequeathments the CDC has had to manage its upgrades in a consider-

the momentum of folly

ably more miserly fashion. The upgrade for this current outbreak is a classic case-in-point: thank Ross for that one, for it was he who snapped up, among other useful electronics, a dozen humongous High Definition Television screens for pennies on the dollar when Circuit City filed for bankruptcy. He then hung the screens from the former auditorium's walls and rafters in such a way as to blackout the already filthy-to-the-point-of-barely-translucent windows and skylights. And he didn't stop there: from other failed businesses he solicited high-end, formerly trendy office furniture, which he artfully arranged with enough attention to both functionality and aesthetics that it reduced Bronwyn to concede, "It looks pretty cool, so long as you don't look too closely," and Hank to start calling him "Dr. Strangedude." And here this morning, as it has each and every morning and afternoon and night for the past fortnight, this *real* War Room bustles with frenetic activity as representative teams from all four subdivisions within the Coordinating Center for Infectious Diseases, in concert with the Geneva-based WHO, track the global spread of the H7N7 infestation and coordinate vaccination efforts in the concerted effort to snuff it out. And it is into this fray that Bronwyn pushes the wheelchair-bound Carl.

"Wow!" Carl effuses, blown-away by the formerly cruddy auditorium's stunning renovation. "Who dressed up this pig?"

"Who else? – Ross," Bronwyn answers, as she brings his wheelchair to a halt a short distance into the room. She then turns towards the center of the vast room and, in an attempt to snag the attention of all its occupants, calls out: "Hey, everybody…" But, what with all of them still enrapt in phone calls or chat room sessions or face-to-face strategy quorums, her efforts prove futile. So she tries again, louder: "People, hey, everyone, can I have your attention, please!" But still nary a one acknowledges her. In fact, out of all the forty or so War Room mongers, it seems the only one who hears Bronwyn is Hank.

"Allow me, Dr. Galloway," Hank says, a hint of pity in his voice as he steps up beside her. Hank then turns towards the room at large and, tucking the tip of his tongue to the roof of his mouth cowboy-style, sends out a whistle so shrill and piercing it leaves everyone no choice but to drop what ever they are doing and turn towards him, their faces chevroned into perturbed and puzzled glares.

"Thank you," Hank says, with a smirk. He then takes their rapt attention and politely redirects towards Bronwyn explaining, "Dr. Galloway has something to say."

"Thank you, Dr. Bruckner," Bronwyn says, with a slight blush. Then, turning back to the roomful of scientists and technicians, she places both hands on Carl's shoulders and announces, "Not to drag you away from your important work, but I'd just wanted to present to you all this season's very first known H7N7 survivor – our very own Dr. Carl Sims!"

With Carl's month-long odyssey already the stuff of legend, the gathered peers give up a heartfelt chorus of hoots and cheers. Amidst the applause, from somewhere out of the center of it all, Stuart's voice can be heard shouting out, "Whoa, and check out the *wheels!*"

Looking up, Carl sees Stuart pumping towards him in his own wheelchair, a beaming smile spread across his face. After turning a quick circle around Carl, Stuart quips, "Cool, all it needs now is a few surf stickers and it will be *almost* as gnarly as mine!" Stuart then pops a wheelie – "Hey, can you do this yet?" – then spins a pirouette while balanced on the rear two wheels.

"Kids' stuff," Carl boasts.

"Yeah, kids' stuff my ass," Stuart retorts, calling Carl's bluff.

Stuart teasingly socks Carl's shoulder, and Carl returns it, followed shortly thereafter by a brief and awkward hug. Genuinely overcome with emotion but rendered slightly uncomfortable by the show of affection, the two pull apart. In the moment thereafter they share a brief glance silently acknowledging what might have been had Hank not interrupted their last meeting in the BSL-4 slammer, thus keeping Stuart from destroying the centrifuged virus with the chlorine bath.

Carl nods, a silent promise to keep Stuart's momentary transgression to himself.

And Stuart accepts the nod with one of his own. Then, changing the subject, Stuart turns to Bronwyn: "Want me to bring the crippled kid here up to date?" he asks, alluding to Carl.

Bronwyn smiles, "Please."

"Alright, here's where we be at…" Stuart begins, leading Carl towards the center of the War Room, pulling their wheelchairs to a stop within ideal viewing of the biggest of the flat screen monitors hanging from the rafters. On the screen is a concise, digital map of the world with national borders and major cities, even mountain ranges and rivers and such rendered in remarkable detail. Several of the cities have red circles around them indicating viral outbreaks.

"As of forty minutes ago, we stand at 434,600 reported cases, most already on various general antivirals as well as Aegis's H7N7-specific antiviral, and most of these cases reported within those fifteen hot zones you see up there on the Ross's War Board."

"Patent pending!" Ross calls out, jokingly, from somewhere across the room.

"Anyway, it should come as no surprise all fifteen hot zones are epicentered in cities our conspirators passed through before our catching up with them."

"I count sixteen," Carl says, directing Stuart's attention towards one red circle with no name in it, located near the center of Africa.

Hank explains: "Yeah, well, for whatever reason, the virus seems to have made the leap to the Lake Victoria region."

"Probably just the first of many secondary outbreak centers," Stuart hypothesizes.

Still staring up at the map and the tiny red circle over Lake Victoria, Carl asks, "So it's still spreading?"

"Oh, yeah, of course; big time. We fully expect infections to double here in the next few days."

"That said, see the green triangles up there?" Ross interjects, directing Carl towards other, differently-colored polygons alighting the War Room's main digital world map. "And the yellow rectangular-shaped thingies?"

"Yeah," Carl replies.

"Those are immunization outposts; *currently-operational* and *soon-to-be* respectively: 140 at present, some three thousand when we're in full swing."

"We're gonna kick some viral ass!" Ross boasts.

"*Ye-ah*, that's what I'm talkin' about," Hank underscores, with he and Ross then sharing a testosterone-fueled high-five.

"Anyway…" Bronwyn interjects, steering the debriefing back towards order, "… we expect infection rates to begin dropping precipitously within the next month or so,"

"Got a death toll yet?" Carl asks.

"189,000 thereabouts," Stuart answers.

"Expected to top out at around one-point-eight million," Hank adds.

"Which is considerably less than the hundred million the Spanish flu took out last time it reared its butt-ugly face," Ross says.

"Or the *billions* this one might have claimed, if not for you," Bronwyn adds, beaming proudly down at Carl.

And Carl smiles back, if somewhat wistfully.

Western Kenya, Northern Tanzania, Southern Uganda

———

Concentric patterns of shimmering waves slip past several hundred feet beneath the floatplane's pontoons. The expanse of water over which it flies is so vast Carl might be excused for mistaking it for open ocean had he, say, just awakened disoriented from yet another flu-induced delirium. But he didn't. In fact, he is fully recovered now, some ten pounds frailer maybe, but rested and feeling strong again. Thus he is well aware this is no *ocean* beneath him, but rather the largest tropical lake on the planet; so large, in fact, it has earned many names from the many peoples who abut it: Ukerewe, Nalubaale, Victoria Nyanza, Lake Victoria. Carl also knows, even if no land can be seen from his window, that this 184,000 square mile catchment is the basin of the Great Rift Valley, wherein the oldest evidence of the *Homo* genus have been found, dating back some 2.3 million years when *Homo hablilis*, with their crude stone tools, first radiated out of the *Australopithecine* taxa. From here three basic migrations would carry the Homo genus to all parts of the world. *Homo hablilis, Homo erectus, Homo rudolfensis, Homo georgicus, Homo ergaster, Homo antecessor, Homo cepranensis, Homo heidelbergensis, Homo neanderthalensis, Homo rhodesiesis, Homo sapiens idaltu,* and *Homo floresiesis* would all have their day in the sun, many simultaneously, and then die off, with only *Homo sapiens sapiens* surviving still to this day. Or so far, anyway.

Why these species died off is difficult to ascertain, but viral or bacterial pandemics are likely explanations. And what exactly will finally snuff out the human line completely — be it a pandemic, meteoric collision, cosmic ray or, perhaps most likely, humankind itself — is equally difficult to predict. All that is certain is that it *will* someday happen; humankind *will* someday cease to be, the Homo genus *will* someday take its last breath then slowly release it, simultaneously laying to rest all of its compiled sin and guilt and envy and hatred and jealousy and worry and dread and joy and love. Whether that fate comes later this year, or five hundred million years from now when our sun becomes a red giant

the momentum of folly

star with a radius large enough to consume Earth's current orbit, or a hundred billion years from now when the Universe has expanded to the point where the massive clouds of hydrogen gas lack the gravity to condense upon themselves in order to attain the requisite ten-million-degree core temperatures needed to ignite nuclear fusion and thus create new stars, rendering our entire universe a hospice/morgue of dead or dying brown stars and their ice-cold satellites, or not until that hypothetical day long, long thereafter when the *everything-there-is* has expanded such as to become so diffuse that neither molecules or individual atoms, nor *any* matter for that matter, possess the gravity to even hold themselves together. Whatever is left of this Universe at that point – be it energy or dark energy or consciousness or nothingness – it certainly won't be peopled with people. However much Nature may abhor a vacuum, there comes a point when the Vacuum wins.

Though the plane can hold twenty-four, Carl is the only passenger. And though this is the regularly scheduled daily flight of *"The Nairobi – Lake Victoria Express!"* this is the airline's first commute in almost five weeks now. This, of course, is due to the United Nations's implementation of mandatory global restrictions on public travel, be it by air, train, bus, boat, car, moped, bicycle, or foot. And this, of course, was all part of the concerted effort to keep the H7N7 virus from spreading. *Hunker down, stay put, avoid public places, wash your hands several times a day, cough into your sleeve and, for goodness sake, don't spit!...* those were some of the injunctions disseminated from the WHO and CDC. And it seems to have paid off, as the virus is clearly on the wane worldwide. Still, they were being extra cautious; in 1918 the governments of the world had been too naïve and lax regarding the Spanish Flu pandemic, and nearly suffered dearly for it. But the current world powers weren't going to allow the same mistake to happen again. The data flowed freely from the WHO and the word was out, and the UN, in its most forceful declaration yet, announced they were going to pounce on this bug, and they fully expected every nation to join in. And pounce they did. In fact it was outright encouraging the way all the disparate nations and peoples pulled together on this; how they all put aside their skirmishes for the time to join together to fight a *real* foe for once. And though no leader would publicly acknowledge it, each harbored the secret hope this momentary unity might allow them to rise above their trite peeves and expensive conflicts with their adversaries once and for all. But this, of course, was not to be. Humanity, after all, is still an ignorant species when it comes to pride and tolerance; still prone to cut off its nose to spite its face. Hence, when the pandemic was over, pretty much everyone suspected what would happen: vengeances would be resume, battles would reignite, blood would spill, children would cry.

The pilots on the plane had been vaccinated; that was the condition of anyone traveling at this point. And Carl, of course, had his own special circumstances — expertise *and* immunity — which allowed him to move about the planet with a freedom few were entitled. Along with bottled water the plane was ferrying some ten thousand servings of *Plumpy Nut*; the tasty, nigh-miraculous peanut, soy oil, milk, sugar, vitamins and minerals concoction well-meaning emergency relief organizations drop like fire retardant onto famine areas everywhere in the world these days. The plane's destination was the Seese Islands of Uganda, a group of the more than 3,000 islands harbored within the lake, and a popular destination for tourists. As with a lot of places, there were people stranded there; nothing too serious, but they had to be fed, and thus this flight. But Carl was just tagging along. He had his own reasons for venturing here.

The plane's pontoons touch down upon the lake's gentle ripples, quickly reducing its speed to a relative crawl. Using the pontoon rudders the pilot turns the plane's snout towards the island's sandy shore, then revs the engines again in order to plow through the floating marsh of hyacinth. Once beached the copilot opens the fuselage door and lowers the gangway ladder. Carl ducks through the plane's hatch, under the hand-painted sign, *The Nairobi — Lake Victoria Express!* Though gaunt and a little pale and a couple of days unshaven, Carl is every bit as healthy as he is lucid again, definitely ready for any pick-up basketball or soccer game that might break out. Standing atop the gangway ladder, he slings his daypack over a shoulder and looks about, as if wondering which direction to head off towards first. The plane's engines shut down. As the roar of both motors quickly fade, the cries of native waterfowl can be heard gliding somewhere overhead. Carl squints skyward in search of the flock, hoping to catch a glimpse of something exotic, but he cannot find even a single bird against the glare of the sun.

The silhouettes of monkeys leap from branch to branch overhead.

"So she *is* American? I suspected so."

the momentum of folly

Carl lowers his attention from the monkeys in the floral canopy above to the backside of the Ugandan missionary — in his forties, sporting a crisp white shirt against jet-black skin — who guides him along this path through the forest, the "short cut" as he explained it. Children, maybe half a dozen of them, some naked, playfully escort them, laughing as they dart in and out of the foliage on either side of the path. Smiling, Carl looks from the kids back up to the missionary, the latter being of the type who needs to make eye contact whenever he is speaking, and thus his neck is craned about as he continues to tell Carl of the stranger who came onto their island some weeks ago, the stranger towards which he is leading Carl.

"She would not speak; not a word the whole time she on the island, but I thought, you know, maybe she is American."

"Was it the baseball cap?" Carl asks, somewhat sarcastically.

"The what?" the missionary asks innocently, having no sense of sarcasm.

"Her *hat*."

"Oh. I don't know. Maybe. She not from here, that is for sure!"

The path begins to fray as the jungle yields to the beach again on the opposite, western side of the island. The missionary slows to a pause, pulls one last branch aside, then nods up ahead.

"There it is. This where she stay."

Carl follows the missionary's nod some thirty meters ahead to where a lone, bamboo bungalow is perched on frail stilts a meter above the gently lapping lakeshore, silhouetted by the fat, orange, late afternoon sun.

"She who you come half way around the world to see?" the missionary asks, incredulously.

"Yep."

"Well, she must be one dear friend!" the missionary laughs.

Carl thinks about it, then smiles. The children rush past like a stampeding herd towards the beach to play. Alluding to them, Carl asks, "Has everyone in your parish received their flu shots?"

"Shots?"

"Vaccinations?"

"Oh, yes, yes; three, no, no, *four* weeks ago now. I feel sick for two days after; fever, chills… Never again. I let God take care of me next time!" the missionary replies, adding as an afterthought, "Is that what she has — the flu?"

Carl nods, leaving it at that.

"*Tsk-tsk,* poor woman!" the missionary sighs, shaking his head in genuine sorrow.

Turning to the missionary, Carl extends his hand. The missionary grabs it and shakes it, accessorizing it with the now globally ubiquitous palm-slide and knuckles-bop. *This too is a virus, ever mutating like fashion or language or music or spiritual belief,* Carl is thinking as they go through the motions of the handshake, this latest of social memes to spread like wildfire across the planet. But it's an epiphany too abstruse to share with even a close friend let alone someone of such a different culture, so Carl keeps it to himself.

"Alright, brother, you be good," the missionary tells Carl in parting, as he turns back to the trail which will take him back across the small island, shouting out to his flock as he goes, "Come, come, children. Crocodiles will eat you for sure; first your arms, then your legs, then your body – just so you can watch and *boo-hoo* as they play futbol with your heads. So, come!"

Carl smiles then returns his attention to the bungalow, just staring at it for a moment before sucking in a courage-mustering breath.

Stepping up to the bungalow's rear side, Carl knocks on the sturdiest piece of bamboo he can find. Nothing. He waits for a few seconds then knocks again. Though again this elicits no response, Carl thinks he may have heard faint coughing emanating from somewhere around the bungalow's opposite side, and so he climbs the three-rung, rope and stick ladder up onto the bungalow's tiny, wrap-around porch. As he makes his way towards the far side he hears the coughing again. Following the sound, he rounds the bungalow's last corner, bringing him to a fairly large, canopied veranda, designed to afford vacationing occupants a relaxing view of the lake. A hand-woven hammock is strung between posts near the veranda's far edge, part of it dangling over the water itself. Judging by the way the hammock hangs, Carl suspects there could just be a human slung in there, though said human – if even alive – would have to be quite frail. The cough rumbles again, louder, this time visibly shaking the hammock and thus confirming life.

"Dr. Williams?" Carl calls out gently.

Though there still is no replay there is, at least, another sign of life from within the hammock as a scrawny, brown arm extends itself towards a rum and coke set on a small, bamboo table beside it. After the glass is pulled back within the fold of the hammock, Carl can hear the slurp of a straw followed by a satisfied if weak sigh.

Carl edges closer to the hammock until he can peek down at Jenna's ravaged body barely filling what had been her snug tank top and curve-hugging safari shorts. If not for her *Cal Bears* baseball cap and slightly out-of-fashion sunglasses Carl might not recognize her at all, so drastic is her deterioration. She sucks again on the straw of her drink, her hollow cheeks narrowing to provide suction.

"Dr. Williams, I presume?" Carl calls out gently, employing subtle humor.

Pulling the straw from her lips, she finally replies: "That's my name, don't wear it out."

However weak and slurred her words might be, Carl is heartened to hear her sarcasm is as healthy as ever. He smiles. "Hello, Jenna."

Though still too taxed to open her eyes, Jenna manages a slight smile of her own. "Ah, White Devil – still alive."

"Still alive."

Jenna raises her glass to toast their mutual survivals. "Cheers then, you're amongst the thirty percent who will survive this scourge."

"You too, it seems."

Jenna takes another draw on her rum and coke, and shakes her head. "Double pneumonia. Rumors of liver damage as well, if you can believe that. It's all just a matter of time."

Confronted with her frank assessment of her fate, Carl finds himself at a rare loss for words which he tries to patch with some trite small talk, "So, how are the missionaries treating you?"

Jenna snorts out a slight chuckle, "Oh, they tolerate me. Bless their hearts." She pauses to take a couple restful breaths before continuing with her line of thought. "I don't dare tell them what I've done, lest they take it as a personal challenge to save me." She takes another breath, then, "God, could you imagine; trying to save *me?*"

Then, what begins as ironic laughter soon develops into a lung-wrenching coughing jag that seems as though it may never end. In order to quell her paroxysms, Jenna reaches for a hypodermic needle lying on the drink table next to a small brown vial. Carl watches with pity as she sticks the needle into her thigh and begins to shoot herself up.

"Morphine?"

Still coughing, but winding down, Jenna shakes her head, "The *real* stuff."

"Heroin?"

"That's what they call me, don't wear it out." As Carl doesn't laugh, she feels compelled to add, "That was *another* joke, Carl. *Ha-ha.* Jesus, where'd your sense of humor go? I'm the one dying, not you."

"Sorry." Carl says, genuinely apologetic.

"Whatever." She then changes the subject back to the little brown vial of heroin, "Yep, got everything I need right here to numb the pain; everything and more," she adds, waving a dismissive hand over the table of other narcotics, then around to include her surroundings, then back to her rum and coke, which she picks up and sips again.

"Why not just give yourself an overdose?"

"And miss out on the big event?" She shakes her head, as if the option somehow insults her. "Never; dying, death – it's the only mystery left. I don't want to be sleepin' through it. I want to greet it at the threshold wide-awake! Well, within reason anyway."

Jenna slides the needle from her thigh, closes her eyes, takes a deep, uninterrupted breath, then allows a calm to wash over her. Carl gently takes the needle from her fingers and sets it back onto the drink table, fully expecting not to hear another word from her. But then she surprises him yet again:

"It's going to be beautiful, Carl," she mutters.

"Death?"

She shakes her head ever so slightly.

"No... *life.* Life here on Earth after..."

Carl waits for the end of her sentence, but it does not come. "After what?"

She takes another breath, eyes clenched tightly. "After *The Cleansing.*"

The Cleansing: so that's what they called their plan. Give it a specious, even hygienic/ antiseptic label and that legitimizes it, that makes genocide conscionable, Carl is thinking, as he watches a self-righteous calm wash over her.

After another long pause, she surprises Carl yet again by mustering the energy to elaborate: "Yours is the first generation in decades, maybe centuries, that actually has reason to be optimistic about the future." She breathes, taking delight, even credit in the world she envisions. "Do you realize how wonderful that is? Do you know how fortunate –"

But her vision of the future is interrupted as a wave of nausea overcomes her. Blanching, she sits upright in the hammock, pulling off her hat and sunglasses, and pausing there to see if her nausea will settle… but it doesn't.

"Pardon me," she says, excusing herself with unnecessary aplomb as she hastily climbs from the hammock.

Carl reaches to help her but she is already out of the hammock and standing –like a scrawny foal unsteadily on first legs – on her own. Carl gently takes her arm in another attempt to assist her balance, but again, almost angrily, she shakes free of him. Grabbing hold of a bamboo rail she begins, as much on her own power as of gravity's, a stumbling descent down the half dozen steps leading into the lake. Stepping off the stairs, she splashes hastily through the knee-deep water, nearly tripping with each weak and clumsy step across the rocky bottom. Then, some fifteen meters or so out from the bungalow, she settles to her hands and knees and begins to dry heave, her flexing, bare midriff and gaping mouth a few inches about the lake's gently rippled surface.

After watching her wretch for some time like this, Carl pulls a factory-sealed, pre-measured, Aegis Pharmaceuticals registered, H7N7 antiviral injector from his pocket. He considers it for a moment; pondering if he should wade out there and inject her without even asking permission. Or should he simply set it on the drink table with her other drugs and leave the decision up to her? Or would it even help by this point, her immune system already ravaged, those rumors of liver damage, et al. Or, best case scenario, what if the antiviral miraculously worked and restored her health and allowed her to live; what then? He would have saved her life only to permit her, to *force* her, to see that her *Cleansing* had failed and that humanity was still hell bent on self-destruction. And from where would she view this realization? Most likely from the defendant's bench at her genocide trial. Free trip to the Haag. Would that be doing her a favor? Would that be *helpful*?

After pondering these likely outcomes, Carl simply slides the injector back into his pocket. Matter settled. He then lifts his attention back to Jenna; an emaciated biped devolved now back onto all fours and silhouetted by the fractured, sinking, orange and crimson African sun, as reflected off the black, wobbling lake surface. As her dry heaves settle some, Jenna raises her head towards the quarter moon set like a jewel within the pale turquoise heavens. Not looking at the moon or the beautiful sky or the radiant sunset or the Eden-esque lake, she releases a long, anguished, defiant, primal howl; a howl that suggests she is no longer an objective, admiring observer of the world, but now fully *part* of it all. To wonder what exactly she is trying to communicate is already to miss the point. Even she doesn't know from where this howl comes or what it is saying; it is a howl, plain and simple – a post-ego post-script, not so much from an individual human as from all life itself. And once she has exhausted every molecule of oxygen from the breath that carried that howl, her head drops, hair dragging in the water, resting, dying. At this point she has no further purpose; no conscious ambition other than to simply fill her lungs once more, if she can – twice, if at all possible – and howl again, and then again, until she can howl no more. That is all there is to do.

The sun is barely an ember by this point, with its warm if distant glow reflected in Carl's face. Though fiery hues still stream at him – whether reflected from off the water or bent around sunset clouds or shooting straight from the hip of the sinking sphere itself – he no longer even needs to squint in order to gaze directly at it. And regarding the silhouette down on all fours there between *that* light and *this* beholder – the silhouette that once had a name, *Jenna*, and some lovers and an achievement or two and weakness for ice-cold beer and at least one grand if unrealized dream – well, there's really not a lot Carl can do for it now, but to respectfully bare witness to its passing.

Stockholm Concert Hall, Sweden, 10 December 2011

A hand gives a cheap ballpoint pen a good workout as it fervently sketches on one of the blank pages near the end of the programme outlining the evening's schedule of presenters and recipients. The hand stretches from out of a pristine white, starched and cufflinked shirt, and the shirt from the fine black sleeve of a formal tuxedo. And though little is known of the as-yet-unseen artist, it's clear he is much more focused on his sketchings than on the grandiose events transpiring, in both Swedish and English, here within the filled-to-capacity concert hall. And the image being drawn, though still very much a work-in-progress, is nonetheless recognizable; it is a crude sketch of a simple billboard, as if sprung from the weeds beside some lonely, rural highway. And the billboard itself is divided into a three-panel display. The first panel contains crude, almost childlike outlines of some endangered species – elephants, tigers, frogs, and polar bears, etc. – under the caption, *"For them."* The center panel depicts a two-child family under a caption that reads, "For us," and, under the *"For it"* caption, a reasonable if lopsided facsimile of the Earth. And currently the hand applies its finishing touches to the caption stretching across the bottom of the billboard, beneath everything else: *"Just two kids. Just two billion. We can live with that."*

The hand pauses, as if pondering how to complete its little project; what final pen strokes to add to make this billboard succinct enough to both terrify and yet inspire hope in whoever might glance up at it. The goal, of course, is to get these passersby curious enough about the cause to inspire them to visit the website – JustTwo.org – displayed there in the lower right hand corner of the billboard. And the goal of this, of course, is to pique their concern enough to get them to reach into their pockets and donate a euro or yuan or buck or peso to the Just Two cause so more billboards can be posted in every city and village and classroom the world 'round so that someday, hopefully soon, every person on the planet will be apprized of the dire consequences of overpopulation and, hence, will know why it is absolutely vital to limit their families to just two children. That is the goal. That is the point of this whole endeavor.

The Nobel Foundation, in a twisted exhibition of esoteric humor, is sometimes referred to as *the house that dynamite built*. This, of course, is because explosives – specifically nitroglycerin and, its more stable incarnation, dynamite – are how Alfred Nobel made his fortune. This all began nearly 180 years ago with Alfred's birth here in Stockholm in 1833, then culminated in the 1860s when he was awarded the patents for those aforementioned explosives, greasing the wheels for the Nobel empire's expansion throughout Europe and across *The Pond* to the just-developing-a-taste-for-warfare United States. So, what might explain the metamorphosis of one of humankind's most infamous war profiteers into one of its most renowned of philanthropists? Well, some opine it was pure and simple *guilt* that served as catalyst to this self-reinvention. Others hint there might have been a woman involved, in this case one by the name of Bertha Kinsky von Chinic und Tettau whom Alfred Nobel hired as a mere housekeeper/personal secretary in 1876, but who quit very shortly thereafter to become an avid peace activist, and who – as author of *Lay Down your Arms* under her new title Baroness Bertha Sophie Felicita von Suttner – became the very first recipient of the Nobel Peace Prize in 1905. Whichever the real explanation for his philanthropic turn – made manifest with the penning of his will and testament in 1893, just three years before his 10 December 1896 death – it must also be said in defense of his character that the vast lion's share of his products were detonated in the peaceful service of humankind, leading one to conclude that possibly it was less a matter of *guilt money* and more a matter of *too much money* that was responsible for the generous Nobel bequeathments so renowned and esteemed today. And isn't it only fitting such a lofty award be presented with extravagant pomp; a week-long party of high praise and humble acceptance speeches, elegant flower arrangements, fine dining, cultured music, and only the finest of wines, and all held within the vast and opulent venue as the Stockholm Concert Hall? Why, of course it is, especially when considering the singular dedication and life-long commitments the brilliant minds being honored put forth in order to achieve their oft-times selfless scientific or peaceful or literary accomplishments. Quite extraordinary the feat. Quite extraordinary the prize. Quite extraordinary the setting.

The aforementioned hand doing the artwork pauses to inspect its crude creation. And though the hand might wish it could draw better, or that it belonged to a better artist, it takes comfort in the fact this sketch is merely a blueprint for what is to come; merely the *concept* drawing to be handed over to professional artists who will be hired with part of the ten million Swedish Krona about to be awarded it in just a few minutes. Of this award there is no doubt: all six Nobel Prizes – be it in Chemistry, Physics, Economics, Literature, the exalted Peace Prize, or, in this case, Medicine/Physiology – were announced back in October, so all the recipients, or teams thereof, know well in advance who they are. And though some might be of the opinion this *knowing-in-advance* renders this culminating evening far less suspenseful than, say, the Academy Awards or the MTV's Best On-Screen Kiss Awards, the Nobel honorees somehow manage to reap satisfaction from the event nonetheless.

The voice of King Carl XVI Gustaf of Sweden reverberates through the concert hall as it announces the next recipient: "Never before in our one hundred and two year history has the Nominating Committee been unanimous in its choice for a Prize..."

As if on cue, a lovely, bare, feminine arm weaves through the artist's tuxedoed arm. Widening, the *feminine* arm is revealed to belong to Angela, never looking more radiantly elegant, and this even with a newborn baby swaddled against her breast. As she turns to her left and beams, it now becomes obvious the aforementioned "artist" doodling in the programme is Carl. He returns her smile, though not with quite the same beaming. His reticence stems from his belief he doesn't quite deserve this honor. After all, Nobel recipients typically receive their deserved accolades only after dedicating entire lifetimes to their science, art, or cause. All Carl did was stumble upon a particularly nasty pathogen, use a bit of his virological expertise, risked his life for a few weeks in order to get it back to the CDC, and, yeah okay, got lucky and saved the world, but should that warrant a Nobel? Of that he's not convinced. Maybe if some other foundation had a category for, say, *Bad Judgment and Dumb Luck*, maybe then he'd be deserving of their award, but certainly not a Nobel.

"Don't look a gift horse in the mouth!" That had been Angela's admonition, delivered as more of an uncontestable edict than as mere advice. And so here they are today; father, mother, and an as-yet-unnamed newborn which, for now, they warmly call "Froggy." Gift horse indeed: a perfect child, a Nobel,

the momentum of folly

ten million SEK, and a smart and beautiful and loving wife worth several times that amount thanks to her having isolated the pathogenic H7N7/A/Alaska/Sims/2011 for the wildly successful, commercially viable antiviral. *War* profiteering? – why, that's old-school, hard-work crap; *pandemic* profiteering is where the big bucks are made these days. And made it she did, for even though her commission was just a fraction of what her CEO reaped when Aegis went public a few months back, her net worth now is such it almost warrants of a foundation of all its own. *Mama didn't raise no fool!* But, owed to the fact she could not have done it without Carl's blood, sweat and tears – especially his *blood* – it is only fitting he be entitled a say in how the fortune is to be spent. All of which brings the focus back to the sketches for the billboards in the programme, which he now tucks into his tuxedo jacket pocket as King Gustaf finally introduces him: "… which is why this year's Prize in Medicine and Physiology –"

But before the King can even utter Carl's name, the entire hall, packed with distinguished guests and honorees, explode to their feet in an eruption of applause and cheers, veritably drowning out the remainder of the King's pronouncement. The King laughs, "You won't even let me say his name. Why, this *is* a first! Ladies and gentlemen distinguished guests all, I present this year's Nobel Prize in Medicine and Physiology to Dr. Carl Sims!" And the applause is nothing short of thunderous as Carl finally rises from his seat and begins taking a few humble, if slightly embarrassed bows.

An hour later the Nobel Awards attendees spill from the towering doorways of the Stockholm Concert Hall, where even the steady Swedish rain cannot dampen their spirits aroused by the culminating evening's events. When Carl, Angela, and Froggy finally emerge they are quickly swarmed by an enthusiastic throng of well-wishers who, though not quite screaming and crying like "tweenagers" in the presence of their latest pop star idol, gush and glad-hand and back-pat nonetheless.

"Congratulations, Dr. Sims!"
"Job well done, my boy, well done indeed!"
"Good on ya, mate!"
"Merci, Mssr. Sims, merci beau coup!"
"Great work. Truly, *truly* great work!"

"You saved the world!" one octogenarian-ish, distinguished-looking German man laughs in awestruck admiration.

"Just doing my job, sir," Carl humbly replies.

"*Just doing your job,* fuck that schista!"

And though this shakes a laugh out of Carl and Angela, the octogenarian proves to them he is far from through with his praise. Holding up his arms he shouts out to the others, "Hey, everyone, I'd like you all to witness this!" And once he has garnered their attention the octogenarian sinks to his knees on the wet marble steps and humbly kisses each of Carl's shoes. Then, upon rising again, he shouts, "This man saved the God-damned world!"

This squeezes another round of laughter and applause from the crowd. But, being that they are mature and respectful, they are not ones to fawn and linger too long, and so soon the throng begins to thin, scattering off into the rainy evening, beneath umbrellas or opened programmes to be used as such, back towards cozy rooms in nearby hotels or awaiting cabs or limos. Now little more than a handful of attendees remain with Carl, Angela, and Froggy there on the expansive, marble portico whose towering roof offers only occasional protection from the gusting downpour. The swaddled infant has just begun to cry, which sends Angela rummaging through her baby bag as Carl tries to keep an umbrella over them all.

"Damn," Angela mutters.

"What?" asks Carl.

"I left her bottle inside."

"Here, give her to me. We'll wait out here for the cab."

Thus begins the awkward extraction of an already fussy baby from her warm and snuggly, womb-mimicking sling against the mother's familiar belly, and equally awkward handover to the cold, wet, relatively untrained arms of the father, which, all very predictably, causes the infant's cries to intensify.

"Mommy will be right back," Angela assures Froggy, sealing the deal with an Eskimo nose rub and a kiss. As Angela turns back towards the Concert Hall the immense doors are held open for her by a Swedish man, just then exiting with friends.

"Forget your Nobel?" the Swedish man jokes wryly to her.

"Yes," Angela jokes back to the Swedish man, then thanks him for holding the behemoth door open for her, "Danke."

the momentum of folly

And with nothing more than that and perhaps the welling of a tear of gratitude in her eyes, Angela slips past the kind strangers and back into the building's foyer. her re-entry is followed by the exodus of a Romanian woman and an English gentleman, who also nod and smile warmly to Angela in passing, then join their Swedish friend – still holding the door open – out on the blustery portico.

"Bloody hell, it's still raining!" the Englishman grumbles, frowning skyward.

"At least it's not cold," the Romanian woman remarks.

"That's because it's *never* cold anymore," the Swede adds, as the three then scurry away down the steps.

It was an innocuous exchange; nothing more than a few trite comments about the weather that *normally*, perhaps as recently as a decade ago, would not have aroused concern. But insofar as these are less naïve times, the comment was a shrill harbinger of the drastic changes of climate that loom ahead. But Carl, overhearing the exchange, tries to remain calm about it all as he continues to sway and bounce his fussing newborn in one arm, all while struggling to keep the umbrella over them both with the other.

"Sssh, sssh, sssh. It's all right. Hush now, mommy'll be right back," he says, trying unsuccessfully to quiet the baby.

"And you thought all the hard work was over!" one of the last lingering pairs of event attendees – this one Japanese – tease Carl as they walk past, arm-in-arm, and off into the rainy night.

"Yeah," Carl confirms, mustering a polite, if strained smile, as he continues to bounce and sway his irritated infant. Suddenly another gust of wind lashes across the portico, dousing them with another sheet of rain and exacerbating Froggy's discomfort. This is quickly followed by another, even stronger gust, which rips Carl's umbrella inside out, rendering it now useless against the intensifying downpour. Carl stuffs the broken umbrella into the nearest trashcan, all the while trying, still unsuccessfully, to comfort the crying infant: "*Sssssh*, it's okay. Just a little rain: rain is our friend. Why, life itself would not be possible without a little rain now and then...."

In an effort to seek more protection, Carl moves them both across the portico around to the leeward side of the building. Rounding the corner he finds another half dozen or so event attendees similarly taking cover from the lashing rain in the downwind hollow of the building as they too await their rides. Carl is surprised to see one of those waiting out in the rain is King Gustaf himself; a head of state, royalty even, just hanging with friends and the common citizenry out in the common rain. Seems unusual but, then again, why wouldn't he? And even though the King – having just presented Carl with the Nobel Prize no more than an hour before – would certainly have recognized the distinguished recipient, Carl opts to keep his distance, allowing the King and his party to enjoy their small talk without having to be pestered by a wailing infant. As it happens, Carl's propinquity to them allows him to overhear much of the group's discussion, and near enough to see that said discussion is fixated on something located directly across the street. Whatever the object is, it has snagged the group's complete and rapt attention, with all now pointing and gazing intently towards it.

One member of the group mentions something he had heard about the object of interest: "Yes, come to think of it, I had heard somewhere it was supposed to occur by year's end!"

"What is it; something like every twelve years or so it happens now, right?" someone else from the King's entourage asks.

"Something like that, yes."

"Amazing timing; that we would just stumble out and witness it!" King Gustaf remarks.

"Then again, it's just an estimate. No one knows the actual numbers; not within a hundred million I would imagine," the first adds.

"Nevertheless," the King says, reeling, "it's remarkable!"

"The more the merrier, eh?"

"*Hmm*," the King responds, unconvinced.

A pair of modest, black limousines pulls up to the curb below.

"Ah, here we are!" one of the entourage says, regarding the limos. And with that the group begins popping open their umbrellas and heading down the steps towards their rides.

"But we'll miss it!" the King objects, half-jokingly.

"Then we'll just have to make a point of catching the *next* one," one of the entourage quips back, as they all proceed down the steps towards their awaiting cars.

With their departure, Carl ambles over to where the King and his entourage had been standing in an attempt to discover what exactly they had been staring towards that caused all the fuss. Still bouncing and swaying Froggy in his arms,

the momentum of folly

Carl relocates from behind one of the huge, marble columns that had previously obstructed his view.

And then he sees it.

Suddenly, recollections of Dr. Jenna Williams come flooding back to him. He recalls her talking about this very thing; about it being the first one she had ever seen; about how Carl's father had put it there intentionally, in deliberate proximity to the Swedish Concert Hall in order to influence those – those luminaries, those world leaders, those academic movers and shakers – in attendance at the Nobels. All in all it had been one of Carl's father's most brazen efforts to warn the world of the single greatest threat confronting it. As to whether or not this effort, and the myriad others like it, would ultimately prove successful or futile, well, only time would tell.

We follow Carl's transfixed gaze across the street and up to the entrance of a modest building where, mounted above the first floor awning, is yet another of the scant handful of Population Clocks scattered across the globe. Through the dark of night and whipping sheets of rain, the "clock's" red, foot-tall, ten-digit, LED numeric display seems all the more surreal. Occupying its left column – the one tallying billions of people – is the number six. This six is followed by a long string of seemingly steadfast nines, interrupted only by an eight in the slowly tumbling hundred's column. This eight hangs in there for some forty seconds before abdicating its spot to yet another nine. This nudges Carl's attention one column to the right to the *flickering-at-a-heartbeat-pace* tens column and, further still, to the hopeless blur that is the ones column, trying its best to register the two and a half new souls added to the human heap every second.

Another gust of wind manages to whip around the marble pillars, slapping Carl and Froggy with yet another sheet of rain, eliciting yet another crying jag from the latter and yet another futile attempt from the former to assuage the infant's suffering with more soft words and hollow assurances, "*Sssh, sssh, sssh –* it's alright, everything's gonna be alright. *Sssh, sssh, sssh...*"

Carl rubs noses with the infant – it worked when Angela did it – and bounces her a few more times. And her cries seem to settle some. He then lifts his troubled gaze back up to the population clock. *And who could resist?* – certainly not Carl. Whether from the rain, or the emotions elicited by the evening's events, or the fact his father had put this "clock" here, or the happenstance of witnessing this momentous occasion while holding his newborn; whatever the reason, Carl's eyes are wet with tears. This welling of tears permit the clock's red LED numbers to reflect clearly, if backwards, off the shiny surface of Carl's pupils. And though the number mirrored therein should come as no surprise to Carl, it proves shocking nonetheless; as that one lone six and its trailing string of nines, flips to 7,000,000,000.

Seven billion people on a planet that can sustain just two billion!

The moment, the number, the arbitrary milestone, comes and goes in a fraction of a second; the 7,000,000,000 becoming 7,000,000,001, becoming 7,000,000,002, and quickly building from there as the population clock's incessant, undaunted, ignorant whirl of red digits tallies the momentum of folly.

the end

About The Author

Robert P. Johnson was born and raised in Oakland, California, then relocated to Lake Tahoe where he ski-bummed, river-guided, and swept chimneys for a decade before moving to "Hollywood." After earning an MFA from UCLA's Department of Film, Theatre and Television, he worked as a screenwriter, winning First Place honors in both the Samuel Goldwyn and Jack Nicholson Screenwriting Awards. He currently lives in Santa Barbara with his wife and two children – just two.